Register Now for
to Your Bo

MW00784154

SPRINGER PUBLISHING COMPANY
CONNECT™

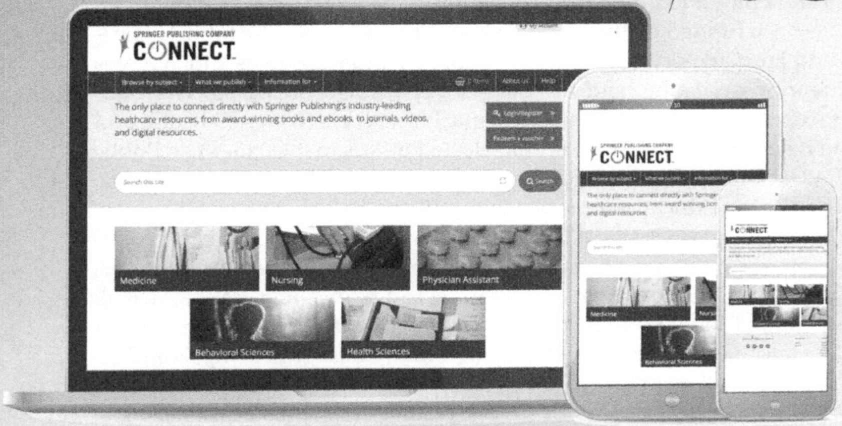

Your print purchase of *Policy and Program Planning for Older Adults and People With Disabilities, Second Edition,* **includes online access to the contents of your book**—increasing accessibility, portability, and searchability!

Access today at:

http://connect.springerpub.com/content/book/978-0-8261-2839-3
or scan the QR code at the right with your smartphone
and enter the access code below.

XCHLT2R7

Scan here for quick access.

If you are experiencing problems accessing the digital component of this product, please contact our customer service department at cs@springerpub.com

The online access with your print purchase is available at the publisher's discretion and may be removed at any time without notice.

Publisher's Note: New and used products purchased from third-party sellers are not guaranteed for quality, authenticity, or access to any included digital components.

CS

Elaine Theresa Jurkowski, PhD, MSW, is a professor at Southern Illinois University Carbondale's School of Social Work, where she teaches courses in health and aging policy, research, and program evaluation and social work practice. Dr. Jurkowski also holds joint appointments with the Department of Public Health and Recreation Professions and SIU's School of Medicine's Family Practice Residency Program. Dr. Jurkowski earned her bachelor's and master's degrees in social work from the University of Manitoba, Winnipeg, Canada, and her PhD from the University of Illinois, Chicago, IL. Dr. Jurkowski's early career experience working as a social worker in a community public health interdisciplinary setting in Manitoba, Canada, exposed her to mental health, disability, vocational rehabilitation, and aging programs. These early experiences, coupled with her training in community health sciences and epidemiology, have shaped her research and practice interests.

Dr. Jurkowski's research has been funded by the National Institutes of Health, the John A. Hartford Foundation, the Health and Human Services Administration, Health Resources and Services Administration, the Administration on Aging, and the Illinois Department on Aging. Her published research articles have focused on the topics of health disparities, access to mental health and healthcare services, aging, and disability issues. She has held elected offices in the American Public Health Association, National Association of Social Workers, the Gerontological Society of America, Association in Gerontology and Higher Education, and the Illinois Rural Health Association. Some of her current research projects include geriatric workforce education and interdisciplinary professional education. She previously coordinated the Certificate in Gerontology on the SIUC campus.

Her work experiences have included consultation within settings in Niger (West Africa), Uganda, Canada, Hong Kong, India, China, Russia, and Egypt. Dr. Jurkowski is also the author of *Policy and Program Planning for Older Adults* (2008), *Implementing Culture Change in Long-Term Care: Benchmarks and Strategies for Management and Practice* (2013), and managing coeditor of *Handbook for Public Health Social Work* (2013), *Implementing Culture Change in Long Term Care: Benchmarks and Strategies for Management and Practice* (2013), and *Aging in Rural Places* (2015), as well as numerous book chapters and professional articles. Dr. Jurkowski's community service includes serving as a member of the board of directors for various not-for-profit healthcare agencies within the southern Illinois area. Dr. Jurkowski also serves as an Advisory Board member to the Southern Illinois Pioneer Coalition Advisory Board.

Policy and Program Planning for Older Adults and People With Disabilities

Practice Realities and Visions

SECOND EDITION

Elaine Theresa Jurkowski, PhD, MSW

SPRINGER PUBLISHING COMPANY
NEW YORK

Springer Publishing Company, LLC
11 West 42nd Street
New York, NY 10036
www.springerpub.com

Acquisitions Editor: Sheri W. Sussman
Compositor: diacriTech, Chennai

ISBN: 978-0-8261-2838-6
ebook ISBN: 978-0-8261-2839-3
DOI: 10.1891/9780826128393

Supplementary podcast discussions of key topics can be accessed at http://connect.springerpub.com/content/book/978-0-8261-2839-3

Instructor's Materials: Qualified instructors may request supplements by emailing textbook@springerpub.com:
Instructor's Manual: 978-0-8261-34974
Instructor's Test Bank: 978-0-8261-3496-7
Instructor's PowerPoints: 978-0-8261-34981

18 19 20 21 22 / 5 4 3 2 1

Library of Congress Cataloging-in-Publication Data
Names: Jurkowski, Elaine Theresa, author.
Title: Policy and program planning for older adults and people with
disabilities : practice realities and visions / Elaine Theresa Jurkowski.
Other titles: Policy and program planning for older adults
Description: Second edition. | New York, NY: Springer Publishing Company, [2019] |
Preceded by Policy and program planning for older adults / Elaine
Theresa Jurkowski. 2008. | Includes bibliographical references and index.
Identifiers: LCCN 2018049248 | ISBN 9780826128386 | ISBN 9780826128393 (ebook ISBN)
Subjects: | MESH: Aged | Disabled Persons | Health Services for the Aged |
Health Services for Persons with Disabilities | Socioeconomic Factors |
Public Policy--legislation & jurisprudence | United States
Classification: LCC HV1461 | NLM WT 31 | DDC 362.6—dc23 LC record available at
https://lccn.loc.gov/2018049248

Printed in the United States of America.

To my parents Lorraine and Eddie Jurkowski whose vision for consumer-based policies and programs inspired this work.

To my dear husband Bill: Thank you for always being there and believing in me!

To all people who are advancing in age with impairments and challenges to their abilities, who can benefit from this work.

Contents

Preface

REALITIES AND VISIONS

Looking around oneself either at the grocery store, at a shopping mall, or in the workplace, a common thread may be seen—a graying population. The first of the baby boom cohort turned 60 in 2006, and by 2030 it is anticipated that 20% or more of the adult population in the United States will be 65 years of age or older. Many of these individuals will also have some form of disability. People with disabilities increasingly are also being viewed in the community, as the community integration movement has now spanned at least 50 years. Consequently, social work, public health, human services, and allied health professionals will be at the forefront of service delivery and policy development. Thus, resources and tools to adequately prepare these individuals for the journey ahead, to meet this changing society, will be vital and critical.

In response to this need, this second edition of *Policy and Program Planning for Older Adults and People With Disabilities: Practice Realities and Visions* has been developed. This textbook offers some innovative features. Essentially, the book takes a public health/population health approach to the development of programs and services for older adults. It attempts to build students' understanding of policy development through a critical analysis and review of policy frameworks and the policy implementation process. Skills to shape policies and programs such as media advocacy, coalition building, and health promotion frameworks will also be addressed within the text. Last, community-based programs and services are addressed. This current edition integrates a variety of media strategies to include websites, YouTube videos, and podcasts. Existing policy texts neglect to triangulate skills, policies, and programs for the reader and neglect to blend a social welfare and public health approach into their conceptual designs.

LAYOUT OF THIS BOOK

This book has been developed with the notion that it will provide the reader with an overview of dimensions impacting policy development, apprise the reader of current mandated policies in the United States that will affect older adults, identify and present tools that are helpful in building both policy and programs for older adults, and showcase programs and services for older adults. Each chapter provides the reader with case studies, websites, YouTube videos, discussion questions, and podcasts as additional resources and reference information. Each chapter also presents some notion of the realities facing older adults and people with disabilities within each topical area, and a summary chapter outlines both realities of today and visions for the future. It is the author's hope that this resource can be valuable for advocates working within the field of aging as they develop programs and policies for our next generation.

Part I of this book lays out a background as to the current and future demographic trends of older adults and makes the case for the reader that there are a variety of philosophical, political, economic, and social factors that affect public policy development. The chapters help the reader explore a range of perspectives that define, shape, and impact the development and implementation of public policy. This section is also intended to prepare the reader to be able to critically analyze public policies related to aging.

Chapter 1 provides a demographic profile of the aging population (60+ years) and people with disabilities, currently, and reviews how these demographics have changed from 1900 until the present time. Demographics are also reviewed from the perspectives of specific health outcomes, gender differences, ethnic composition, and rural/urban dimensions. The chapter concludes by looking at how these specific demographic changes will shape challenges for the future and gaps to be addressed through policy and program developments.

The second chapter takes the reader through a historical review of policy, economic, political, and social changes that have occurred both on the American and global fronts for older adults and people with disabilities. It reviews such dimensions within 10-year increments, highlighting major innovations or developments from 1900 to 2018. The chapter concludes by challenging the reader to consider factors that have led to innovations in science and technology as opposed to aging-related policies and lays the groundwork to begin to explore philosophical paradigms that impact policy development.

Chapter 3 provides an overview of different philosophical paradigms that impact the development of policy proposals and eventually drafted or legislative bills. The chapter also explores various factors and policy frameworks that impact the implementation of aging policy. Philosophical paradigms include: blaming the victim, elitism, social welfare as a right, econometric perspectives, cause versus function, cronyism, and window of opportunity, to name a few. These philosophical frameworks help the reader understand the development of aging- and disability-related policies and programs, while the policy frameworks help the reader understand the implementation process related to aging policy. Implementation strategies will include frameworks such as street-level bureaucrats, incrementalism, rationalism, and window of opportunity. An important perspective of this chapter is that the reader is exposed to the view that a range of perspectives ranging from extreme liberal to conservative impact the development and implementation of public policy.

The fourth chapter of the book, and the last in Part I, lays out a variety of tools and government documents available and how these are used to provide evidence and rationale for public policy development and analysis. Sources include Congressional Universe Congress.gov, Government Printing Office (GPO) documents, Government Accountability Office (GAO) documents, and various databases available through the national database sources. This chapter also makes the linkage between using data and evidence to support policy and program development decisions. Some exercises are provided at the conclusion of the chapter to help the reader understand and utilize these sources.

Part II of this text will provide an overview to major federal policies and programs that impact older adults and people with disabilities. Some historical developments leading up to the actual development and implementation of the policies are also examined. Policies include Social Security, Medicare, the Older Americans Act, the Americans with Disabilities Act, the Community Mental Health Centers Act, the Affordable Care Act, the Caregiver Support Act, and Elder Justice Act are addressed in this section.

Chapter 5 provides a backdrop to our current Social Security Program, provides an overview to some models for Social Security programs in Europe and Canada, and explores the genesis of the Social Security program in the United States. The contents of the original Social Security Act will be explored and compared to the current-day titles and programs mandated through the current Social Security Act. Chapter 6 reviews the history of Medicare and reviews some of the changes in Medicare legislation over time. It also provides an overview of the current services available through Medicare Parts A, B, C, and D.

The Older Americans Act has seen a growth of programs, legislative resources, and a series of amendments since its inception into law in 1965. Chapter 7 reviews some of the history leading up to the signing, the original components of the act, amendments that have occurred over time, including the most recent amendments of 2016, which will serve as a guidepost until 2021. The chapter concludes with a discussion about Aging and Disability Resource Centers. The use of Aging and Disability Resource Centers (ARDC's) has been a widely utilized model of service delivery for resources that address the needs of older adults and people with disabilities since the first edition of this book was written, Chapter 7 also addresses how the ARDC's have been used as a strategy to inform the general public about programs and services, which have been mandated by the various legislative initiatives addressed through Part II of this textbook.

Chapter 8 provides an overview to the Americans with Disabilities Act and examines how this landmark piece of legislation impacts the lives of older adults. Mobility impairments and other impairments associated with disability and chronic conditions have posed major barriers and challenges to people as they age and develop mobility or sensory limitations. Within the area of mobility and sensory deficits and challenges, older adults as well as people with disabilities have greatly benefited from the work and accomplishment of the disability and independent living movements.

Chapter 9 reviews mental health legislation and its impacts for older adults/people with disabilities living within the community. It also explores President Bush's Freedom Commission Initiative and explores how this legislation affected older adults'/people with disabilities lives in the United States.

The Patient Protection and Affordable Care Act (ACA) are addressed in Chapter 10. A new addition to this edition, the chapter reviewers the 10 titles of the ACA and provides the reader with some understanding of how the legislation plays a role in the lives of older adults and people with disabilities.

Chapter 11 reviews the Elder Justice Act, an outgrowth of the ACA, and helps the reader understand the implications of Adult Protective Services and the role they play in the lives of older adults and people with disabilities. This chapter also examines some of the legislation that affects grandparents raising grandchildren, such as child welfare components. Elder abuse is addressed and gaps in services and public policy are also presented in this chapter. The incidence and prevalence of elder abuse is probably largely underreported. While efforts are being made to understand the magnitude of the problem, limited resources hamper progress. The Older Americans Act has some resources in place to deal with the education of providers and screening/detection of individuals who have been at risk of abuse; however, Adult Protective Services plays a key role also in this intervention process. The role of one's cultural beliefs and help-seeking behavior also plays a significant role. Challenges in uncovering this silent epidemic face the healthcare provider, programs, and services.

Legal issues, including those related to power of attorney, enduring power of attorney, end-of-life care issues, are also examined in Chapter 11. It also presents dilemmas in public policy development relative to how these are implemented. In addition, legal services provided to older adults as a result of the Older Americans Act and Elder Justice Act are explored, and challenges within the realm of legal issues outlined.

Chapter 12 explores the Caregiver Support Act and the role it plays in providing supports to caregivers who are addressing the needs of older adults and people with disabilities. It provides a history of caregiver support and also addresses the specific resources available to help address the unique challenges that a caregiver faces. It also addressees the unique dilemmas grandparents raising grandchildren face when straddling aging and child welfare policies. This chapter also provides an overview of the current status of grandparents raising grandchildren, as well as some background on the literature, and it provides an awareness of issues that grandparents face as primary caregivers. A literature review examines some of the current issues and services needed. Resources and services designed to meet the needs of grandparents raising grandchildren are discussed, and programmatic responses identified through the national resources. Lastly, some best practice interventions are outlined for review.

Chapter 13 examines housing policies that play a role for older adults and people with disabilities. The chapter also explores various models of community living and residential options for older adults. Traditional models of long-term care, home- and community-based, will be examined and innovative approaches presented, such as consumer-directed approaches. This chapter examines the current status of the long-term care system, seeks to provide different residential models of care for people as they require community-based settings or settings with supports, and addresses issues that will face the long-term and community-based care settings in the future.

Chapter 14 examines policies related to substance use/misuse and the role substance use/misuse has played in the lives of older adults and people with disabilities. It also addressed the current opioid crisis and how this has evolved for people within our target group categories.

Part III provides some tools for the reader to use to be more adequately equipped to prepare program initiatives that flow from policy appropriations. The tools also are designed to prepare the practitioner or reader with some skills to more effectively advocate for policy change. This section helps bridge some of the skills and tools used both within the disciplines of social work and public health and begins to expand the boundaries of public policy development.

Chapter 15 addresses health behavior models and lays out the premise that understanding and programming with some concept of health behavior in mind will strengthen community-based programs and improve the return on investment in these programs. Health behavior models addressed within this chapter will include four specific models, including the "health belief model," "stages of change," and "theories of reasoned action." An overview of these models and their components will be presented and reviewed. These will then be examined relative to aging/disability policies and the implementation of specific programs. The chapter concludes with making a case for the importance of using health behavior models in the development of aging programs and provides some "best practice" examples.

Chapter 16 provides an innovative tool for policy advocates, which is the use of media and advocacy strategies for change. This chapter provides an overview of the social marketing process and media/advocacy strategies inherent in the process of developing advocacy campaigns for creating public awareness. A variety of specific constituent groups are addressed, and media strategies are presented. Strategies include the use of preparing sound bites, developing fact sheets, letter writing campaigns, use of the Internet, infomercials, "trinket techniques" (T-shirts, bumper stickers, visors, etc.), and social media.

The focus of tools presented in Chapter 17 is on coalitions and coalition building. This chapter provides an overview of coalitions, and their development and use as a technique for policy development or program implementation.

Chapter 18 outlines and reviews tools used in the needs assessment process. This chapter outlines the use of needs assessment tools and how either one, or all five strategies discussed in this chapter are used in the development of community, agency, state, or national priorities. Strategies include community forums, social indicators, key stakeholders, service statistics, and surveys.

The third part of this text concludes with Chapter 19, which attempts to pull together each of the chapters in this section on tools and make the linkage between the first three parts and the last part of this book. This chapter provides the reader with a short overview of how the tools presented are salient in the process of program development and sets the stage for the concluding part of this text.

The last part of this text (Part IV) outlines specific aging/disability areas that provide unique programming needs from aging/disability policies, and specific components that flow from federally mandated policies. Chapter 20 concludes by laying out realities, proposing visions for the future and summarizing a top 10 list of challenges for the future.

1. Designing paradigms to meet the demographic and social needs of our graying population through evidence-based approaches.
2. Social Security—boom or bust?
3. Medicare: Will there be a pot at the end of the rainbow for preventive services?
4. Understanding health behavior and planning with this understanding in mind.
5. Using the media, advocacy, and coalitions for social change.
6. Home- and community-based care.
7. Mental health programs, services, and issues.
8. Health programs, services, and issues.
9. Long-term care.
10. Diversity and special populations.

This text also offers various unique features, which include some of the following:

- The book is presented in four parts, addresses philosophical paradigms underlying policy making, addresses current policies impacting older adults, describes tools and strategies for policy making and program planning, and presents programs and services to address the needs of older adults.
- The book addresses some unique areas such as evidence-based policy development, the media, and coalition building.
- The book presents materials on the Older Americans Act Reauthorization Act of 2016.
- The book provides strategies for learning and the development of "flip classrooms" such as the use of discussion questions, YouTube video resources, podcasts, and additional resource materials.

In addition, this book addresses specific strategies and tools that can be useful in the development of renewed social policy for older adults or people with disabilities and equips the reader with tools and strategies to impact public health or health policies and programs. The reader is apprised of current legislative efforts that impact older adults/people with disabilities in practice settings, or that impact program development. It also provides a conceptual or philosophical framework that guides the development of social policy. Tools, strategies, and resources that shape social policy efforts are also addressed, followed by programs and services currently in place. Since the text is sole authored, a linkage between chapters is possible, which lends itself to continuity throughout the text.

A graying society is a reality—thus we can be prepared to plan, or we can plan to fail. Planning promotes engagement, thus rendering a healthy community and a foundation for our generations to come.

Elaine Theresa Jurkowski

Qualified instructors can access ancillary materials by emailing textbook@springerpub.com.

Acknowledgments

The completion of a project such as a manuscript or book cannot be possible without the support and helping hands of many people. This entire book would not be possible without the vision and support of Sheri W. Sussman, Senior Editor at Springer Publishing for her vision and unwavering support through this process. Sheri, along with her assistant Mindy Chen were invaluable in terms of their support and attention to details.

This book also would not have been possible without the input from many of my students, especially, students within the Certificate in Gerontology program and School of Social Work at Southern Illinois University Carbondale. Many students (too many to name individually), helped shape the ideas that went into this work. Although many students have contributed insights and asked questions which evolved the various chapters of this book, there are some students that should be acknowledged by name for their help with literature searches, media artifacts, and technical details, such as Terry Tippet Jr., George Lowery, Ashunti Jackson, Fatoumata Saidou Hangadoumbo, M. Helen Hogue, Eric Eblin, and Teresa Corisco Eblin. Arwen McElhany deserves mention for her attention to the conversion of files, data management, and electronic media. Brian Chainy was unwavering with his technical support for the podcast series.

I would also like to acknowledge my colleagues and writing group of doctoral and MSW students, who provided sources of input and offered valuable suggestions for the manuscript itself.

Most of all, I would like to acknowledge my family for their patience, understanding, unconditional support, and never wavering belief in my potential. Bill and "our girls" deserve acknowledgment for the many hours they spent ignored at home while I was absorbed in the research and writing associated with publishing this book.

Introduction

It is a pleasure to present the second edition of *Policy and Program Planning for Older Adults and People With Disabilities*. This edition integrates materials on people with disabilities, as a result of the merge between the Administration on Aging (AoA) and the Administration for People with Disabilities in 2012. On April 18, 2012, a new entity known now as the Administration for Community Living (ACL) was operational under the leadership of Kathleen Greenlee, the Administrator for the ACL. This administration currently under the umbrella of the Health and Human Services Secretariat (HHS) carries an annual budget of over 1.8 billion dollars (FY2016) and provides services from cradle to grave essentially. ACL's Principal Deputy Administrator serves as Senior Advisor to the HHS Secretary for Disability Policy.

The ACL is structured to provide general policy coordination while retaining programmatic operations specific to the needs of each population served. ACL is divided into the following units:

- Office of the Administrator
- AoA
- Administration on Intellectual and Developmental Disabilities (AIDD)
- Center for Consumer Access and Self-Determination (CCASD)
- Center for Management and Budget (CMB)
- Center for Policy and Evaluation (CPE)

The AoA is led by the Assistant Secretary for Aging, who is directly supported by the Deputy Assistant Secretary for Aging. Reporting directly to the Deputy Assistant Secretary for Aging are the following offices:

- Office of Supportive and Caregiver Services
- Office of Nutrition and Health Promotion Programs
- Office of Elder Justice and Adult Protective Services
- Office of American Indian, Alaskan Native, and Native Hawaiian Programs
- Office of Long-Term Care Ombudsman Programs

The Administration on Disability is headed by a Commissioner, who reports directly to the ACL Administrator, and a Deputy Commissioner who also serves as Director of Independent Living. Reporting directly to the Commissioner and Deputy Commissioner are the following offices:

- AIDD
- Independent Living Administration

Reporting directly to the Deputy Administrator of the Center for Integrated programs are the following offices:

- Office of Healthcare Information and Counseling
- Office of Consumer Access and Self-Determination
- Office of Integrated Care Innovations

Reporting directly to the Deputy Administrator of the CMB are the following offices:

- Office of Budget and Finance
- Office of Administration and Personnel
- Office of Grants Management
- Office of Information Resources Management

Reporting directly to the Director of the CPE are the following offices:

- Office of Policy Analysis and Development
- Office of Performance and Evaluation

Reporting directly to the Director of the National Institute on Disability, Independent Living, and Rehabilitation Research are the following offices:

- Office of Research Sciences
- Office of Research Evaluation and Administration

Figure I.1 provides an organizational chart of the entire Administration, to help navigate the entire scope of services and entities covered by the ACL. A listing of regional offices supporting these operations can be found in Appendix A.

The overall goal of merging Administrations was to better meet and serve communities that include the diversity of people growing older and people living with some types of impairments or disabilities. The ACL believes that communities cannot thrive without a variety of voices and perspectives. Healthy communities value the inclusion of all people, including the growing populations of older people and people with disabilities. Independent living and aging in place are vital to keeping intact the rich diversity that makes our community strong (ACL, 2015, retrieved from www.acl.gov). This vision is a dramatic departure from the previous lens that many services were delivered from—a medical model of service provision—and moves toward a community-based model that embraces self-determinism, personhood, and least restrictive environments. While these principles and values have been embraced by the disability communities for decades, they are steadily influencing the aging arena. The merge between Administrations into the ACL, will only reinforce the principles and values that most people would probably prefer—dignity, self-determination, and autonomy within the least restrictive settings.

The previous version of this book focused on the services specific to the AoA and other policy entities that touched upon the lives of older adults. With the recent merge between the AoA and the Administration on Disabilities, this second edition includes materials related to people with disabilities specific to the older adult and aging population. This second edition also makes an attempt to bring the content to life or practice through integrating case students throughout the materials. These cases, which are introduced at the outset of the book, are woven throughout the chapters with the hopes of helping the reader anchor how policies and programs impact individuals, communities, and organizations in direct practice. The chapters conclude with discussion questions to help with peer and classroom discussions. Instructors making use of these materials for their classroom settings can also take advantage of an instructor's guide that includes test bank questions, discussion questions, and exercises, as well as, PowerPoint materials for each chapter. We hope that you enjoy the journey into the realm of policies and programs for older adults and people with disabilities!

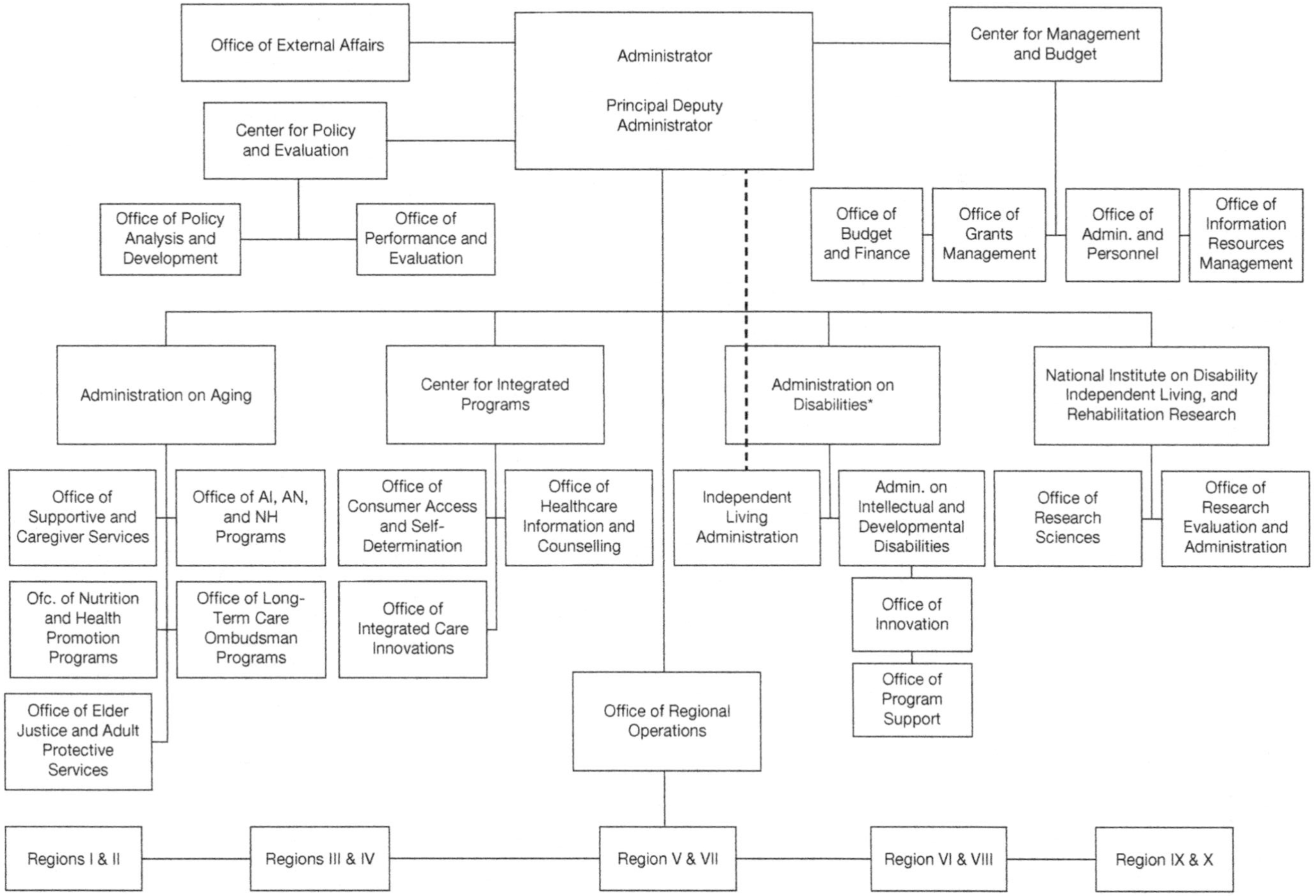

* The Administration on Disabilities is headed by a Commissioner, who reports directly tothe Administrator, and a Deputy Commissioner/Director of Independent Living. In this dual role, the Deputy Commissioner/Director of Independent Living serves as a member of the Administrator's senior leadership and reports directly to the Administrator in carrying out the functions of the Director of Independent Living consistent with Section 701A of the Rehabilitation Act.

Figure I.1 Organizational chart for the Administration for Community Living.

Source: https://acl.gov/about-acl/organization/organizational-chart

INTRODUCING THE CASES PRESENTED THROUGHOUT THIS BOOK

Throughout this book, a series of cases are introduced and used to showcase the theory and detail presented in each chapter. The use of these vignettes helps the reader to better understand the content and dynamics of social policy specific to older adults and people with disabilities. In addition, it helps the reader better understand how specific federal policies play out in terms of programs, services, and individual functioning. This introduction is designed to help the reader find a quick and easy reference guide while working with the materials presented in this book. Each of the cases are based upon real situations, however, the names have been altered to protect one's anonymity.

Susan: Susan is a 57-year-old woman who has sustained a work-related injury that has affected her knees and mobility. In addition to her own mobility impairment, she lives with her older parents, Irma and Gus. Gus was diagnosed with early stages of Alzheimer's disease about 10 years ago, and it has progressed to the point where he is mobility impaired and needs constant supervision. Irma is a brittle diabetic and cannot handle the care needs of her husband—she relies on Susan for help. They lived on a farm, but have now moved to a metropolitan area with Susan. Susan has five adult siblings, but she is the only one who lives with their parents. Susan is able to work at a full-time job as a result of the Americans with Disabilities Act.

Theresa: Theresa is a 47-year-old professional gerontologist who currently works within the Policy and Program Planning division of a state Department of Aging and Community Living. The disability services portfolio has recently been added to the former Department of Aging and Theresa is assigned to deal with the policy and programmatic changes. Theresa has an MSW and a Certificate in Gerontology.

Erica: Erica is a researcher working at a Geriatric Workforce Enhancement Program in Madison, WI. This recently funded Health Resources and Services Administration (HRSA) program is designed to work on building an intraprofessional geriatric workforce within the state of Wisconsin.

Margie: Margie, 70 years of age and native to California, moved to a rural property in Oregon with her late husband Carey approximately 4 years ago, to a rural property. The home they built home is fairly isolated and sits on 80 acres of wooded land. The couple moved to Oregon permanently around the time that Carey had been diagnosed with stage 4 cancer. The couple had decided that they wanted to exercise a "Dignity with Death" option if need be when Carey was at a stage in his terminal illness. Carey passed away a year and a half ago, and now Margie is confronted with living in a beautifully wooded area with limited resources that she can access for her physical and emotional needs.

Betty: Betty recently celebrated her 95th birthday and lives in her own home in rural California, in a small town known as Grimes, which boasts a population of 375 people. The movie *Paper Moon* was filmed in Grimes in the late 1970s, and it is still the talk of the town. Betty still drives her own car, although does not pursue night driving anymore due to her macular degeneration. She has chickens on her property and barters eggs for other goods and services such as milk and yard chores. Betty's children do not live near her, although her closest son lives about 65 miles away in Elk Grove, CA.

Angela and Joseph: Angela (83) and Joseph (86) are currently living in Houston, TX; however, they have worked in many corners of the world as a result of Joseph's distinguished career in the Air Force. Upon retirement from the Air Force, Joseph joined the National Aeronautics and Space Administration (NASA) and worked as an aeronautical engineer until his retirement at 69 years of age. Angela stayed at home while their three children were in school and then worked as a jewelry clerk at a local jewelry store.

Ida: Ida, a resident of a Medicaid-funded long-term care facility in Denton, TX, has lived with symptoms of multiple sclerosis since she was 52 years of age. Now 80 years of age, Ida is a widow, and her stepchildren look after her needs. Her stepchildren are spread throughout the Dallas area, and her daughter June and four grandchildren reside in Washington state.

Gerry: Gerry was born with cerebral palsy and hydrocephalus, and was hospitalized for several months following his birth. During the first year of his life, a shunt was surgically implanted into his skull. However, the shunt needs to be replaced periodically. Gerry is on Social Security Disability, and receives funding monthly. Gerry lives in a rural community, attends master's-level classes in Rehabilitation Studies at a local university, and mobilizes himself with an electric wheelchair. He boasts that he is 38 years of age—one year younger than Jack Benny!

Lorraine: Lorraine is a 96-year-old woman who has survived the Holocaust and currently lives in Fort Myers, FL. Lorraine moved into an assisted living facility 2 years ago after she lost her driving privileges and had been reported to be falling within her home. Lorraine needs assistance with shopping for groceries and household chores such as laundry and cleaning her apartment. She has also been having some flashbacks recently from her days in the Holocaust. Her unemployed son has also been receiving frequent donations from Lorraine, which appear to be more than a casual occurrence.

Joan: Joan currently lives in Ohio, and manages independently, despite a car accident that left her with a severe head injury 36 years ago. Joan became a parent shortly after her head injury, and she often suffers from aphasia. She currently lives in her own home with her adult son.

Mary: Mary recently celebrated her 70th birthday and currently lives in Lexington, KY. She attended a Historically Black College/University program where she obtained her MSN and then an MSW. Mary also has the Power of Attorney for her four older sisters who reside in Lexington and Cincinnati, OH.

Nora: Nora is both a caregiver to her 87-year-old father and disabled due to an orthopedic injury while riding a bicycle. Her recent knee replacement surgery has left her with less mobility in her right knee than she had prior to her surgery. Being a caregiver to her father leaves her with limited emotional resources at the end of a day. Nora's father is legally blind, suffers from Crone's disease, and has had a series of mini strokes. They live together in the three bedroom family home, and receive in-home services to support Nora in her caregiving role. Nora's father also attends a day program 3 days per week. Nora's mother passed away 10 years ago, and she also helps in the caregiving role for her two grandsons. Nora's father was emotionally distant to her while growing up and she is an only child.

List of Figures

List of Tables

List of Podcasts

Part I

Understanding Policy and Program Development

This part lays out a background as to the current and future demographic trends of older adults and people with disabilities (Chapter 1), making the case for the reader that there are a variety of philosophical, political, economic, and social factors that affect public policy development. The chapters help the reader explore a range of perspectives that define, shape, and impact the development and implementation of public policy. This part is also intended to prepare the reader to be able to critically analyze public policies related to aging. Chapter 2 compares and contrasts the changes that have happened in society over time, as well as policy development within the realm of aging and disability arenas. The policy overview journey sets out with a glimpse of factors that play a role in policy development (Chapter 3) and concludes with a model for policy development that helps guide a reader through this book (Chapter 4).

1

Background and Demographic Profile of People Growing Older and/or People With Disabilities

LEARNING OBJECTIVES

At the end of this chapter, readers will:

1. *Be familiar with some of the demographic trends affecting people as they age.*
2. *Be familiar with some of the demographic trends for people with disabilities.*
3. *Be familiar with cultural and socioeconomic challenges for older adults and people with disabilities.*
4. *Be familiar with the challenges demographic trends pose for older adults and people with disabilities.*

Theresa is a 47-year-old professional gerontologist who currently works within the Policy and Program Planning Division of a state Department of Aging and Community Living. She has been tasked with preparing a white paper on policy and program planning initiatives and a strategic plan, which will serve as a roadmap for the department for the next decade, and also assist with workforce development initiatives, which will be funded in partnership with the Health Resources and Services Administration-funded Geriatrics Workforce Enhancement Program (GWEP). With Theresa's skill set recently acquired from her Certificate in Gerontology, she is eager to set out upon this task and eager to collaborate with her colleague Erica from the local GWEP. Theresa's first step is to understand the demographic landscape of the aging arena.

PREPARING FOR THE "BOOM"

America is graying at a faster rate than ever before. In addition to the graying population, we are also recognizing that many of these boomers are living within the community with impairments and "disabilities." In 2006, the first baby boomer turned 60 and became eligible for Older Americans Act services. In addition, this same group of people have benefitted from the Americans with Disabilities Act (ADA), which celebrated its

© Springer Publishing Company DOI:10.1891/9780826128393.0001

25th anniversary in 2015. Baby boomers are a distinct group, with attitudes and values unlike those of the seniors who have preceded them. This group of people, advancing in age, thrives on choice, seeks out information, is consumer-oriented and demanding, and wants individual independence. Are we prepared to deal with the policy and program needs this group presents and needs? Are we ready to address the gaps in services that this group demands of us? How will human service, public health practitioners, and policy makers be prepared for community and individual needs? What are the realities for current services, and what visions will be presented from baby boomers for new or revised services? What paradigms shape services that are currently in place, and how can we revise these services using tools for program planning and policy development? This book addresses these questions and challenges readers to address these issues while thinking "outside the box."

Before we can address these issues, an exploration of the current demographic face in America is necessary. What does our landscape of people advancing in age and people with disabilities look like? How do we anticipate the impact these demographic changes will have in shaping our social and community needs?

THE CHANGING DEMOGRAPHIC STRUCTURE AND AGING POPULATION

Life expectancy has dramatically increased over the past century. At the turn of the 20th century (1900), life expectancy was 47 years (Pickett & Hanlon, 1995). In 1958, the life expectancy of adults increased to 68 years, and by 1991, the life expectancy was 76 years, while in 2003 life expectancy in the United States was 77.6 years (Centers for Disease Control and Prevention [CDC], 2005a). In 2016, the life expectancy had risen to 81.1 years for women, while men lagged behind at 76.1 years (CDC, 2017). For a person who attained the age of 65, life expectancy in the United States would be an additional 18.0 years for males or 20.6 years for females (OECD, 2018). This life expectancy rate in the United States is low compared to countries such as Iceland (18.7 years for males; 21.3 years for females), or Japan (19.6 years for males; 24.4 years for females; OECD, 2018). Other countries that exceed these life expectancy ages include Sweden, France, and Switzerland (OECD, 2018).

Hand in hand with these changes, there has been an increase in the number of elderly living within the United States over the past century. In 1900, 4% of the population was over 65 years of age, while it reached 12.7% by 1997 (nearly triple), and by 2017 people over the age of 65 comprised 15.6% of the population (U.S. Census Bureau, 2017a). Although, the U.S. Census Bureau estimated that by the year 2060, at least 23% of the population would be over 65 years of age (Vespa, Armstrong, & Medina, 2018), other forces have kept this population growth in check. Table 1.1 presents these demographic changes over time.

Interestingly, approximately one out of about every eight Americans falls into the older adult population. The number of older Americans has increased by nearly 11% since 1900, compared to a 9% increase in the 45-to-64 population (Administration for Community Living, 2016; U.S. Census Bureau, 2002, 2012). As the clock ticks away, every 8 seconds a Baby Boomer turns 60 (U.S. Census Bureau, 2018a). Figure 1.1 provides an overview of this demographic shift.

The population of people who are 60 years of age and older is expected to double by 2060. The 85 and older group is expected to grow faster than any other group (Federal Interagency Forum on Aging-Related Statistics, 2006, 2016a). In 2017, people who fell into

Table 1.1 Demographic Changes of an Aging Population in the United States Over Time

Year	Percentage of the Population 65 Years of Age or Older
1900	4.0
1920	4.6
1940	6.8
1980	11.3
1990	12.4
2000	12.0
2005	12.3
2010	15.0
2015	15.3
2017	15.6

Source: U.S. Bureau of the Census, 1900, 1920, 1940, 1980, 1990, 2000, 2005, 2010, 2015, 2017 (assorted years).

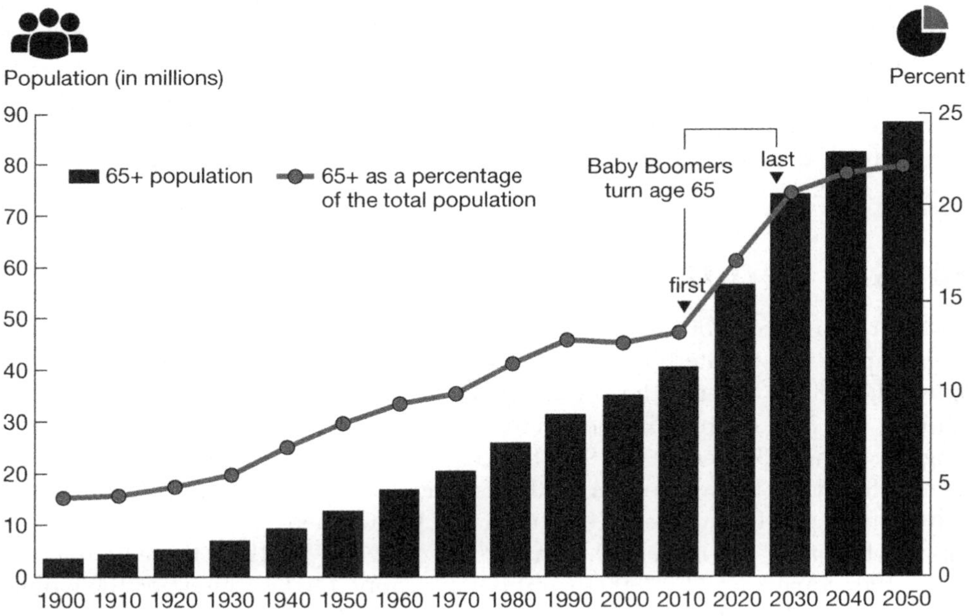

Figure 1.1 Baby boom generation and its affect on U. S. population age 65 and over, 1900 through 2050.

Sources: West, L. A. Cole, S. Goodkind, D. & He, W. (2014). *65+ in the United States: 2010* (Current Population Reports, P23-212). Washington, DC: U.S. Government Printing Office; Federal Interagency Forum on Agency Related Statistics. (2016). Population Aging in the United States: A Global Perspective. Retrieved from https://agingstats.gov/images/olderamericans_agingpopulation.pdf

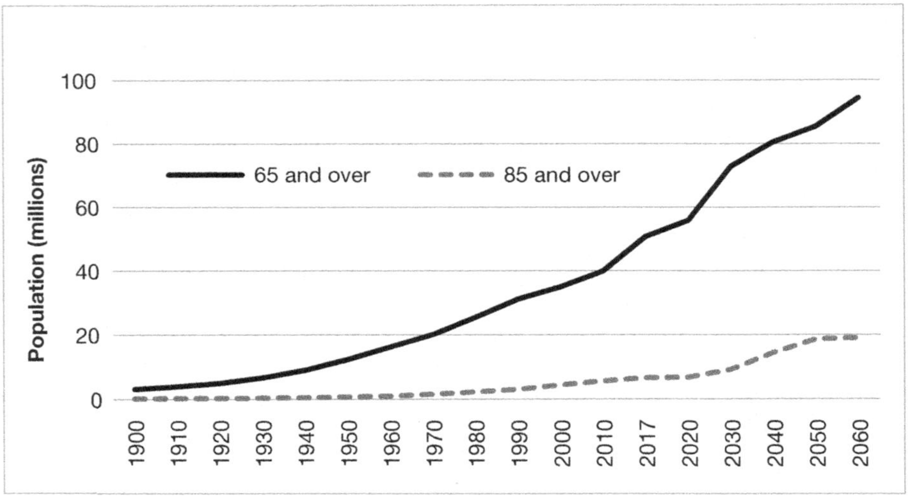

Figure 1.2 Population breakdown by age group.

Note: Data for 2020 to 2060 are projections of the population. Data refer to resident populations and noninstitutionalized individuals.

Source: U.S. Census Bureau, National Census and Projections, 2017.

the age group 85 and older represented 12.7% of the older adult population and represented a 33.8% growth from 2000 (U.S. Census Bureau, 2011, 2018b). In the 2000 U.S. Census, there were 50,454 centenarians, while 2010 recognized an increase of 5.5% in this category and a total of 53,364 centenarians living in the United States (U.S. Census Bureau, 2018a). By 2017, it was estimated that there were 86,248 centenarians living in the United States (U.S. Census Bureau, 2018a). See Figure 1.2. Thus, our population profile appears to be growing older and grayer.

CHANGES IN OUR POPULATION PROFILE

It has been estimated that the fastest growing group of older adults is the 85-year and older group. It is estimated by the U.S. Census Bureau that approximately 19 million people will be 85 or older in the United States by 2060 (see Figure 1.3).

During the 20th century in the United States, there was a significant gender shift among the aging (65+ years). In 1900, the U.S. Census Bureau reported that there were 108.5 men for every 100 women. In 1950, this ratio declined slightly; however, there were still more men per 100 women (102.3 men per 100 women). In 1960, there were equal numbers of women per men (100 men per 100 women). By 1980, there were only 69.7 men per 100 women, and by 1990 the ratio had dropped to 64.1 men per 100 women, as shown in Table 1.2. By 2005, this ratio has increased to 74.5 men per every 100 women at 65 years of age or older. The good news is that this gap was slightly narrowed by 2017, and the number of men per 100 women at 65 years of age and older increased to 79.7 (U.S. Census Bureau, 2018b). This figure dramatically changes as people age, and at the 85-year-old and older category, we find 54.4 males per 100 females (U.S. Census Bureau, 2018b). However, this is an increase from 2000 and 1990, which recognized ratios of 50.5 and 45.6 respectively (U.S Census Bureau, 2018b).

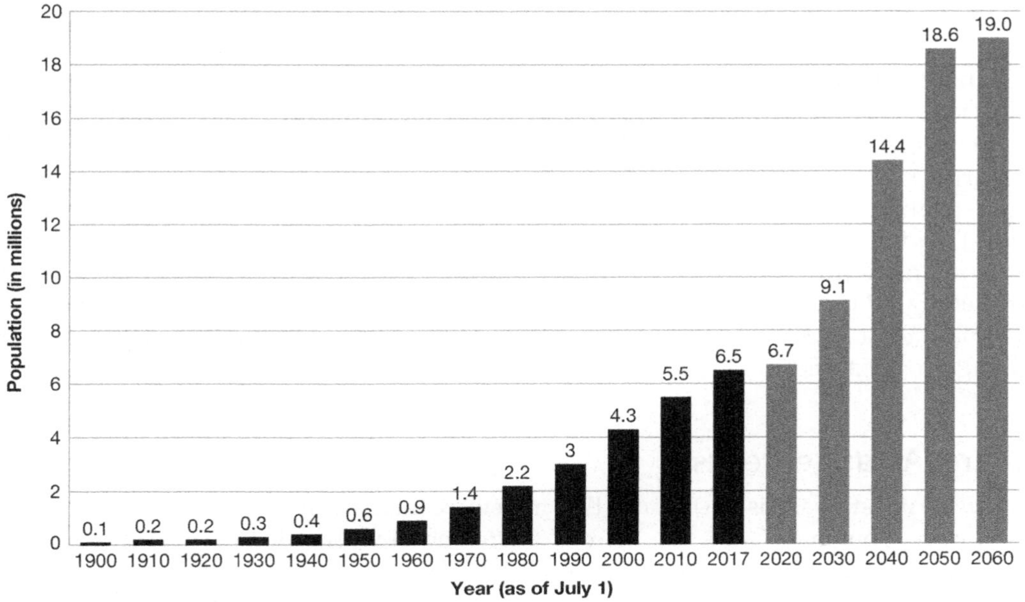

Figure 1.3 Number of persons age 65 and over, 1900 to 2060 (numbers in millions).

Note: Chart shows the large increases in the older population from 0.1 million people in 1900 to 6.5 million in 2017 and projected to 19.0 million in 2060.
Note: Increments in years are uneven.

Source: U.S. Census Bureau, 2017 Population Estimates and Projections.

Table 1.2 Changes in Population Profile: Males and Females

Year	Number of Males per 100 Females
1870	111.4
1900	108.5
1950	102.3
1960	100
1980	69.7
1990	64.1
2000	76.3
2010	80.2
2014	78.5
2017	79.7

Source: U.S. Bureau of the Census, 1870, 1900, 1950, 1960, 1980, 1990, 2000, 2010, and 2017 (assorted years).

These dramatic shifts in numbers, especially over the past 40 years, will leave more women living alone and widowed, while men will be more likely to remain married or attended by women. Other implications of these statistics will include the need to target income support mechanisms and social support programs for widowed and single women. This will have multiple effects on policies related to Supplemental Security Income (SSI), disability insurance (DI), and Medicare, especially funding. Statistically, more older adult men are married (70%) than are older adult women (46%), and more women are widowed (33%) than men (11%). Only 5% of men and 6% of women are found to be single (never married). While in 2005, 8% of both groups are separated or divorced, by 2017 this number had risen to 16% for women and 14% for men (ACL, 2018). Figure 1.4 provides an illustration of these statistics and the changes over a decade.

Living Arrangements

As to marital status, it is no surprise that men were more likely to live with spouses (72%) than were women (48%), while more women tended to live alone or with nonrelatives (34%) than were their male counterparts (20%). Women were also more likely to live with other relatives (16.8%) than were men (6.1%) in 2005. In comparison, by 2015 (the latest available data for this parameter) the numbers had not changed significantly: 6.0% of men and 16.4% of women (FIFARS, 2016) lived with other relatives. Figure 1.5 provides an illustration of these data (ACL, 2018).

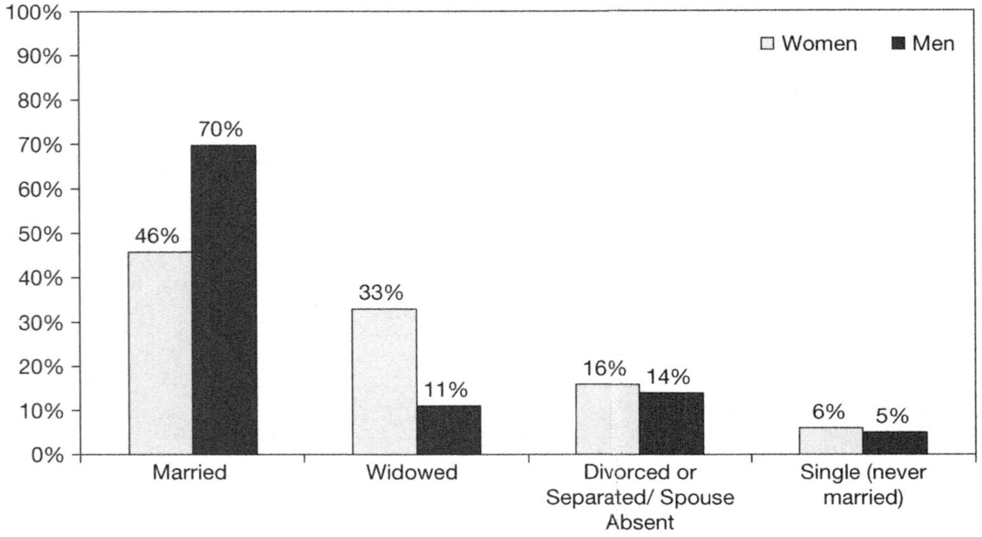

Figure 1.4 Marital status of persons age 65 and over, 2017.

Note: Chart shows the gender differences as men are more likely to be married (70% to 46%) and women more likely to be widowed (33% to 11%).

Source: U.S. Census Bureau. (2017a). *Current population survey, annual social and economic supplement. Table 1: Educational attainment of the population 18 years and over, by age, sex, race, and Hispanic origin: 2017.* Retrieved from http://www.census.gov/data/tables/2017/demo/education-attainment/cps-detailed-tables.html

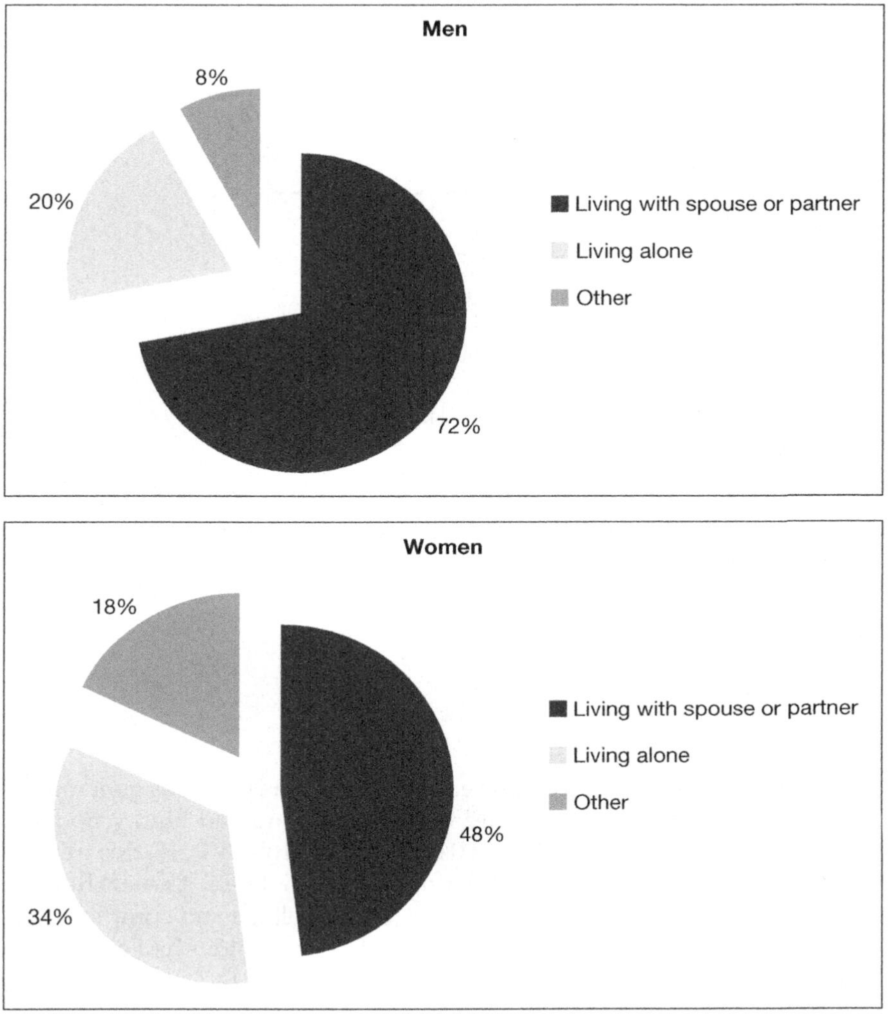

Figure 1.5 Living arrangements of persons age 65 and over, 2017.

Source: U.S. Census Bureau. (2017a). *Current population survey, annual social and economic supplement. Table 1: Educational attainment of the population 18 years and over, by age, sex, race, and Hispanic origin: 2017.* Retrieved from http://www.census.gov/data/tables/2017/demo/education-attainment/cps-detailed-tables.html

A number of interesting trends have occurred between 1970, 2005, and 2017 among both men and women with regard to living alone. The number of men living alone has steadily increased among men aged 65 to 74 years of age (11.3% in 1970 to 16.1% in 2005 and 17.9% in 2017). Men living alone in the 75-and-over age category have also steadily risen from 19.1% in 1970 to 23.2% in 2005 and to 24.1% in 2017. The percentage of women between the ages of 65 and 74 living alone has slightly dropped (31.7% in 1970 versus 28.9% in 2005 and 26.9% in 2017). The age group that has had the most drastic rise in women living alone is the 75-and-over category (37% in 1970 as compared with 49.9% in 2004, and 44.6% in 2017; U.S. Census Bureau, 2017b, 2017c). Figure 1.6 provides an overview of these data.

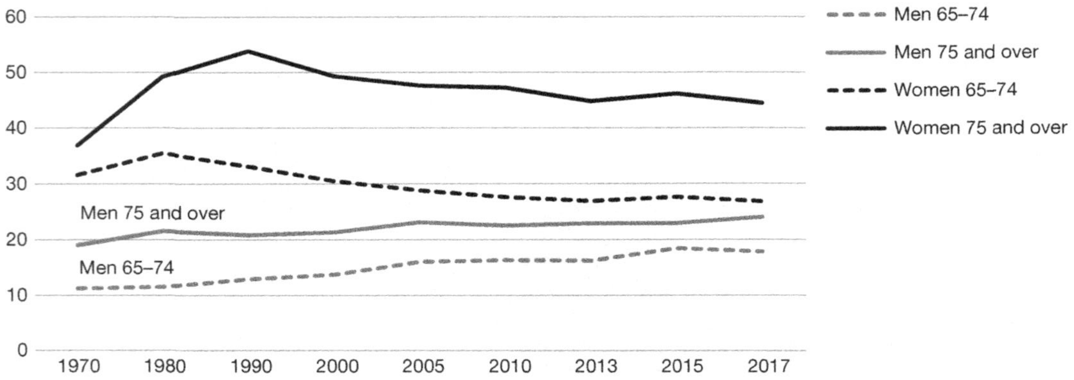

Figure 1.6 Percentage of population age 65 and over living alone, by sex and age, selected years, 1970 to 2017.

Note: Reference population: These data refer to the civilian noninstitutionalized population.

Source: U.S. Census Bureau. (2017a). *Current population survey, annual social and economic supplement. Table 1: Educational attainment of the population 18 years and over, by age, sex, race, and Hispanic origin: 2017.* Retrieved from http://www.census.gov/data/tables/2017/demo/education-attainment/cps-detailed-tables.html

Education Level

Today older adults are increasingly more educated than the previous generation. In 1965, only 23.5% of adults 65 years of age and older had completed high school degrees as compared to 48.2% in 1985 and 73.1% in 2004 (FIFARS, 2016). By 2017, this trend increased to 86% of people over the age of 65 completing high school (U.S. Census Bureau, 2017a). Similarly, there has been an increasing trend to attend college and complete a bachelor's degree. In 1965, only 5% of older adults 65 years of age and older had completed a bachelor's degree, as compared to 9.4% in 1985 and 18.7% in 2004. By 2017, 30% of people over the age of 65 had completed at least a bachelor's degree. (U.S. Census Bureau, 2017a). Figure 1.7 provides an illustration of these data.

Despite improvements in the overall education level of older adults over the past few decades, disparities still exist across ethnic groups. In 2007, non-Hispanic Whites were more educated than Blacks, Asians, and Hispanics. Whites aged 65 years and older were more likely than any other group to complete high school (81.1%) and a bachelor's degree (20.5%), than Blacks (57.4% completing high school and 10.3% completing a bachelor's degree) or Hispanics (42.2% completing high school and 8.9% completing a bachelor's degree). These variations in education level pose implications for the development of innovative resources, teaching tools, and training initiatives that may need to be tailored for the various educational levels.

A decade later, these educational gaps narrowed significantly. In 2017, high school completers among Whites had jumped an additional 10% to 91% from 81%. Asians had 79% high school completers, and 74% of African Americans completed high school in 2017 as compared to 57.4% in 2007. Hispanics could boast of 58% high school graduates in the 65+ cohort in 2017 as compared to 42.2% a decade earlier. Figure 1.8 provides an overview of these data.

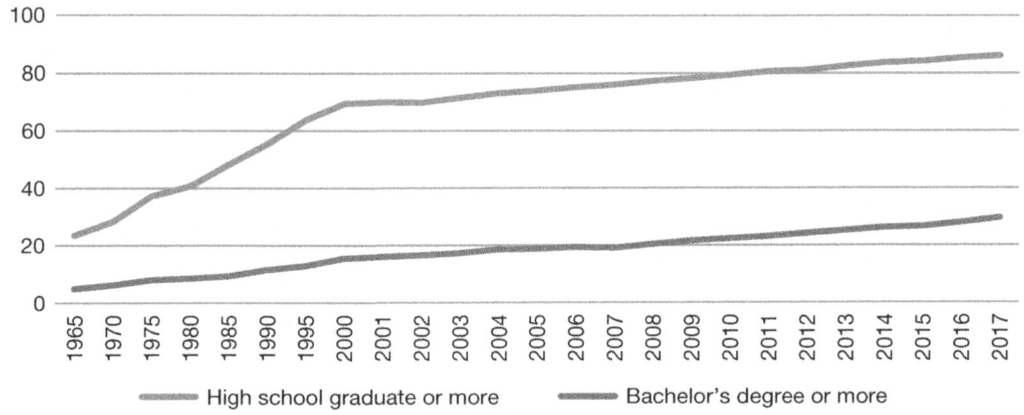

Figure 1.7 Educational attainment of the population age 62 and over, 1965 to 2017.

Note: A single question that asks for the highest grade or degree completed is used to determine educational attainment. Prior to 1995, educational attainment was measured using data on years of school completed. Reference population: These data refer to the civilian noninstitutionalized population.

Source: U.S. Census Bureau. (2017a). *Current population survey, annual social and economic supplement. Table 1: Educational attainment of the population 18 years and over, by age, sex, race, and Hispanic origin: 2017.* Retrieved from http://www.census.gov/data/tables/2017/demo/education-attainment/cps-detailed-tables.html

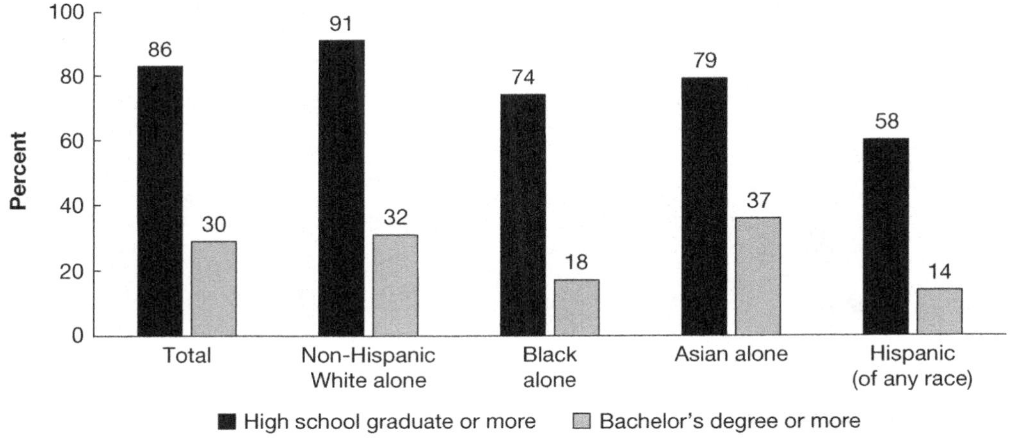

Figure 1.8 Educational attainment of the population age 65 and over, by race and Hispanic origin, 2017.

Note: The term "non-Hispanic White alone" is used to refer to people who reported being White and no other race and who are not Hispanic. The term "Black alone" is used to refer to people who reported being Black or African American and no other race, and the term "Asian alone" is used to refer to people who reported only Asian as their race. The use of single-race populations in this chart does not imply that this is the preferred method of presenting or analyzing data. The U.S. Census Bureau uses a variety of approaches. Reference population: These data refer to the civilian noninstitutionalized population.

Source: U.S. Census Bureau. (2017a). *Current population survey, annual social and economic supplement. Table 1: Educational attainment of the population 18 years and over, by age, sex, race, and Hispanic origin: 2017.* Retrieved from http://www.census.gov/data/tables/2017/demo/education-attainment/cps-detailed-tables.html

Economic Well-Being

Over the past several years there has been much debate about privatizing the Social Security program. Although there may be a portion of the population within a high-income bracket that could afford to invest money for their future (38% of people over the age of 65 years have incomes of $75,000 or more), over one fourth of families with the head of the household over 65 years of age (26%) are families living below $35,000 per year (see Figure 1.9). When one further explores this issue and examines the distribution of income among people 65 years of age and older, it is found that 66% of this group are receiving less than $35,000 per year (see Figure 1.10). These limited funds make survival difficult within one's retirement years without some financing alternatives such as "reverse mortgages" and other creative financing options.

When considering sources of income for people 65 years of age and over, it appears that there is a trend toward reliance upon Social Security income, more so in 2015 (33%) than in 1962 (31% support). Pensions were also increasingly important (20% of income in 2015) as compared to 1962 (9% pension income). Asset income in 2015 accounted for 9% of total income as compared to 16% of total income in 1962. Table 1.3 provides an overview of these data.

This trend has been changing over the past decades. In 1974, the median household income for people 65 years of age and older was $23,817 (expressed in 2016 dollars), while the median household income in 2016 was $58,559 (ACL, 2018). Income for this aging population came from five major sources, with Social Security still supporting the majority of people within this age group (84%). This was followed by asset income (63%), private pensions (37%), earnings (29%), while government employee pensions accounted for 16% of household income assets (ACL, 2018).

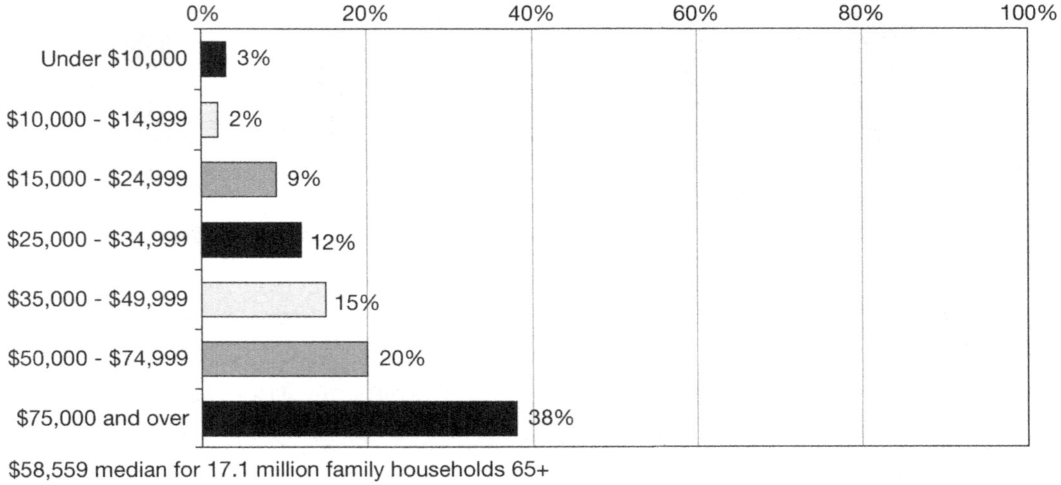

Figure 1.9 Family households with householder age 65 and over, 2016.

Note: Percentages may not add to 100 due to rounding.

Source: Administration for Community Living. (2018). *Profile of older Americans: 2017 profile.* Retrieved from https://www.acl.gov/sites/default/files/Aging%20and%20Disability%20in%20America/2017OlderAmericansProfile.pdf

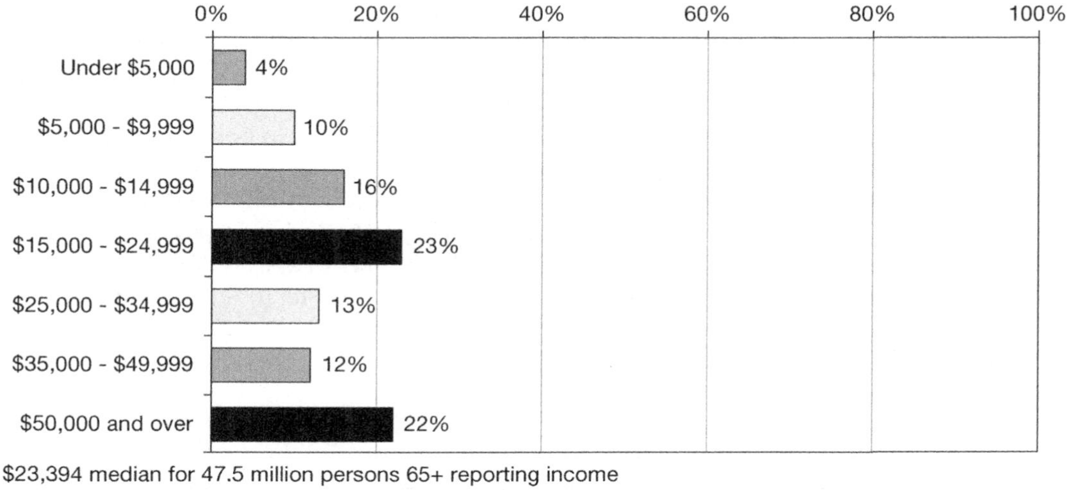

Figure 1.10 Persons age 65 and over reporting income, 2016.

Note: Percentages may not add to 100 due to rounding.

Source: Administration for Community Living. (2018). *Profile of older Americans: 2017 profile.* Retrieved from https://www.acl.gov/sites/default/files/Aging%20and%20Disability%20in%20America/2017Older AmericansProfile.pdf

Table 1.3 Sources of Income for Adults 65+ Years of Age (Represented by Percent Values)

Source	1962	1976	1980	1990	2000	2004	2015
Social Security	31	39	39	36	38	39	33
Asset income	16	18	22	24	18	13	9
Pensions	9	16	16	18	18	13	20
Earnings	28	23	19	18	23	26	34
Other	16	4	4	4	3	2	4
Total	100	100	100	100		100	100

Notes: Income is aggregated by source for selected years, 1962 to 2004, represented as percentages. The definition of "other" includes, but is not limited to, public assistance, unemployment compensation, worker's compensation, alimony, child support, and personal contributions.
Data refer to noninstitutionalized populations.

Sources: Social Security Administration, 1963 Survey of the Aged, 1968 Survey of Demographic and Economic Characteristics of the Aged.

Sources from Administration for Community Living (2018):
U.S. Census Bureau, Current Population Survey, Annual Social and Economic Supplement, FINC-01. Selected Characteristics of Families by Total Money Income in 2016; PINC-01. Selected Characteristics of People 15 Years Old and Over by Total Money Income in 2016, Work Experience in 2016, Race, Hispanic Origin, and Sex; and U.S. Census Bureau, Income and Poverty in the United States: 2016, Current Population Reports, P60-259, issued September 2017. Social Security Administration, "Fast Facts and Figures about Social Security, 2017."

Despite these concerns about income, older adults 65 years of age and older are not actually the most prevalent group living in poverty over time. When compared to individuals younger than 18 years of age or people aged 18 to 64, more of the youngest age group were noted to be in poverty (18.0%) than were other age groups. Although one would think that the older adults would be more prone to living in poverty, by 2016, 18% of children were living in poverty as compared to about 9% of adults 65+ years of age (ACL, 2018; FIFARS, 2016; U.S. Census Bureau, 2016). Among individuals over the age of 65, the oldest group of people were the most likely to be living in poverty, based on the latest available data in 2014 (ACL, 2018). People 85 years of age and older were noted to have 12.7% of their cohort living in poverty, as compared to 10% for all individuals 65 years of age and older. Over the past decade these trends have not changed much. Figure 1.11 shows these data.

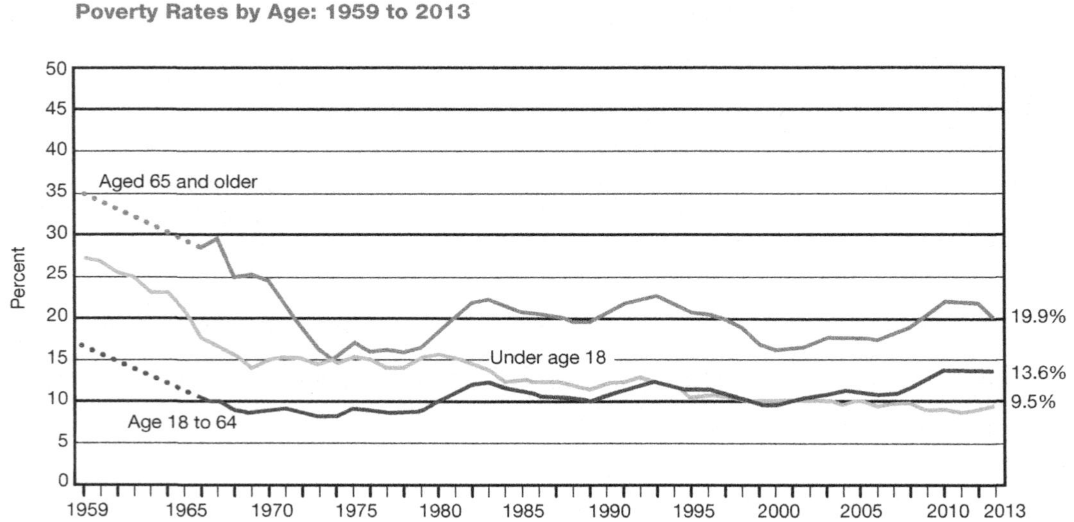

Figure 1.11 Percentage living in poverty—a comparison across the life span.

Note: Data for people aged 18 to 64 and 65 and older are not available from 1960 to 1965.

Source: DeNavas-Walt, C. & Proctor, B. (2014). *Income and Poverty in the United States: 2013* (Current Population Reports, P60-249). Retrieved from https://www2.census.gov/library/publications/2014/demographics/p60-249.pdf

Racial variation was seen among those living in poverty in 2016. For example, in 2016, older non-Hispanic White men were less likely to live in poverty than African American, Hispanic, or Asian men. Only 6% of older non-Hispanic White men lived in poverty compared to 16% of older African American men, 14% of older Hispanic men, and 10% of older Asian men. The same contrasts also held true for women, as older non-Hispanic White women were represented in poverty by 8% as compared to African American women being represented 20%, older Hispanic women by 20%, and Asian women by 13%. The stark difference between older men and older women of color living in poverty may be an issue to consider with regard to policy to address this gender gap (U.S. Census Bureau, 2017d).

Changes in Rural Population

Although there has been a well-documented shift from agrarian/rural-based population to urban settings, the proportion of people living in rural settings (areas of fewer than 9,999 people) has remained relatively stable over since the 1990s. At the turn of the 20th century, 39.8% of the population lived in rural settings. This percentage increased steadily until 1950, when nearly three fourths of all Americans lived in rural settings (71.2%). Between 1950 and 1960, nearly 50% of people living in rural settings migrated to urban settings, dropping from 71.2% to 37.5%. The percentages have remained relatively stable over the last 40 years with slight decreases in rural populations from year to year. In 2016, 17.5% of the total rural population were 65 years of age or older (U.S. Census Bureau, 2016).

The rural demographic portrait becomes more descriptive, particularly with regards to the proportion of people living in rural areas who are 65 years of age and over and who live in very small rural communities (fewer than 2,500 people). Table 1.4 outlines this demographic shift.

This demographic picture is further compounded by those who were foreign-born and are living in rural areas, as shown in Table 1.5. These are foreign-born people who immigrated to the United States and are living in Frontier Rural Communities (referred to areas of fewer than 2,500 people) or who live in rural communities (2,500–9,999). While there has been a decrease (over 50%) of foreign-born people living in rural areas (59.8% in areas of <2,500 people; 14.3% in areas of 2,500–9,999 in 1900 vs. 24.8% Frontier Rural in 1990 and 6.0% in rural communities with a population of 2,500–9,999, respectively), there have been more women than men 65 years of age and older and more foreign-born people residing in smaller rural centers.

Table 1.4 Shift in Percentage of People Living in Rural Settings

Year	Percentage of the Population Living in Rural Settings
1900	59.8
1950	71.2
1960	37.5
1970	33.5
1980	32.7
1990	30.8
2000	24.6
2010	17.2
2016	17.5

Source: U.S. Bureau of the Census, 1900, 1950, 1960, 1970, 1980, 1990, 2000, 2005, 2010, 2016 (assorted years) 2016, Current population estimate survey.

Table 1.5 Percentage of People Foreign Born

Year	<2,500	2,500–9,999	%65+	Males	Females	Rate: Males/Females
1900	59.8	14.3	9.2	8.8	9.7	108.5
1910	53.7	24.3	8.9	8.1	9.9	105.3
1920	48.6	25.4	9.7	9.0	10.5	104.7
1930	43.8	26.6	12.0	11.6	12.5	107.7
1950	43.5	27.7	26.3	26.2	26.5	100
1960	30.1	7.4	32.6	33.4	31.9	100
1970	26.5	7.0	32.0	31.5	32.3	82.4
1980	26.3	6.4	21.2	18.6	23.4	69.7
1990	24.8	6.0	13.6	10.9	16.3	64.1
2000	22.4	5.7	10.7	4.2	6.5	65.6
2010	21.2	5.6	10.2	4.1	6.3	64.5
2015	20.9	5.6	10.1	4.1	6.2	64.4

Sources: Gibson, C. J., & Lennon, E. (1999). *Historical census statistics on the foreign-born population of the United States: 1850–1990* (Population Division Working Paper No. 29). Washington, DC: U.S. Census Bureau; U.S. Census Bureau. (2005). *Census 2000 special tabulations (STP-159).* Washington, DC: Author; United States Census Bureau Population Estimates, 2015.

The number of foreign-born people residing in small rural areas or Frontier Communities (fewer than 2,500) who are over 65 years of age raises some serious concerns about the need for services, which may need to be culturally sensitive and culturally diverse. These services may also need to address such issues as cultural expectations around help-seeking behaviors, the role of religion and mortality, the aging process, loss of independence, and expectations around social supports. Language barriers may also play a role in the delivery of services and access to services within rural communities (see Table 1.5.)

Trends in Morbidity and Mortality

Over the last century there have been dramatic changes in the facts of morbidity for older adults. These changes are due to technological advances, changes in quality of life and living conditions, and advances in medicine. In 1900, the leading cause of death for people 40 years of age and older was tuberculosis, while for women it was childbirth (Picket & Hanlon, 1995). According to the National Health Interview Survey (NHIS; CDC & NHIS, 1997), the leading cause of morbidity in 1994 for people 65 years of age and over was arthritis (50 per 100). Hypertension was the second leading cause of morbidity (36 per 100), followed by heart disease (32 per 100). The first editions of this text (published in 2007) suggested that the changes in morbidity lead to a need for renewed public health, health promotion, and health education strategies. New approaches were thought to be necessary to accommodate these health promotion efforts, which have recently been identified within the Older Americans Act amendments of 2006 and subsequently followed up within amendments in succeeding years. Updates from the Federal Interagency Forum on Aging-Related Statistics (2016a) indicate that the rates of morbidity and mortality is not increasing, but slightly decreasing. Thus, the focus on health literacy and health promotion efforts does appear to be making an inroad with the control of morbidity and mortality for older adults (see Table 1.6 and Figure 1.12).

Recently, there has been a change in perceptions about health among older adults. In 2014, 21.7% of the population 65 and older rated their health as fair to poor, as compared to 9.7% for the general population. However, there was a difference between general perceived health status of African Americans, 13.2% of whom reported their health as fair to poor, and only 9.4% of Whites who reported their health as fair to poor (CDC, 2014). These statistics show a growing percentage of the population over the age of 65 who perceive themselves to be in poor health and an increase in disparity between people of color (CDC, 2014). These data serve to illustrate the importance of interventions to target diverse groups. The differences in perceived health status will also have an impact on health promotion programs to target older adults and reach minority groups in meaningful ways (see Figure 1.13).

One's perceived health status is also compounded by difficulties reported with carrying out activities of daily living (ADLs) by people 65 and older. Respondents in the 2014 National Health Interview Survey (CDC, 2014) who identified themselves as being over 65 years old and were living independently within their community reported difficulties

Table 1.6 Rates of Morbidity

Type of Illness	Rate per 100 in the Population (65+)
Arthritis (2013–2015)	49.6 per 100
Hypertension (2015–2016)	63.1 per 100
Heart disease	29.4 per 100
Hearing	29 per 100
Cataracts	17 per 100
Orthopedic impairments	15 per 100

Source: Barbour, K. E., Helmick, C. G., Boring, M., & Brady, T. J. (2017). Vital signs: Prevalence of doctor-diagnosed arthritis and arthritis-attributable activity limitation—United States, 2013–2015. *Morbidity and Mortality Weekly Report, 66*(9), 246–253. Retrieved from http://www.cdc.gov/mmwr/volumes/66/wr/mm6609e1.htm; Fryar, C. D., Ostchega, Y., Hales, C. M., Zhang, G., & Kruszon-Moran, D. (2017). *Hypertension prevalence and control among adults: United States, 2015–2016* (NCHS Data Brief No. 289). Hyattsville, MD: National Center for Health Statistics. Retrieved from http://www.cdc.gov/nchs/data/databriefs/db289.pdf; Centers for Disease Control and Prevention, National Center for Health Statistics. (2013). *Summary health statistics for the U.S. population, the National Health Interview Survey, 2012*. Hyattsville, MD: U.S. Department of Health and Human Services.

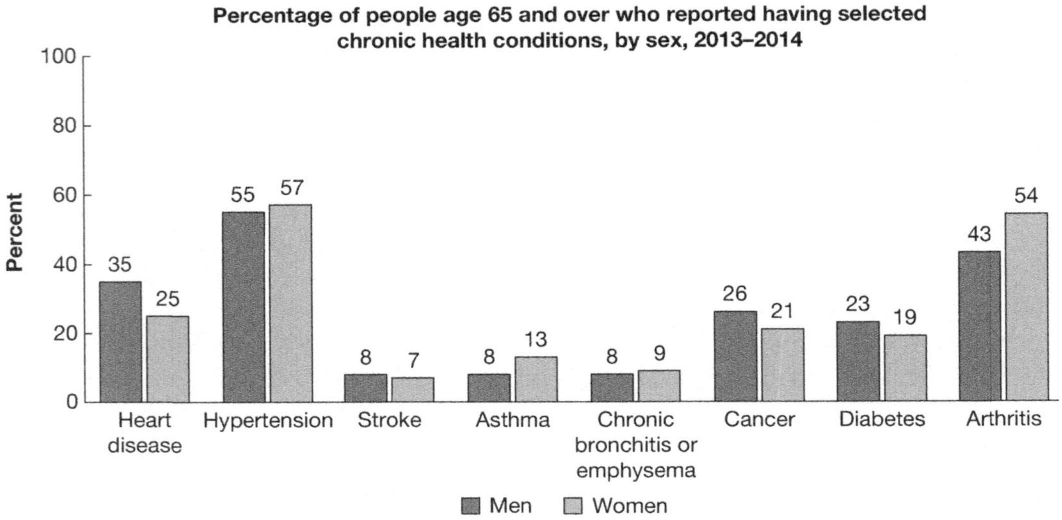

Figure 1.12 Health status related to chronic conditions of older adults.

Note: Data are based on a 2-year average from 2013 to 2014.

Source: Centers for Disease Control and Prevention, National Center for Health Statistics (2014). Summary health statistics for the U.S. population, the National Health Interview Survey, 2014. Hyattsville, MD: U.S. Department of Health and Human Services. Retrieved from https://ftp.cdc.gov/pub/Health_Statistics/NCHS/NHIS/SHS/2014_SHS_Table_A-11.pdf

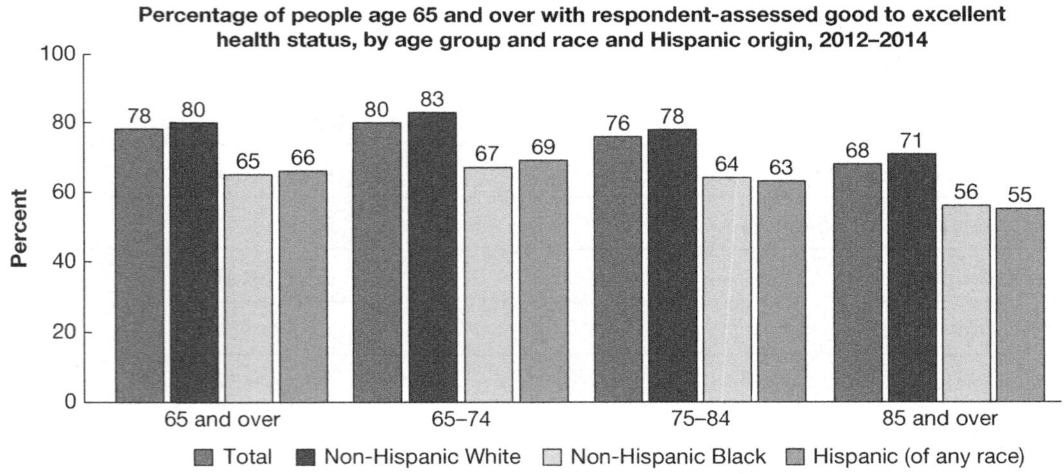

Figure 1.13 Perceived health status—comparing for ethnic diversity.

Note: Data are based on a 3-year average from 2012 to 2014. Total includes all other races not shown separately. See data sources for the definition of race and Hispanic origin in the National Health Interview Survey. Reference population: These data refer to the civilian noninstitutionalized population.

Source: Centers for Disease Control and Prevention, National Center for Health Statistics (2014). Summary health statistics for the U.S. population, the National Health Interview Survey, 2014. Hyattsville, MD: U.S. Department of Health and Human Services. Retrieved from https://ftp.cdc.gov/pub/Health_Statistics/NCHS/NHIS/SHS/2014_SHS_Table_A-11.pdf

with carrying out both ADLs and instrumental activities of daily living (IADLs). These are reflected in greater detail in Tables 1.7, 1.8, 1.9, and 1.10). ADLs, characterized as bathing, dressing, feeding, mobility, toileting, and transferring were reported as problematic for 14% of the noninstitutionalized population who were over 65 years of age. These figures have not changed radically over the past decade, and this number changed slightly (by 1%) and as recently as 2015 represents 15% of the older adult population (Administration for Community Living, 2016). According to the CDC, 37.9% of people 65 years of age or older report having a disability that impacts their ADLs. In addition, although treated, 94% of people in the same age category report taking medication for high blood pressure.

Furthermore, 6.4% of the population reported having difficulty with IADLs. These activities included meal preparation, shopping, managing money, taking medication, doing housework, and using the telephone. These difficulties translate into needs for services to allow people to remain in their homes and communities. Increasingly, people

Table 1.7 Older Adults With Difficulties in Physical Functioning (Age Adjusted Percentages)

Area of Functioning	18–44 Years	65–74 Years	75+
Any physical activity	4.9	28.3	47.0
Cannot walk ¼ mile	1.6	14.3	27.0
Difficulty climbing 10 stairs without rest	1.2	10.1	20.1
Difficulty standing for 2 hours	2.7	18.0	30.4
Difficulty stooping, bending, or kneeling	2.6	17.0	28.6
Difficulty reaching over one's head	0.7	3.6	7.8
Difficulty grasping or handling small objects	0.5	3.1	5.1
Difficulty lifting or carrying 10 pounds	1.1	7.2	15.3
Difficulty pushing or pulling large objects	1.9	10.4	20.4

Source: Centers for Disease Control and Prevention, National Center for Health Statistics (2014). *Summary health statistics for the U.S. population, the National Health Interview Survey, 2014.* Hyattsville, MD: U.S. Department of Health and Human Services. Retrieved from https://ftp.cdc.gov/pub/Health_Statistics/NCHS/NHIS/SHS/2014_SHS_Table_A-11.pdf

Table 1.8 Older Adults (65+) With Difficulties in Physical Functioning, by Insurance Type (Age Adjusted Percentages)

Area of Functioning	Private	Medicare and Medicaid	Medicare Only	Other	Uninsured
Any physical activity	33.2	62.4	36.6	43.2	54.5
Cannot walk ¼ mile	17.7	38.6	20.9	20.2	12.1
Difficulty climbing 10 stairs without rest	12.0	33.2	15.5	14.2	22.9
Difficulty standing for 2 hours	20.7	43.6	24.1	28.4	15.1
Difficulty stooping, bending or kneeling	20.0	42.3	21.4	23.3	28.3
Difficulty reaching over one's head	4.4	15.5	5.2	6.7	–
Difficulty grasping or handling small objects	3.0	8.7	4.5	5.6	–
Difficulty lifting or carrying 10 pounds	7.9	32.8	11.4	9.7	19.1
Difficulty pushing or pulling large objects	11.7	38.4	15.5	14.2	30.0

Source: Centers for Disease Control and Prevention, National Center for Health Statistics (2014). *Summary health statistics for the U.S. population, the National Health Interview Survey, 2014*. Hyattsville, MD: U.S. Department of Health and Human Services. Retrieved from https://ftp.cdc.gov/pub/Health_Statistics/NCHS/NHIS/SHS/2014_SHS_Table_A-11.pdf

Table 1.9 Overview of Physical Functioning in the United States in 2014

Selected Characteristic: Family Income	Age 18 and Over	Any Physical Difficulty (Frequencies)	Any Physical Difficulty (Percentages)
Total	239,688	36,172	14.2 (0.23)
Sex			
Male	115,541	13,181	11.1 (0.31)
Female	124,148	22,990	16.9 (0.34)
Age (years)			
18–44 Years	112,149	5,521	4.9 (0.25)
45–64 Years	82,605	14,471	17.5 (0.46)
65–74 Years	26,362	7,453	28.3 (0.87)
75 Years and Over	18,573	8,726	47.0 (1.14)
Race			
One Race	235,831	35,606	14.1 (0.23)
White	190,462	29,130	13.9 (0.26)
African American	29,355	4,873	17.4 (0.65)
American Indian or Alaska Native	1,948	413	21.3 (3.56)
Asian	13,733	1,111	9.3 (0.72)
Native Hawaiian or Other Pacific Islander	333	79	31.9 (6.77)
Two or More Races	3,858	566	17.1 (1.94)
African American, White	760	69	17.0 (5.12)
American Indian or Alaska Native, White	1,590	373	21.2 (3.38)
Hispanic or Latino Origin and Race			
Hispanic or Latino	36,571	3,919	14.0 (0.56)

(*continued*)

Table 1.9 Overview of Physical Functioning in the United States in 2014 (*continued*)

Selected Characteristic: Family Income	Age 18 and Over	Any Physical Difficulty (Frequencies)	Any Physical Difficulty (Percentages)
Mexican or Mexican American	22,326	2,276	14.5 (0.77)
Not Hispanic or Latino	203,117	32,252	14.3 (0.26)
White, Single Race	157,364	25,622	14.0 (0.29)
African American, Single Race	27,875	4,726	17.6 (0.67)
Education			
Less than a High School Diploma	27,612	8,179	24.9 (0.80)
High School Diploma or GED	52,697	10,799	18.1 (0.55)
Some College	59,919	10,068	16.5 (0.49)
Bachelor's Degree or Higher	67,940	5,836	9.3 (0.37)
Current Employment Status			
Employed	146,624	7,930	7.5 (0.40)
Full-Time	117,112	5,153	6.3 (0.58)
Part-Time	27,205	2,505	10.8 (0.78)
Unemployed but has Worked Previously	79,316	25,437	24.9 (0.57)
Unemployed and Never Worked	13,623	2,779	22.2 (1.34)
Family Income			
Less than $35,000	69,793	18,034	23.7 (0.49)
$35,000 Or More	144,503	14,433	10.5 (0.27)
$35,000–$49,999	28,044	4,342	14.7 (0.63)

(*continued*)

Table 1.9 Overview of Physical Functioning in the United States in 2014 (*continued*)

Selected Characteristic: Family Income	**Age 18 and Over**	**Any Physical Difficulty (Frequencies)**	**Any Physical Difficulty (Percentages)**
$50,000–$74,999	35,733	4,311	11.7 (0.59)
$75,000–$99,999	27,053	2,557	10.1 (0.63)
$100,000 Or More	53,673	3,224	7.8 (0.49)
Poverty Status			
Poor	31,383	7,713	27.2 (0.78)
Near Poor	42,675	9,518	21.0 (0.59)
Not Poor	152,199	16,834	10.4 (0.26)
Health Insurance Coverage			
Under 65			
Private	129,666	7,963	5.5 (0.24)
Medicaid	23,239	5,888	25.8 (0.90)
Other	9,095	3,336	27.1 (2.37)
Uninsured	31,587	2,662	9.0 (0.55)
65 and Over:			
Private	22,525	7,216	33.2 (0.93)
Medicare and Medicaid	2,951	1,835	62.4 (2.28)
Medicare Only	15,536	5,488	36.6 (1.22)
Other	3,513	1,451	43.2 (2.58)
Uninsured	313	140	54.5 (6.33)
Marital Status			
Married	126,926	16,776	118 (0.31)
Widowed	14,312	6,445	20.7 (1.75)
Divorced or Separated	26,802	6,710	20.8 (0.77)
Never Married	53,788	4,370	15.2 (0.66)
Living With a Partner	17,497	1,801	14.3 (1.27)

(*continued*)

Table 1.9 Overview of Physical Functioning in the United States in 2014 (*continued*)

Selected Characteristic: Family Income	Age 18 and Over	Any Physical Difficulty (Frequencies)	Any Physical Difficulty (Percentages)
Place of Residence			
Large MSA	130,402	16,731	12.7 (0.30)
Small MSA	73,885	11,803	14.9 (0.44)
Not MSA	35,402	7,638	18.3 (0.73)
Region			
Northeast	41,490	5,499	11.6 (0.46)
Midwest	55,095	8,621	14.8 (0.50)
South	89,270	14,810	15.5 (0.40)
West	53,834	7,242	13.41 (0.49)
Hispanic or Latino Origin, Race, and Sex			
Hispanic or Latino, Male	18,309	1,419	10.9 (0.76)
Hispanic or Latino, Female	18,262	2,501	16.8 (0.79)
Not Hispanic or Latino:			
White, Single Race, Male	76,277	9,643	11.3 (0.39)
White, Single Race, Female	81,087	15,979	16.5 (0.44)
African American, Single Race, Male	12,626	1,537	12.9 (0.83)
African American, Single Race, Female	15,249	3,189	21.1 (0.93)

GED, General Education Diploma; MSA, Metropolitan Statistical Areas.

Note: Represents the percentages (with standard errors) and frequencies (number in thousands) of individuals in the United States living with difficulties in physical functioning among individuals ages 18 and over in the United States, 2014.

Source: National Center for Health Statistics. (2016). *Health, United States, 2015: With special feature on racial and ethnic health disparities*. Hyattsville, MD: Centers for Disease Control and Prevention.

Table 1.10 Overview of People Living With Disabilities in the United States (2014)

Selected Characteristic	Age 18 and Over	ADLs	IADLs
Total	239,684	2.1 (0.07) 5,322	4.0 (0.10) 9,950
Sex			
Male	115,539	1.8 (0.09) 2,102	3.2 (0.11) 3,648
Female	124,145	2.4 (0.09) 3,220	4.7 (0.13) 6,303
Age (Years)			
18–44 Years	112,146	0.8 (0.06) 871	1.5 (0.08) 1,642
45–64 Years	82,604	1.9 (0.10) 1,542	3.8 (0.15) 3,112
65–74 Years	26,210	3.5 (0.24) 929	6.4 (0.31) 1,679
75 Years and Over	18,724	10.6 (0.51) 1,981	18.8 (0.76) 3,518
Race			
One Race	*236,024*	*2.1 (0.07) 5,214*	*4.0 (0.10) 9,716*
White	190,508	1.9 (0.07) 3,887	3.8(0.11) 7,733
African American	29,458	3.9 (0.22) 1,044	5.9 (0.26) 1,585
American Indian or Alaska Native	2,078	3.7 (0.87) 64	5.4 (1.03) 98
Asian	13,665	2.1 (0.24) 213	2.9 (0.29) 292
Native Hawaiian or Other Pacific Islander	316	2.9 (1.13)*	8.0 (3.20)*
Two or More Races	*3,659*	*4.0 (0.71) 109*	*7.7 (0.96) 235*
African American, White	90	4.7 (2.30) 11	8.3 (2.62) 35
American Indian or Alaska Native, White	1,487	4.4 (1.08) 62	10.6 (1.80) 153
Hispanic or Latino Origin and Race			
Hispanic or Latino	36,571	2.6 (0.18) 648	3.9 (0.22) 1,025

(continued)

Table 1.10 Overview of People Living With Disabilities in the United States (2014) (*continued*)

Selected Characteristic	Age 18 and Over	ADLs	IADLs
Mexican or Mexican American	22,625	2.5 (0.26) 350	3.7 (0.30) 539
Not Hispanic or Latino	203,113	2.1 (0.07) 4,674	4.1 (0.11) 8,926
White, Single Race	157,459	1.8 (0.08) 3,301	3.8 (0.12) 6,855
African American, Single Race	27,941	4.0 (0.22) 1,015	5.9 (0.27) 1,520
Education			
Less than a High School Diploma	27,164	4.1 (0.22) 1,409	7.4 (0.29) 2,498
High School Diploma or GED	54,688	2.7 (0.15) 1,633	5.0 (0.20) 3,037
Some College	57,708	2.0 (0.12) 1,128	4.2 (0.21) 2,397
Bachelor's Degree or Higher	65,986	1.2 (0.10) 674	2.5 (0.15) 1,362
Family Income			
Less than $35,000	64,836	3.7 (0.16) 2,687	7.6 (0.22) 5,504
$35,000 Or More	138,067	1.5 (0.08) 1,706	2.4 (0.10) 2,904
$35,000–$49,999	25,876	1.9 (0.17) 523	3.5 (0.23) 937
$50,000–$74,999	33,830	1.4 (0.13) 447	2.3 (0.17) 744
$75,000–$99,999	25,789	1.6 (0.21) 341	2.6 (0.25) 534
$100,000 Or More	52,581	1.2 (0.14) 394	2.1 (0.19) 689
Poverty Status			
Poor	29,228	4.9 (0.28) 1,234	9.9 (0.42) 2,513
Near Poor	41,335	3.1 (0.17) 1,391	6.1 (0.23) 2,731
Not Poor	146,714	1.4 (0.07) 2,045	2.5 (0.09) 3,663
Health Insurance Coverage			
Under 65			
Private	129,633	0.4 (0.04) 601	0.9 (0.05) 1,276

(*continued*)

Table 1.10 Overview of People Living With Disabilities in the United States (2014) (*continued*)

Selected Characteristic	Age 18 and Over	ADLs	IADLs
Medicaid	22,740	5.5 (0.32) 1,225	9.7 (0.41) 2,170
Other	8,497	3.7 (0.46) 381	7.6 (0.64) 841
Uninsured	31,333	0.6 (0.10) 178	1.4 (0.14) 415
65 and Over			
Private	22,018	4.4 (0.30) 890	9.7 (0.48) 1,961
Medicare and Medicaid	2,943	22.6 (1.61) 646	32.7 (1.97) 943
Medicare Only	15,867	7.3 (0.46) 1,099	12.4 (0.66) 1,858
Other	3,483	7.2 (0.91) 236	11.3 (1.10) 383
Uninsured	359	10.3 (4.50)* 21	10.4 (0.29)* 26
Place of Residence			
Large MSA	130,586	2.2 (0.10) 2,787	3.8 (0.13) 4,853
Small MSA	73,795	2.1 (0.12) 1,601	4.2 (0.18) 3,272
Not MSA	35,303	2.3 (0.19) 935	4.5 (0.29) 1,825
Region			
Northeast	42,170	2.0 (0.14) 926	3.4 (0.19) 1,553
Midwest	54,254	1.7 (0.13) 965	4.0 (0.21) 2,262
South	89,395	2.3 (0.12) 2,172	4.2 (0.17) 3,916
West	53,865	2.4 (0.15) 1,260	4.2 (0.21) 2,219
Hispanic or Latino Origin, Race, and Sex			
Hispanic or Latino, Male	18,308	2.0 (0.24) 246	2.8 (0.27) 368
Hispanic or Latino, Female	18,262	3.1 (0.24) 402	4.8 (0.30) 657
Not Hispanic or Latino			
White, Single Race, Male	76,265	1.6 (0.11) 1,351	3.1 (0.14) 2,564

(*continued*)

Table 1.10 Overview of People Living With Disabilities in the United States (2014) (*continued*)

Selected Characteristic	Age 18 and Over	ADLs	IADLs
White, Single Race, Female	81,195	2.0 (0.11) 1,949	4.4 (0.16) 4,292
African American, Single Race, Male	12,596	3.3 (0.31) 373	4.2 (0.33) 498
African American, Single Race, Female	15,346	4.4 (0.31) 642	7.0 (0.37) 1,022
Hispanic or Latino Origin, Race, and Poverty Status			
Hispanic or Latino			
Poor	7,759	4.2 (0.41) 231	6.7 (0.58) 394
Near Poor	10,251	2.8 (0.36) 188	4.0 (0.39) 290
Not Poor	15,504	1.4 (0.20) 149	2.5 (0.30) 248
Not Hispanic or Latino			
White, Single Race			
Poor	12,929	4.7 (0.41) 574	11.5 (0.74) 1,397
Near Poor	21,951	2.9 (0.24) 783	6.5 (0.33) 1,789
Not Poor	108,067	1.3 (0.08) 1,527	2.5 (0.11) 2,920
Black or African American, Single Race			
Poor	6,237	6.3 (0.59) 329	10.3 (0.69) 551
Near Poor	6,447	4.9 (0.50) 310	7.9 (0.64) 497
Not Poor	12,254	2.7 (0.33) 264	3.1 (0.33) 321

*$p \leq .05$.

ADLs, activities of daily living; IADLs, instrumental activities of daily living.

Represents the percentages (with standard errors) and frequencies (number in thousands) of individuals in the United States living with a limitation in ADLs and IADLs among individuals ages 18 and over in the United States, 2014.

Source: National Center for Health Statistics. (2016). *Health, United States, 2015: With Special Feature on Racial and Ethnic Health Disparities*. Hyattsville, MD.

are living in communities who require assistance with basic ADLs and services to promote functional status and healthy living. Given that current health policies support only services that are "medically necessary," a challenge for health educators and health promotion experts going forward will be the development of health policy provisions to include health education and health promotion programs.

THE CHANGING DEMOGRAPHIC STRUCTURE OF THE OLDER ADULT POPULATION WITH DISABILIES AND IMPAIRMENTS

One would be remiss without considering the functional status of older adults and their status as it related to disability and impairments. In 2016, the American Community Survey reported that 15% of people over the age of 65 reported living with a disability; 23% experienced some form of ambulation difficulty, and 8% experienced problems with self-care. In addition, 9% experienced some cognition difficulties along with vision impairments that limited functioning (7%). Hearing impairments impacting functioning was also reported by 15% of the noninstitutionalized population. More than a third (35%) of the older adult population reported any type of disability that impacted their functioning (Figure 1.14).

Theresa and Erica now feel that they have a handle on some of the demographic changes that have occurred over time for people growing older. As they ponder this material and begin discussions about where to go next in their planning process, they realize they need to continue to understand the social, political, and cultural landscape that will support social policies and program initiatives. Although they are working at a state-based level, they will need to understand how these variables will shape and define both policy development and program changes. To this end, they have decided to embark on a journey to first understand the factors that impact social policy and ultimately programs and services and resources.

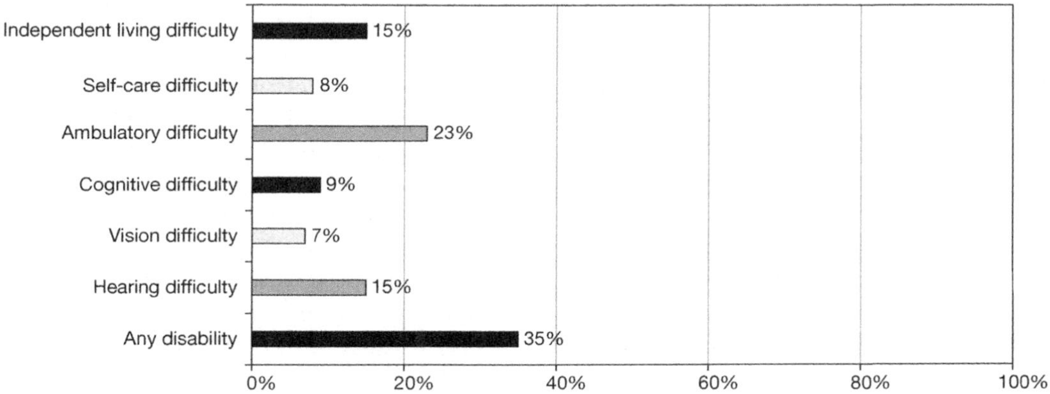

Figure 1.14 Percentage of persons age 65 and over with a disability, 2016.

Note: Chart shows the percentage of older persons with disabilities.
Among people age 65 and over, 35% have at least one disability.
Other disabilities range from 7% with a vision difficulty to 23% with an ambulatory difficulty.

Source: U.S. Census Bureau, American Community Survey.

CHANGES WITHIN THE SOCIAL, POLITICAL, AND CULTURAL EXPECTATIONS OF COMMUNITIES

Up to this point, this chapter has highlighted some of the current health programs and policies in place and changes in demographic trends for older adults living within American society. In addition, substantial changes within the social, political, and cultural expectations of communities over the past century pose challenges for policies and programs serving older adults.

Socially, healthcare has been impacted by numerous changes in gender roles and expectations over the last century (Kinsella & Gist, 1998). Women, especially women advancing in age, continue to be active members of the community and maintain a high degree of civic engagement long into retirement. Many have retired after having had careers and having been self-supporting for many years. (Government Accounting Office, 2016, 2015, 1997). Women have also begun to outnumber men as they grow older. Along with this demographic shift, there are growing numbers of women who are independent of their husbands or in same sex/gender relationships. These social changes have generated new social policy needs for women (GAO, 2014, 2012, 1998).

As noted, there has been an increased mobility to urban centers from rural communities and a shift from agrarian to industrial communities. Despite this movement, many of the older foreign-born population and minorities have remained in rural communities, especially people with more severe functional impairments and disabilities. Coupled with smaller and more mobile families, this situation will lead to the need for alternative care models for people in rural areas as they grow older and for service paradigms that will address the unique needs of rural communities.

Emerging service models that include community care and assisted living care models will serve as alternatives to traditional care of elders (Kovner & Jonas, 1999; Kronenfeld, 2000). Many of the traditional cultural expectations for families have eroded as a result of cross-cultural or interracial marriages, smaller families, and more mobile family units. These changes to the social structure of families are resulting in a need for differences in service composition for the older adult.

The shift from family to community support systems is another social change that will impact healthcare services (Atchley, 2000). Support provided by extended families and large families caring for the elderly has evolved into greater reliance on informal systems including the faith community and formal systems such as local community-based service and philanthropic organizations. This shift leads to implications for the delivery of social programs through faith-based initiatives associated with local religious communities. Funding appropriations for such programming will need to be supported through some mechanism, either private donations or through some legislative mandate (GAO, 2014; Lee & Estes, 2001). Despite this reliance upon the faith-based community for supports and services, younger people living with a disability may not be as inclined to seek services from the faith-based networks, nor may they align with these networks. Thus, this may create differences in the ways consumers will seek services and in their expectations of services. The merge of the Administration on Aging and Administration on Disabilities may also limit resources available and shortchange services to one group or another.

In summary, demographic changes; educational levels; income levels; and shifts in social, cultural, and service expectations of communities will contribute to changes in social services, programs, and policy initiatives as we move further into the 21st century. These will pose challenges to the aging arena and to policies and programs for the aging.

CHALLENGES FOR AGING AND DISABILITY POLICIES AND PROGRAMS

Several issues emerge as realities within the context of policy development and program planning for older adults, as we have seen in this chapter. These issues include changes in living arrangements, education levels, economic well-being, and rural population settings; trends in morbidity and mortality; and changes within the social, political, and cultural expectations of communities. As the stigma of mobility impairment has changed since the 1990s and the passage of the ADA, older adults are increasingly remaining in communities. These changes lead to challenges to the current realities of our policies on aging and service delivery network. Communities and service providers will also be challenged to prepare for the onslaught of baby boomers, who will challenge paradigms and will be consumer-driven. The realities of our system will require professionals working within the field of aging to challenge the current contexts, take a hard look at what exists in reality, and develop strategies to envision an innovative set of interventions, services, and policy/legislative initiatives (Binstock, 1998, Derthick, 1979, Hiller & Barrow, 1999). Such an approach will demand a new skill set that may be foreign to the current workforce. Such skills will include an in-depth understanding of what factors and contexts impact legislative initiatives, paradigms that affect the development of legislation, and data that may influence or contribute to policy development. Tools such as coalition building, media advocacy, and theoretical perspectives on health behavior are also going to be critical in this endeavor. Finally, building an awareness of what programs and services currently exist will also be a part of this process. Hence, all these considerations lay the groundwork for the remainder of this text, which is divided into three distinct parts and designed to address each of the skill areas required to enable reflective practitioners to build on their skills and be effective program and policy advocates in the aging arena.

REALITIES AND VISIONS

In summary, health policies related to aging in the United States have focused on in-kind medical services, supportive state and local services, and antipoverty benefits. Despite the availability of programs and services resulting from health policies, many programs have focused upon "medically necessary" services and have lacked a health promotion, health education, or community-based focus (Torres-Gil, 1998; Torres-Gil & Villa, 2000). A challenge for health professionals working with the elderly will be to lobby for social policies that will offer health education and health promotion options to maintain a healthy elderly population. The benefits of such advocacy efforts will include the development of a more active and healthy elderly population leading to cost containment and the preservation of current benefits and programs available to the elderly living in the United States.

With this information in hand, Theresa feels ready to embark upon the next leg of the journey in her new role, that is, to better understand the policy making process and factors that contribute and play a role. Erica is eager to work with Theresa because of the anticipated overall benefits of enhancing the workforce's capacity to delivery programs and services as a result of strengthening public policies to support older adults and people living with disabilities.

DISCUSSION QUESTIONS

1. How does the changing demographic profile of older adults over the past decades lend itself to the need for changes in social policies?
2. How do the changes in demographics for minorities suggest a need for policy changes to address the needs of ethnic, racial, and gender minorities when shaping social policies and programs?
3. Given the demographic trends to date, what social policy arenas do you think will need to be addressed over the next decade at the federal and state levels?
4. How do these demographic changes play a role in the professional development and training in your discipline and the professional disciplines of others?

REFERENCES

Administration for Community Living. (2016). *A profile of older Americans: 2016*. Retrieved from https://www.acl.gov/sites/default/files/Aging%20and%20Disability%20in%20America/2`016-Profile.pdf

Administration for Community Living. (2018). *Profile of older Americans: 2017 profile*. Retrieved from https://www.acl.gov/sites/default/files/Aging%20and%20Disability%20in%20America/2017OlderAmericansProfile.pdf

Atchley, R. (2000). *The social forces of aging: An introduction to social gerontology*. Belmont, CA: Wadsworth Publishing.

Barbour, K. E., Helmick, C. G., Boring, M., & Brady, T. J. (2017). Vital signs: Prevalence of doctor-diagnosed arthritis and arthritis-attributable activity limitation—United States, 2013–2015. *Morbidity and Mortality Weekly Report, 66*(9), 246–253. Retrieved from http://www.cdc.gov/mmwr/volumes/66/wr/mm6609e1.htm

Binstock, R. H. (1998). Health care policies and older Americans. In J. S. Steckenrider & T. M. Parrott (Eds.), *New directions in old-age policies* (pp. 13–35). Albany, NY: State University of New York.

Centers for Disease Control and Prevention (2016, January). *Chronic Disease Overview*. Retrieved from http://cdc.gov/chronicdisease/overview/index.htm

Centers for Disease Control and Prevention. (2017). *Mortality in the United States, 2016*. Retrieved from http://www.cdc.gov/nchs/products/databriefs/db293.htm

Centers for Disease Control and Prevention. (2018). *Healthy aging data*. Retrieved from http://nccd.cdc.gov/DPH_Aging/default.aspx

Centers for Disease Control and Prevention, National Center for Health Statistics. (2005). *Life expectancy hits record high*. Retrieved from http://www.cdc.gov/nchs/pressroom/05facts/lifeexpectancy.htm

Centers for Disease Control and Prevention, National Center for Health Statistics. (2006). *1997 National Health Interview Survey*. Retrieved from ftp://ftp.cdc.gov/pub/Health_Statistics/NCHS/Survey_Questionnaires/NHIS/1997/qsamadlt.pdf

Centers for Disease Control and Prevention, National Center for Health Statistics. (2013). *Summary health statistics for the U.S. population, the National Health Interview Survey, 2012*. Hyattsville, MD: U.S. Department of Health and Human Services.

Centers for Disease Control and Prevention, National Center for Health Statistics. (2014). *Summary health statistics for the U.S. population, the National Health Interview Survey, 2014*. Hyattsville, MD: U.S. Department of Health and Human Services. Retrieved from https://ftp.cdc.gov/pub/Health_Statistics/NCHS/NHIS/SHS/2014_SHS_Table_A-11.pdf

Centers for Disease Control and Prevention, National Center for Health Statistics. (2016). *National Health Interview Survey, Table P-1. Respondent-assessed health status, by selected characteristics: United States, 2016*. Hyattsville, MD: U.S. Department of Health and Human Services. Retrieved from http://ftp.cdc.gov/pub/Health_Statistics/NCHS/NHIS/SHS/2016_SHS_Table_P-1.xlsx

DeNavas-Walt, C. & Proctor, B. (2014). *Income and Poverty in the United States: 2013* (Current Population Reports, P60-249). Retrieved from https://www2.census.gov/library/publications/2014/demographics/p60-249.pdf

Derthick, M. (1979). *Policy making for social security*. Washington, DC: The Brookings Institute.

Federal Interagency Forum on Aging-Related Statistics. (2006). *Older Americans update 2006: Key indicators of well-being. Federal interagency forum on aging-related statistics*. Retrieved from https://agingstats.gov/docs/PastReports/2006/OA2006.pdf

Federal Interagency Forum on Aging-Related Statistics. (2016a). *Older Americans 2016: Key indicators of well-being*. Retrieved from https://agingstats.gov/docs/LatestReport/Older-Americans-2016-Key-Indicators-of-WellBeing.pdf

Federal Interagency Forum on Agency Related Statistics. (2016b). *Population aging in the United States: A global perspective*. Retrieved from https://agingstats.gov/images/olderamericans_agingpopulation.pdf

Fryar, C. D., Ostchega, Y., Hales, C. M., Zhang, G., & Kruszon-Moran, D. (2017). *Hypertension prevalence and control among adults: United States, 2015–2016* (NCHS Data Brief No. 289). Hyattsville, MD: National Center for Health Statistics. Retrieved from http://www.cdc.gov/nchs/data/databriefs/db289.pdf

Government Accounting Office. (1997). *Social Security reform: Implications for women's retirement income*. GAO/HEHS-98-42. Retrieved from https://www.gao.gov/assets/230/225143.pdf

Government Accounting Office. (1998). *Social Security reform: Raising retirement age improves program solvency but may cause hardship for some*. GAO/T-HEHS-98-207. Retrieved from https://www.gao.gov/assets/110/107545.pdf

Government Accounting Office. (2012). *Retirement security: Women still face challenges*. GAO-12-699. Retrieved from https://www.gao.gov/assets/600/592726.pdf

Government Accounting Office. (2014). *Retirement security: Trends in marriage and work patterns may increase economic vulnerability for some retirees*. GAO-14-33. Retrieved from https://www.gao.gov/assets/670/660202.pdf

Government Accounting Office. (2015). *Retirement security: Most households approaching retirement have low savings*. GAO-15-419. Retrieved from https://www.gao.gov/assets/680/670153.pdf

Government Accounting Office. (2016). *Retirement security: Low defined contribution savings may pose challenges*. GAO-16-408. Retrieved from https://www.gao.gov/assets/680/676942.pdf

Gibson, C. J., & Lennon, E. (1999). *Historical census statistics on the foreign-born population of the United States: 1850–1990* (Population Division Working Paper No. 29). Washington, DC: U.S. Census Bureau.

Hiller, S., & Barrow, G. (1999). *Aging, the individual and society*. Belmont, CA: Wadsworth Publishing.

Kinsella, K., & Gist, Y. (1998). *Gender and aging* (International Brief No. 98-2). Washington, DC: U.S. Census Bureau.

Kovner, A., & Jonas, S. (1999). *Health care delivery in the United States*. New York, NY: Springer Publishing Company.

Kronenfeld, J. J. (2000). Social policy and health care. Social policy and the elderly. In J. Midgley, M. B. Tracy, & M. Livermore (Eds.), *The handbook of social policy* (pp. 222–236). Thousand Oaks, CA: Sage.

Lee, P. R. & Estes, C. L. (2001). *The nation's health* (6th ed,). Boston, MA: Jones and Bartlett.

National Center for Health Statistics. (2013). *Morbidity and mortality data for older adults*. Retrieved from www.nchs.gov

National Center for Health Statistics. (2016). *Health, United States, 2015: With special feature on racial and ethnic health disparities*. Hyattsville, MD: Centers for Disease Control and Prevention.

OECD. (2018). *Life expectancy at 65 (indicator)*. Retrieved from http://data.oecd.org/healthstat/life-expectancy-at-65.htm

Pickett, G., & Hanlon, J. (1995) *Public health administration and practice*. St. Louis, MO: Times Mirror Publishing.

Torres-Gil, F. M. (1998). Policy, politics, aging: Crossroads in the 1990s. In J. S. Steckenrider & T. M. Parrott (Eds.), *New directions in old-age policies* (pp. 75–87). Albany, NY: State University of New York.

Torres-Gil, F. M., & Villa, V. (2000). Social policy and the elderly. In J. Midgley, M. B. Tracy, & M. Livermore (Eds.), *The handbook of social policy* (pp. 209–220). Thousand Oaks, CA: Sage.

United Nations. (2017). *UN statistics: Populations by age and sex 2000–2015*. Retrieved from www.UNSTAT.org

United Nations Statistics Division (2018). *Demographic statistics database*. Retrieved from http://data.un.org/Data.aspx?d=POP&f=tableCode%3a22

U.S. Census Bureau. (2002). *Demographic trends in the 20th century*. Washington, DC: Author. Retrieved from http://www.census.gov/prod/2002pubs/censr-4.pdf

U.S. Census Bureau. (2005). *Census 2000 special tabulations (STP-159)*. Washington, DC: Author.

U.S. Census Bureau. (2012). *A look at the 1940 census*. Washington, DC: Author. Retrieved from http://www.census.gov/newsroom/cspan/1940census/CSPAN_1940slides.pdf

U.S. Census Bureau. (2016). *Percent of the total population who are 65 years and over—United States—urban/rural and inside/outside metropolitan and micropolitan area: Total population. 2012-2016 American community survey 5-year estimates*. Retrieved from https://factfinder.census.gov/faces/tableservices/jsf/pages/productview.xhtml?pid=ACS_16_5YR_GCT0103.US26&prodType=table

U.S. Census Bureau. (2017a). *Current population survey, annual social and economic supplement. Table 1: Educational attainment of the population 18 years and over, by age, sex, race, and Hispanic origin: 2017*. Retrieved from http://www.census.gov/data/tables/2017/demo/education-attainment/cps-detailed-tables.html

U.S. Census Bureau. (2017b). *Table AD3. Living arrangements of adults 65 to 74, 1967 to present*. Retrieved from http://www2.census.gov/programs-surveys/demo/tables/families/time-series/adults/ad3-65-74.xlsx

U.S. Census Bureau. (2017c). *Table AD3. Living arrangements of adults 75 and over, 1967 to present*. Retrieved from http://www2.census.gov/programs-surveys/demo/tables/families/time-series/adults/ad3-75andover.xlsx

U.S. Census Bureau. (2017d). *Poverty status in 2016*. Retrieved from http://www.census.gov/data/tables/time-series/demo/income-poverty/cps-pov/pov-34.2016.html

U.S. Census Bureau. (2018a). *Annual estimates of the resident population by single year of age and sex for the United States: April 1, 2010 to July 1, 2017*. Retrieved from http://factfinder.census.gov/faces/tableservices/jsf/pages/productview.xhtml?pid=PEP_2017_PEPSYASEXN&prodType=table

U.S. Census Bureau. (2018b). *Annual estimates of the resident population for selected age groups by sex for the United States, states, counties, and Puerto Rico Commonwealth and Municipios: April 1, 2010 to July 1, 2017*. Retrieved from https://factfinder.census.gov/faces/tableservices/jsf/pages/productview. xhtml?pid=PEP_2017_PEPAGESEX&prodType=table

Vespa, J., Armstrong, D. M., & Medina, L. (2018). *Demographic turning points for the United States: Population projections for 2020 to 2060* (Current Population Report P25-1144). Washington, DC: U.S. Census Bureau. Retrieved from http://www.census.gov/content/dam/Census/library/publications/2018/demo/P25_1144.pdf

West, L. A. Cole, S. Goodkind, D. & He, W. (2014). *65+ in the United States: 2010* (Current Population Reports, P23-212). Washington, DC: U.S. Government Printing Office.

2

Social, Political, Economic, and Demographic Factors and Historical Landmarks Impacting Aging and Disability Public Policy

LEARNING OBJECTIVES

At the end of this chapter, readers will:

1. *Be familiar with the demographic and social factors that influence and shape aging and disability policy over time.*
2. *Become aware of policy changes over the past century within disability and aging public policy.*
3. *Be aware of the contrast between advances in science and technology and public policy related to people growing older and people with disabilities.*

> *Theresa and Erica spent time in deliberation about what were some of the best strategies to identify trends in policy development within both the aging and disability arenas. In order to examine the progress and impact that have occurred within both arenas, they decided to compare developments of policy dimensions over the past century to developments within science, technology, and our social environment. In this quest, they reviewed landmarks of U.S. and world history highlighted in this chapter as they tried to compare and contrast these dimensions.*

THE ROLE OF HISTORICAL LANDMARKS IN SHAPING SOCIAL TRENDS AND PUBLIC POLICIES

Landmarks serve as essential tools to help us recall specific historical events in time and mark specific historical junctures. Historical landmarks are also integral in the development of social trends and social policies. As landmark events have occurred throughout history, we witness the evolution of new trends and the development of specific social mores, values, and institutions. Along with these specific institutions we also witness the development of new trends in social welfare, technology, science, and social life. Historical landmarks, such as the development of the "talking pictures"

 DOI:10.1891/9780826128393.0002

in Hollywood, enabled women to expand their roles beyond the wife and mother. World War II, an event that saw the exodus of the male workforce to fight for freedom, opened up opportunities for women to enter and engage in the workforce. The upshot of this historical landmark also saw the making of social welfare policy designed to help women maintain their role within their homes if they chose to do so, such as through the Aid to Families with Dependent Children (AFDC) legislation. Historical landmarks, science, and technology have played significant roles in the evolution of social policies; however, aging and disability policies may not have made as many strides as other areas throughout history. This next segment explores the relationship between historical landmarks and aging/disability policies, presents developments within science, technology, and historical landmarks (Glennon, 1995), and compares some of these historical landmarks to those of labor, gender, and racial and ethnic developments (Day, 2006) over the same course of time.

THE RELATIONSHIP BETWEEN HISTORICAL LANDMARKS AND AGING AND DISABILITY-RELATED POLICIES

Social policy can be dramatically influenced by trends in social issues, the political climate, and labor/economic perspectives during a given time frame. All three factors play a role in the social fabric of one's culture or the prevailing culture in communities (Compton, 1980). It is interesting to examine the development of aging policy vis-à-vis other economic, social, and cultural trends that took place over the course of time. We begin to see the initial steps that make up some of our current aging policies evolve in the United States in 1920 with the passing and enactment of the Civil Service Retirement Act. Prior to 1920, although other countries worldwide had begun to make strides toward evolving some legislation for social security and a mandatory retirement age, the United States did not actually pass any such legislation until at least a decade later. Commencing with the 1920s, we began to see the development of legislation for retirement benefits; however, aging policy does not mirror other policy development initiatives or social developments that took place during the past century. In contrast, policies began to develop to address and support people with disabilities long before the development of aging-related policies. In addition, history has demonstrated that there have been more developments within the area of policies to support people with disabilities than for people who are growing older. This chapter addresses a brief overview of these policies. A more thorough discussion and presentation of these policies can be found in Appendix A.

TRENDS IN POLICY, SOCIAL, AND POLITICAL INFLUENCES AND LANDMARKS IN THE UNITED STATES

The Roaring '20s: 1920–1929

Aging Policy Landmarks

The pioneer efforts to develop a retirement system for government employees emerged with the passing of the Civil Service Retirement Act in 1920, which included members of the U.S. Congress and uniformed and civil servants. While we see just the emergence of a society to care for the aged, which seems like a bare essential, we see burgeoning developments elsewhere within American society. This same time period was characterized with major developments within the fields of technology and science.

Disability Policy Landmarks

Although the first federal vocational rehabilitation program was established in 1918 for soldiers returning from World War I with disabilities, this piece of legislation was expanded in 1920 to include civilians as well. The Fess-Smith Civilian Vocational Rehabilitation Act created a vocational rehabilitation program for civilians with disabilities and reached both civilians and soldiers.

Industry/Technology and Social Landmarks

During the 1920s, widespread availability of petroleum and electricity occurred, along with the advent of many new products such as refrigerators, vacuum cleaners, wristwatches, foam rubber, disposable tissues, and frozen foods. During this era, Charles Lindbergh made his historic transatlantic flight, which was a first step toward revolutionizing travel. This first solo flight for Lindbergh was also unique in that it did not have a fleet of resources to travel as "ground" support beneath him. Technology had also advanced the movie industry, and the first feature-length "talking picture" was released—*The Jazz Singer* starring Al Jolson. Women viewed this era also as a time of social experimentation and enjoyed dances like the Charleston. Their sexual freedom may have been encouraged by the popularity of Freud. Yet despite these developments, women realized that securing the right to vote (1920) did not improve their economic position or lead to any improvements in social policies to advance women.

Labor Landmarks

The labor movement was trying to organize; however, unionist efforts were resisted through the "trickle down" economic policy. In 1926, the United States Senate passed a law to allow unions to organize. Jane Addams, the "mother of social work," and Elizabeth Gurley Flynn, among others, became founding members of the American Civil Liberties Union (ACLU) in 1920.

Racial and Ethnic Discrimination Landmarks

Legislation on other fronts included the Immigration Act (1921), which attempted to levy controls on the diverse nature of society and attempted to "maintain the racial preponderance of the basic strain of people." Racial/ethnic groups such as Blacks, Hispanics, Native Americans, and Asian Americans were systematically discriminated against by legislative efforts. Quotas were set for immigration based upon one's national origin, and the Immigration Act set quotas to restrict people of African descent (1924).

Poverty Landmarks

In terms of poverty, a perception existed that all would share in prosperity as the economic climate improved; however, with the stock market crash in 1929, this illusion was shattered. The New York Stock Market crash of 1929 led to what is known as the Great Depression.

The Dirty '30s: 1930–1939

Aging Policy Landmarks

The "dirty thirties," or the time span characterized by the Great Depression, saw the development of hallmark legislation impacting older adults in the United States: the Social Security Act of 1935. This piece of legislation was passed and signed into legislation by President Franklin D. Roosevelt to ensure that protection into old age was a right for older workers in America, and to establish social insurance programs. Some of the titles signed as components of the Social Security Act established provisions for Old-Age Insurance (OAI) programs, Workers' compensation programs, and unemployment compensation. In addition, the Social Security Act provided for public health programs such as maternal and child health services, vocational rehabilitation programs, and public health clinics. Public assistance programs such as Aid to the Blind (AB) and Aid to Dependent Children (ADC) were also components of the Social Security Act.

In addition, the Railroad Retirement Act, signed into law in 1937, was enacted to ensure that pensions or annuities were available for retired railroad employees and their spouses. President Roosevelt, who had been instrumental in passage of the Social Security Act, was reelected in 1936.

Provision for widows and children through the Old-Age, Survivors and Disability Insurance (OASDI) Trust Fund was added in 1939, thus providing some financial support for those left behind once a retired worker was deceased. On face value, this amendment could have been perceived to have been costly by the House and Senate when moving through the legislative process. However, OASDI was presented as an insurance program based on the myth that benefits would be based upon some actuarial contribution. Although the formulary presents itself as being progressive, women are not necessarily the benefactors, and those who were the most poor were least likely to benefit from this provision.

Disability Policy Landmarks

Earlier in this segment we noted that The Social Security Act became U.S. law; however, it also provided federally funded old-age benefits and funds to states for assistance to blind individuals and disabled children. The Act also extended existing vocational rehabilitation programs.

In 1936, the Randolph–Sheppard Act (20 U.S.C. § 107 et seq.), a federal law, ensured that blind individuals a priority in operation of vending facilities on federal property. Although this enabled people with visual impairments to be small business owners, it also expanded employment options for people who were visually impaired. (This specific law was amended and updated significantly in 1974 through Pub. L. No. 93–651.) The notion of employment opportunities for the visually impaired was expanded in 1938 with the passage of the Wagner–O'Day Act, which mandated that U.S. federal agencies purchase products from workshops for people with visual impairments.

Industry/Technology and Social Landmarks

The Indian Reorganization Act (1934) was responsible for partially repealing the Dawes Act and restoring tribal rights. Native Americans began to acknowledge their roots and embrace their birthrights to their tribal organizations. The act put a halt to the allotment of tribal lands to White people and also put an end to the forced assimilation of Native Americans into the dominant White culture. It also enabled Native Americans to develop their own constitution for tribal councils and the development of tribal business councils.

While the United States was working toward devising opportunities to improve the lives of older adults, events were brewing on the international scene that led to the decline of economic growth. Hitler assumed leadership in Germany in 1933, and his rise to power led to the onset of World War II (1939). The resulting war effort saw an end to the economic slowdown and depression of the decade; however, it laid the groundwork for a number of changes politically and economically, as countries developed new political alliances throughout the world to combat Hitler and restore a more peaceful order to the world.

Labor Landmarks

During the 1930s, labor unions were legalized and empowered using the 1928 National Labor Relations Act (also known as the Wagner Act). In this decade, a coalition began to emerge between unions and the Democratic Party. Unions gained momentum and force during this decade.

Racial, Ethnic, and Gender Landmarks

The Social Security Act effectively (if not intentionally) limited participation of many Blacks and some other minorities from coverage by excluding domestic and agricultural workers, many of whom belonged to these groups. In addition, women for the most part were also excluded from Social Security, except as widows.

In the Tuskegee study on syphilis, African American veterans and men serving in the military were recruited by their healthcare providers to participate in what they were told was treatment for "bad blood." In reality, the study was examining the course of syphilis, and rather than receiving treatment they were simply given a placebo.

President Roosevelt appointed a "Black Cabinet" including Mary McLeod Bethune, A. Phillip Randolph, and Robert Weaver. Bethune also founded the National Council of Negro Women in 1935 in New York City. This endeavor brought together spokespeople from over 25 organizations with the goal of improving the lives of back women and the communities that they resided in.

Poverty Landmarks

Despite the passage of the Social Security Act, and the goal to provide a safety net from poverty for older adults, this goal was not met for various groups such as those identified and the reasons cited in the previous paragraph. During this time frame poverty was rampant, and Roosevelt's New Deal programs were thought to be temporary, including the Federal Emergency Relief Act (FERA), the National Industrial Recovery Act (NIRA), the Public Works Administration (PWA), and the Civil Works Administration (CWA).

The War-Torn '40s: 1940–1949

Aging Policy Landmarks

During the 1940s, we see the first visage of a state agency on aging. The state of Connecticut was the first to establish a state-based agency on aging. It was called the State Commission on the Care and Treatment of Chronically Ill, Aged, and Infirm.

Disability Policy Landmarks

Although some may argue that no significant developments specific to disability policy or legislation took place during the 1940s, some specific advances did occur. In 1940, Jacobus founded The National Federation of the Blind was founded in 1940 by Jacobus tenBroek, progenitor of the white cane laws and the rights of the blind to have a voice as consumers and in addressing their own needs.

Also in 1940, The American Federation of the Physically Handicapped was founded by Paul Strachan. This group was the first cross-disability national (American) political organization to urge an end to job discrimination and lobby for the passage of related legislation and initiatives to benefit people with physical disabilities. Members also called for a National Employ the Physically Handicapped Week, which in 1945 was proclaimed by Congress as the first week in October of each succeeding year.

In 1943, the LaFollette–Barden Vocational Rehabilitation Act added physical rehabilitation to the goals of federally funded vocational rehabilitation programs. Formerly, vocational rehabilitation was strictly defined to narrowly limit services specific to employment, but provisions of this Act added funding for certain care services if these would enhance employability.

After World War II (1946), President Truman signed another landmark piece of legislation, the National Mental Health Act, which called for the establishment of a National Institute of Mental Health. In the same year, The Hill–Burton Act (also known as the Hospital Survey and Construction Act) became law in the United States and authorized federal grants to states for the construction of hospitals, public centers, and health facilities for rehabilitation of people with disabilities.

Also in 1946, The National Mental Health Foundation was founded by American conscientious objectors from World War II who served as attendants at state mental institutions rather than serving in the war. The Foundation exposed the abusive conditions that took place within these facilities and became a major impetus toward the deinstitutionalization movement.

During this era, a number of advances were also made to support the World War II veterans who returned with mobility impairments. Although the focus was on physical disability, eventually these initiatives did impact people growing older with mobility impairments. In 1947, The President's Committee on National Employ the Physically Handicapped Week was held in Washington, DC, with a goal of breaking the stigma against returning veterans who had acquired a disability during their performance of honorable service. During this promotional week, publicity campaigns, coordinated by state and local committees, emphasized the competence of people with disabilities and used movie trailers, billboards, and radio and television advertisements to showcase the strengths and capacities of people with disabilities and convince the public that hiring the disabled was good business.

The consumer arm of disability advocacy organizations saw its beginnings in 1947 with the creation of The Paralyzed Veterans of America, and in 1948 with the establishment of the National Paraplegia Foundation. Together, these two organizations played lead roles in advocating for disability rights and advancing disability oriented legislation.

Industry/Technology and Social Landmarks

On the international scene after World War II ended, the United Nations was established in 1945 in response to the universal feeling that there should be some mediating body in place to ensure that the world would not face another global war. The United Nations split Palestine into two nations in 1947, resulting in Israel and Palestine. Other significant events on the international front included India's independence from Britain through the influence of Mohandas Gandhi. Gandhi's leadership called attention worldwide to the notion of nonviolent negotiation strategies.

Labor and Racial Discrimination Landmarks

There were a number of advances politically, but this did not mean necessarily that these advances were felt by minority groups or oppressed populations. Labor unions consolidated their power both economically and politically, which resulted in post–World War II compromises that led to an increase in both prices and wages. Discrimination against Blacks and women was rampant, despite the active roles these two groups played during World War II or President Truman ordering the armed services to desegregate in 1948. There was a rise in activity of civil rights groups and increased African American migration to the North in response to people advocating for and seeking their civil rights.

Gender-Related Landmarks

Although women entered the workforce in large numbers during World War II, they were driven out afterward and were encouraged to enjoy their time at home. Thus, during this decade, what would later be known as "Cleaver" phenomenon (named for a popular television program) began to emerge; it encouraged women to be the "head of their home" as domestic engineers and homemakers. This resulted in the growing market targeting women as consumers. The decade drew to a close with the postwar baby boom.

The Golden Age: 1950–1959

Aging Policy Landmarks

During the 1950s, developments within the aging arena began to emerge. This decade witnessed the first National Conference on Aging held in Washington, DC, sponsored by the Federal Security Agency. In 1956, a special staff on aging was assigned to coordinate responsibilities for the field of aging within the office of the Secretary of the Department of Health, Education, and Welfare. In 1958, Representative John E. Fogarty introduced a bill in Congress calling for a White House Conference on Aging. In 1959, the Housing Act was passed, which authorized a direct loan program, making nonprofit rental projects available for the elderly at low interest rates. In addition, the U.S. Senate Special Committee on Aging was created.

Some amendments to the Social Security Act were also passed during this decade. In 1950, incapacitated fathers were included as recipients of aid through the AFDC program. In 1956, people with mental illness were classified as disabled for the purpose of receiving disability support and Old-Age Security and Disability (OASDI) through the Old-Age Security Insurance (OASI) program.

Disability Policy Landmarks

The Social Security Act Amendments of 1950 created a public assistance program for people who are "totally and permanently disabled." Each state determined eligibility standards and assistance levels in accordance with the Act, which provided for federal financial assistance. These Social Security Amendments also established a federal-state program to aid people permanently and totally disabled in America.

The Vocational Rehabilitation Act was revised in 1954 and established a system of state vocational rehabilitation agencies. These Vocational Rehabilitation Amendments were passed that authorized federal grants to expand programs available to people with physical disabilities. In addition, with the Social Security Amendments of 1954 (Pub. L. No. 83–761), included a freeze provision for workers who were forced by disability to leave the workforce. This legislation protected their benefits by freezing their retirement benefits at their predisability level.

The Social Security Amendments of 1956 (Pub. L. No. 84–880) created the Social Security Disability Insurance (SSDI) program for disabled workers aged 50 to 64. The Social Security Amendments of 1958 extended Social Security Disability benefits to dependents of disabled workers in America.

In 1958, two significant pieces of legislation would have a major impact on the quality of life of not only the hearing impaired and developmentally delayed but, over the long haul, also for people growing older. Public Law 85–905, which authorized loan services for captioned films for the deaf, paved the way for Title III of the Americans with Disabilities Act (ADA) of 1990. The second piece of legislation, Public law 85–926, provided federal support for training teachers of children with mental retardation.

During this era (1950), Mary Switzer was appointed the Director of the U.S. Office of Vocational Rehabilitation, where she emphasized independent living as a quality of life issue. Although this is not necessarily legislative action, Ms. Switzer's philosophy promoting person-centered services and the importance of the least restrictive environment undergirds the Administration for Community Living today and plays a significant role in shaping legislation for people growing older and/or people with disabilities.

Another landmark, that occurred in 1953, The President's Committee on National Employ the Physically Handicapped Week became the President's Committee on Employment of the Physically Handicapped, a permanent organization reporting to the President and Congress. This action also led to showcasing the importance of integrating people with disabilities within society at every corner possible.

Industry/Technology and Social Landmarks

As a society, the United States experienced a number of social advances. As people left their agricultural homesteads, movement toward urban centers forced housing expansions into the suburbs, where the need for nearby shopping centers led to the development of shopping malls.

The Geneva Accords of 1954 split Vietnam into two parts, one Communist and one noncommunist. This split would eventually lead the United States into the Vietnam War.

The development of psychotropic medications provided new help to people with mental illness. This development led to the vision and goal that people with severe persistent mental illnesses could live outside institutions and become a part of the community.

During this decade, most homes were furnished with televisions, revolutionizing the entertainment patterns for families. Other lifestyle developments included the appearance of sugar-free soft drinks (1952) and the debuts of *MAD* magazine (1952) and the Barbie doll (1959).

Racial, Ethnic, and Gender Landmarks

The rise of civil rights activism became pivotal during this decade with the first groundbreaking case challenging the notion of segregation. *Brown v. Topeka Board of Education* (347 U.S. 483, 1954). In their ruling on this case the Supreme Court ordered the desegregation of the public school system, which would lead the way for groundbreaking desegregation movements within local communities through their school systems. This movement was further augmented one evening in 1955 in Montgomery, Alabama, when Rosa Parks, a Black woman, refused to give up her bus seat to White passengers and move to the segregated back section of the bus; an event that crystallized opposition to the practice of segregation.

The Age of Technology Explosion: 1960–1969

Aging Policy Landmarks

The Social Security program went through a number of changes during the 1960s. In 1960, Social Security amendments made a number of changes in the law, including: (a) eliminating age 50 as a minimum age to qualify for disability benefits, and (b) liberalizing the retirement test and requirement for fully insured status.

In addition, on July 14, 1965, the Medicare health insurance program for the elderly was legislated, along with Medicaid (a health insurance program for the poor). The Older Americans Act was passed and signed into law by President Johnson in 1965.

In 1961, the first White House Conference on Aging took place, under the Eisenhower administration (Wooley & Peter, 2018). Following this White House Conference, in 1962, more than 160 bills were introduced in Congress that related to the aged and aging. Of these, eight were enacted.

The passage of the Older Americans Act also led to a number of amendments during this decade. For example, in 1967, amendments to the Older Americans Act extended its provisions for 2 years and directed the Administration on Aging to undertake a study of personnel needs in the aging field. Another change took place in 1969 when amendments to the Older Americans Act extended its provisions for 3 years and authorized the use of Title III funds to support area-wide model projects. Another advance within the civil rights arena, was the Age Discrimination Act of 1967, signed into law by President Johnson.

The Administration on Aging was placed in a newly created Department of Social and Rehabilitative Services. The face of human services changed dramatically when John F. Kennedy was elected as president of the United States (1960). This introduction of social democracy led to the appointment of two presidential commissions—the President's Commission on Mental Health and the President's Commission on Mental Retardation. Unfortunately, some of Kennedy's vision may not have been fully materialized by the time of his assassination in 1963, but many of the recommendations were carried out by the Johnson administration.

Disability Policy Landmarks

One of the most significant landmarks during this era was The Social Security Act of 1965, which established the Medicare and Medicaid programs under Titles XVIII and XIX. The initial purpose of Title XIX was to improve access to and the quality of medical care for all low-income people; it did not provide services solely based on disability. States were required to provide certain services to individuals who were categorically needy; states could offer optional services and choose to cover individuals who were medically needy. Medicare and Medicaid were established through passage of the Social Security Amendments of 1965, providing federally subsidized healthcare to disabled and elderly Americans covered by the Social Security program. These amendments also changed the previous definition of disability under Social Security Disability program from "of long continued and indefinite duration" to "expected to last for not less than 12 months." Although less significant, during this era The Social Security Amendments of 1960 eliminated the restriction that disabled workers receiving Social Security Disability benefits must be 50 or older.

Other significant legislation at the federal level included Pub. L. No. 88–164 (1964), also called the Community Mental Health Act, authorizing funding for developmental research centers in university-affiliated facilities and community facilities for people with mental retardation—the first federal law directed to help people with developmental disabilities (DD).

This era also marked a turning point for philosophical perspectives regarding people with disabilities, and moved the landscape from one of custodial care, to person-centered care. Birnbaum's seminal paper, "The Right To Treatment" appeared in 1960 in the *American Bar Association Journal*, marking the first published use of the term *sanism* (sanity) in reference to a person with mental illness. Blatt and Kaplan (1966) published *Christmas in Purgatory: A Photographic Essay on Mental Retardation*, which graphically documented poor living conditions at American state institutions for people with DD. Further to these two seminal publications, Wolfensberger's work *The Origin and Nature of Our Institutional Models* (1969) hypothesized that society characterized people with disabilities as deviant, subhuman, and burdens of charity, which resulted in the adoption of a "deviant" role as opposed to one of strength, dignity, and worth.

The Vocational Rehabilitation Amendments of 1965 authorized federal funds for construction of rehabilitation centers, expansion of existing vocational rehabilitation programs, and the creation of the National Commission on Architectural Barriers to Rehabilitation of the Handicapped. In 1963, South Carolina passed the first statewide architectural access code in America, which was a precursor to the Architectural Barriers Act. The Architectural Barriers Act (1968) required all federally owned or leased buildings to be accessible to disabled people. Among other provisions, it required access to toilet facilities for people with disabilities.

The Voting Rights Act of 1965 provided sweeping protections for minority voting rights, and it allowed those with various disabilities to receive assistance "by a person of the voter's choice," as long as that person was not the disabled voter's boss or union agent.

The Lanterman–Petris–Short (LPS) Act of 1967, (Cal. Welf & Inst. Code, sec. 5000 et seq.), was signed into law by then-governor of California Ronald Reagan (although it did not go into full effect until July 1, 1972). The Act in effect ended all hospital commitments by the judiciary system in California, except in the case of criminal sentencing, for example, convicted sexual offenders, and those who are "gravely disabled," defined as unable to obtain food, clothing, or housing. It did not, however, impede the right of voluntary commitment. It also expanded the evaluative power of psychiatrists and created provisions and criteria for holds. This act set the precedent for modern mental health commitment procedures throughout the United States.

In comparison to aging legislation, the disability movement pushed for advances in legislation on a variety of fronts. These fronts, which included community living options, vocational options, citizenship, and building design, all help promote community living, independence, and personhood.

Industrial/Technological and Social Landmarks

Additional landmarks included the Cuban missile crisis (1962) and the United States' commitment, as advisors, to the Vietnam War (1963). Racial parity was on its way with the enactment and passage of the Civil Rights Act (1964), a result of the rise in the civil rights movement. In 1963, the Community Mental Health Act was passed. This and the Great Society legislation of President Lyndon B. Johnson changed social work and the face of human services.

Several landmark civil rights efforts occurred during this decade. Martin Luther King Jr.'s "I Have a Dream" speech symbolized the movement for civil rights and paved the way for laws and cultural norms accepting people regardless of race, color, or creed. Regardless of gains within the aging arena, several events occurred that led to an impact on social development. Martin Luther King was assassinated at the Lorraine Motel in Memphis, Tennessee, the day after delivering his "I've Been to the Mountaintop" speech.

Technology and science passed a new frontier as United States astronauts from the Apollo XI mission landed on the moon on July 21, 1969.

On the political front, farm workers began to organize, and gender also began to be an issue in legislation. In an effort to embarrass the supporters of civil rights legislation, opponents included gender in the legislation. Although the power of the inclusion of gender was not immediately recognized, it later became the basis of several lawsuits. The "pill" and sexual revolution were also in full swing.

Poverty Landmarks

The war on poverty was declared in 1964. Within 1 year, 1,000 community action centers opened. These community action centers became the training grounds for many community organizers who became active in many of the movements that followed.

The Decade of Presidential Resignation: 1970–1979

Aging Policy Landmarks

The 1970s mark a decade of development within the aging arena in the United States. The second White House Conference on Aging convened in Washington, DC. Some of the major resolutions during this decade included the following:

The Supplemental Security Income (SSI) program was created in 1972 and was implemented to provide economic supplements to low-income individuals in their old age and to care for widows or children of the deceased. SSI benefits were available to beneficiaries if money had been paid into the system for the requisite number of quarters.

In 1973, The Older American Comprehensive Service Amendments established area agencies on aging, and amendments authorized model projects for senior centers.

The Domestic Volunteer Service Act provided for foster grandparent programs. This is the first acknowledgment of grandparents' role.

The Comprehensive Employment and Training Act (CETA) provided job training for those facing barriers to employment, including older workers. CETA became an employment agency for temporary public service jobs, thus creating a labor opportunity for talented older workers.

The Age Discrimination Act of 1975 was passed and signed into law by President Nixon. Some of the hallmarks of this legislation include penalties to employers who discriminate against older workers on the basis of their age.

Disability Policy Landmarks

The Urban Mass Transportation Act of 1970 addressed legislative needs of people in wheelchairs utilizing public transportation opportunities. The law required all new American mass transit vehicles be equipped with wheelchair lifts, but the American Public Transportation Association delayed implementation for 20 years. Regulations were finally issued in 1990 along with the ADA, 1970. The Rolling Quads organization was started by Edward Roberts at UC Berkeley in California, and was instrumental in changing the mindset of people living with disabilities. This group's activism led to accessible campuses and community-based settings, as well as the independent living movement.

The Developmental Disabilities Services and Facilities Construction Amendments became law in 1970. These amendments contained the first legal definition of DD. They also authorized grants for services and facilities for the rehabilitation of people with DD and state DD Councils.

The Physically Disabled Students Program (PDSP) was founded by Edward Roberts, John Hessler, Hale Zukas, and others at UC Berkeley in 1970. With its focus on community living, political advocacy, and personal assistance services, it became the nucleus for the first Center for Independent Living, founded in 1972. While this program, in and of itself, was not specific legislation, it paved the way for advocacy and legislation that would promote independence and community living.

The U.S. District Court, Middle District of Alabama, decided in *Wyatt v. Stickney* (1971) that people in residential state schools and institutions had a constitutional right "to receive such individual treatment as would give them a realistic opportunity to be cured or to improve their mental condition." Disabled people were no longer to be locked away in custodial institutions without treatment or education.

In terms of vocational training and rehabilitation, the Fair Labor Standards Act of 1938 (Pub. L. No. 75–718) was amended to bring people with disabilities (other than blindness) into the sheltered workshop system in 1971.

Education for people with disabilities was advanced during this era, particularly in 1975 through the passage of the Education for All Handicapped Children Act (IDEA). In *Pennsylvania Association for Retarded Citizens (PARC) v. Commonwealth of Pennsylvania*, 334 F. Supp. 1257 (E.D. Pa. 1971), the U.S. District Court, Eastern District of Pennsylvania, ruled that it was the obligation of the state of Pennsylvania to provide free public education to mentally retarded children, which it was not doing at that time. This decision struck down various state laws used to exclude disabled children from the public schools. In *Mills v. Board of Education*, 1972, the U.S. District Court in the District of Columbia decided that every child, regardless of the type and severity of his or her disability, was entitled to a free public education. Advocates cited these decisions during public hearings, and these cases led to the passage of the Education for All Handicapped Children Act of 1975.

In 1972, The Center for Independent Living was established by Edward Roberts and associates in Berkeley, California with funds from the Rehabilitation Administration, and it is recognized as the first Center for Independent Living. This organization sparked the Independent Living Movement.

The Social Security Amendments of 1972 created the SSI program. The law relieved families of the financial responsibility of caring for their adult disabled children.

Also in 1972, demonstrations were held by disabled activists in Washington, DC, to protest President Richard M. Nixon's veto of the Rehabilitation Act. Among the demonstrators were Disabled in Action, Paralyzed Veterans of America, and the National Paraplegia Foundation. This led to the Rehabilitation Act of 1973. Section 504 of the Act states "No otherwise qualified handicapped individual in the United States, shall, solely by reason of his [sic] handicap, be excluded from the participation in, be denied the benefits of, or be subjected to discrimination under any program or activity receiving federal financial assistance." This was the first U.S. federal civil rights protection for people with disabilities.

A federal district court ruled in *Souder v. Brennan* (1973) that patients in mental health institutions must be considered employees and paid the minimum wage required by the Fair Labor Standards Act of 1938 whenever they performed any activity that conferred an economic benefit on an institution. Following this ruling, institutional peonage was outlawed, as evidenced in Pennsylvania's Institutional Peonage Abolishment Act of 1973.

The Federal-Aid Highway Act of 1973 authorized federal funds for construction of curb cuts. The Architectural and Transportation Barriers Compliance Board, established under the Rehabilitation Act of 1973, enforced the Architectural Barriers Act of 1968.

The Education for All Handicapped Children Act (Pub. L. No. 94–142; 1975; renamed the Individuals with Disabilities Education Act [IDEA] in 1990), declared that handicapped children could not be excluded from public school because of their disability, and that school districts were required to provide special services to meet the needs of handicapped children. The law also required that handicapped children be taught in a setting that resembles as closely as possible the regular school program, while also meeting their special needs and established Parent and Training Information Centers to help parents of children with disabilities exercise their rights under the law.

The Developmental Disabilities Assistance and Bill of Rights Act (1975; Pub. L. No. 94–103) established protection and advocacy (P & A) services and provided federal funds to programs serving the developmentally disabled.

The Community Services Act (1975) created the Head Start Program. It stipulated that at least 10% of program openings were to be reserved for disabled children.

In *Disabled in Action of Pennsylvania, Inc. v. Coleman* (1976), known as the Transbus lawsuit, Disabled in Action of Pennsylvania, the American Coalition of Cerebral Palsy Associations, and others were represented by the Public Interest Law Center of Philadelphia. They successfully filed suit to require that all buses purchased by public transit authorities receiving federal funds meet transbus specifications (making them wheelchair accessible).

The Lanterman Developmental Disabilities Act (AB 846), also known as the Lanterman Act, is a California law, initially proposed by Assembly member Frank D. Lanterman in 1973 and passed in 1977, that gives people with DD the right to services and supports that enable them to live more independent and normal lives. The Lanterman Act declares that persons with DD have the same legal rights and responsibilities guaranteed all other persons by federal and state constitutions and laws, and charges the regional center with advocacy for, and protection of, these rights. Legal Services Corporation Act Amendments of 1977 added financially needy people with disabilities to the list of those eligible for publicly funded legal services.

In *Lloyd v. Regional Transportation Authority* (1977), the U.S. Court of Appeals, Seventh Circuit, ruled that individuals have a right to sue under Section 504 of the Rehabilitation Act of 1973 and that public transit authorities must provide accessible service. However, the U.S. Court of Appeals, Fifth Circuit, in *Snowden v. Birmingham Jefferson County Transit Authority* undermined this decision by ruling that authorities need to provide access only to "handicapped persons other than those confined to wheelchairs."

Title VII of the Rehabilitation Act Amendments of 1978 established the first federal funding for consumer-controlled independent living centers and created the National Council of the Handicapped under the U.S. Department of Education.

In *Southeastern Community College v. Davis* (1979), the U.S. Supreme Court ruled that under Section 504 of the Rehabilitation Act of 1973, programs receiving federal funds must make "reasonable modifications" to enable the participation of otherwise qualified disabled individuals. This decision was the Court's first ruling on Section 504, establishing reasonable modification as an important principle in disability rights law.

In *Rogers v. Okin* (1979), the United States Court of Appeals for the First Circuit ruled that a competent patient committed to a psychiatric hospital has the right to refuse treatment in nonemergency situations.

The Education for Handicapped Children Act (1973) mandates that public schools provide students with disabilities a "free appropriate public education (FAPE)" in the "least restrictive environment." The Act requires educators to develop an "individual education plan (IEP)" for each child receiving special education services. Part B of the Act provides federal financial assistance to states and local education agencies to meet the mandates.

The DD Services and Facilities Construction Amendments of 1970 gave states responsibility for planning and implementing comprehensive services for people with severe disabilities, calling for DD Councils in each state to plan, and coordinate activities.

The Social Security Amendments of 1972 (Pub. L. No. 92–603) authorized the SSI program, a consolidated, federally administered cash benefits program for needy individuals and couples who are aged or blind or have a disability. Children under the age of 18 with disabilities, including children who are blind, become eligible for benefits provided their disabilities are comparable in severity to those of adult recipients.

The Developmental Disabilities Assistance and Bill of Rights Act (1973; Pub. L. No. 106–402) reauthorized the DD Services and Facilities Construction Amendments of 1970 and provides formula grants to state-based DD Councils. This act also authorizes the University-Affiliated Facilities and establishes state P & A systems to protect the rights of individuals with DD.

The Rehabilitation Act of 1973 (Pub. L. No. 93–112) was rewritten, providing stronger emphasis on people with severe disabilities. This act requires vocational rehabilitation agencies to develop an "individualized written rehabilitation program (IWRP)" with each individual receiving services. Section 504 of the act protects individuals with disabilities from discrimination in all federally assisted programs and activities. Sections 501 and 503 protect people with disabilities from employment discrimination by federal agencies or federal contractors.

The Housing and Community Development Act of 1974 created the Community Development Block Grant (CDBG) program, authorizing funds for removal of existing architectural barriers and in construction of public facilities. Urban areas are required to prepare a Housing Assistance Plan that reflects the needs of individuals with disabilities.

Industry/Technology and Social Landmarks

The rise of technology led to innovations and changes in communication through computers. Industry was brought into the computer era, and businesses began to systematize administrative and data management procedures.

In 1973, *Roe v. Wade*, which legalized abortion, was part of the growth of the women's movement. This also led to the empowerment of women and opened up many opportunities for women.

Poverty was addressed through the food stamp program, which nationalized and established eligibility standards. The poor also saw an end to their "voice" through President Nixon's dissolution of the ability for legal aid recipients to file class action lawsuits against governmental agencies.

The Era of Economic Entrenchment: 1980–1989

Aging Policy Landmarks

During the 1980s, the aging arena once again experienced a number of new developments. Commencing in 1981, amendments to the Older Americans Act extended the program for 3 years, through September 30, 1984. In 1984, additional amendments to the Older Americans Act clarified the roles of state and area agencies on aging in coordinating community-based services and in maintaining accountability for the funding of national priority services (legal, access, and in-home services). In 1985, *A Compendium of Papers Honoring the Twentieth Anniversary of the Older Americans Act* was compiled by the U.S. House of Representatives Select Committee on Aging. In 1987, amendments to the Older Americans Act authorized new initiatives on mental health, elder abuse, home healthcare for the frail elderly, and outreach to eligible SSI recipients.

Disability Policy Landmarks

The Omnibus Budget Reconciliation Act (1981; Pub. L. No. 97–35) authorized Medicaid to waive certain federal requirements so that states can provide personal care and other home and community-based services to individuals who would otherwise receive care in an institutional setting.

The Tax Equity and Fiscal Responsibility Act (TEFRA; 1982; Pub. L. No. 97–248) allows states to cover home care services under Medicaid for children with disabilities, even when family income and resources exceeded that of the state's financial eligibility standards.

The Rehabilitation Act Amendments (1984; Pub. L. No. 98–221) established the Client Assistance Program (CAP), a formula grant program for states designed to inform individuals with disabilities who are receiving rehabilitation services how to access available benefits and ensure protection of individual rights through legal, administrative, or other remedies.

The Education for Handicapped Children Act (1988) was expanded to include Part H, a formula grant program, to assist states in developing early intervention services for infants and toddlers with disabilities.

The Employment Opportunities for Disabled Americans Act (1986; Pub. L. No. 99–643) made permanent the work incentives provision, Sections 1619 (a) and 1619 (b) of the Social Security Act, authorizing special SSI benefits and continued Medicaid coverage for people with disabilities who are working and whose income exceeds "substantial gainful activity" levels. Medicaid coverage is extended to people with disabilities who may lose SSI or Section 1619(a) benefits due to excess earnings but who are unable to afford healthcare coverage equal to coverage under Medicaid.

The Protection and Advocacy for Individuals with Mental Illness Act (PAIMI, 1986) established a formula grant program for statewide mental health advocacy services to be operated directly by or through contract with the state P & A agency to protect and advocate for the rights of people with mental illness and to investigate incidents of abuse and neglect.

The Omnibus Budget Reconciliation Act of 1987, known as the Nursing Home Reform Act, requires states to conduct Preadmission Screening and Resident Review (PASRR) of individuals with disabilities (mental illness, intellectual disabilities, DD) prior to admission to a nursing facility to determine if they actually need nursing facility level of care, even if the individual is not Medicaid eligible. PASRR requires that individuals with disabilities be provided specialized services while in a nursing facility. If nursing facility level of care is not required but an individual requires specialized services, the state must provide for or arrange for the specialized services in an appropriate setting.

The Technology-Related Assistance for Individuals with Disabilities Act (1988; Pub. L. No. 100–407) established grant programs to encourage the development and distribution of assistive technology for people with disabilities.

The Fair Housing Amendments Act (1988; Pub. L. No. 100–430) expanded the Fair Housing Act of 1968 to prohibit discrimination based on disability or on familial status (presence of child under age of 18, and pregnant women); it establishes new administrative enforcement mechanisms, revises and expands Justice Department jurisdiction to bring suit in Federal district courts. In connection with prohibitions on discrimination against individuals with disabilities, the Act contains design and construction accessibility provisions for certain new multifamily dwellings.

The Omnibus Budget Reconciliation Act of 1989 (OBRA 89; Pub. L. No. 101–239) defines the Medicaid Early Periodic Screening, Diagnosis, and Treatment (EPSDT) program, a comprehensive and preventative child health program for individuals under the age of 21. OBRA requires that any medically necessary healthcare service be provided to an EPSDT recipient, even if the service is not available under the State's Medicaid plan for the rest of the Medicaid population.

Industry/Technology and Social Landmarks

On the international scene, President Ronald Reagan and General Secretary Mikhail Gorbachev of the Soviet Union signed the historic Intermediate-Range Nuclear Forces (INF) arms treaty (1987). This arms treaty led to alliances between the two superpowers of the world—the United States and the Soviet Union.

In 1988, the Canada–United States Free Trade Agreement (CUSFTA) was signed, phasing out a range of trade restrictions and increasing trade between the two countries. The CUSFTA was later expanded to include Mexico through the North American Free Trade Agreement (NAFTA).

Racial, Ethnic, and Gender Landmarks

From a racial/ethnic perspective, an increased recognition of affirmative action and hiring goals also led to the increased presence of women in the labor market and nontraditional sectors. Sandra Day O'Connor is a good model for women in nontraditional roles, as she was appointed the first woman Supreme Court Justice (1982).

Poverty Landmarks

Despite these advances, there was an increased rate of poverty, particularly, among people with disabilities and people with severe persistent mental illness. Some may argue that the decreased support to social programs through "Reaganomics" impacted poverty, since spending for social services was reduced by 50% or more; however, massive cuts to federal and social programs began following the passage of the Gramm–Rudman–Hollings Act (GRH) in 1986. Protected programs, which received only moderate or modified cuts in fiscal spending, included OASDI, AFDC, Child Nutrition, Food Stamps, Medicaid, SSI, Veterans' compensation and pensions, and Medicare and Social Services block grants, to name a few. Unprotected programs included, Head Start programs, rural development programs, and many services for the elderly and disabled. Unfortunately, GRH failed miserably at the reduction of spending because it did not address some of the tax policies that led to deficits in spending for existing programs.

The Era of Globalization: 1990–1999

Aging Policy Landmarks

In 1992, amendments to the Older Americans Act (Pub. L. No. 102–375) included the addition of Title VII, the Vulnerable Elders Rights Protection Title, and funded efforts to increase education on how healthy lifestyles reduce the risk of chronic health problems in later life. These were major advances to the Older Americans Act and laid the groundwork for showcasing the importance of prevention programs for maintaining one's health.

The Balanced Budget Act of 1997 affected older adults through the enrollment of eligible Medicaid retirees into managed care health insurance programs. This act enabled individual states to force Medicaid recipients to enroll in managed care organizations (MCOs) or with primary care case managers (PCCMs).

Disability Legislation Landmarks

The ADA (Pub. L. No. 101–336) passed in 1990. The ADA provided comprehensive civil rights protection for people with disabilities, closely modeled after the Civil Rights Act and Section 504 of the Rehabilitation Act of 1963, and mandated that local, state, and federal governments and programs be accessible, that employers with more than 15 employees make "reasonable accommodations" for workers with disabilities and not discriminate against otherwise qualified workers, and that public accommodations and commercial facilities make "reasonable modifications" to ensure access for disabled members of the public and not discriminate against them (see Chapter 8 for a more detailed discussion of the ADA).

The Mental Health Parity Act (MHPA) of 1996 (Pub. L. No. 110–343) required that large group health plans not impose annual or lifetime dollar limits on mental health benefits.

Although geared toward children rather than older adults, the Education for All Handicapped Children Act was amended and renamed the IDEA in 1990. This Act contains a permanently authorized grant program that provides federal funding to the states;

all states that receive these federal funds are required to provide a "free, appropriate public education" to all children with disabilities in the "least restrictive environment."

In 1992, amendments to the Rehabilitation Act of 1973 were infused with the philosophy of independent living. In 1992, two landmark court decisions impacted people living with mental illness. In *Foucha v. Louisiana*, the U.S. Supreme Court ruled that the continued commitment of an insanity acquitted patient who was not suffering from a mental illness was unconstitutional.

The American Indian Disability Legislation Project was established in 1993 to collect data on Native American disability rights laws and regulations.

The Persian Gulf War Veterans Act of 1998 (Pub. L. No. 105–277) required the Secretary of Veterans Affairs to determine, based on National Academy of Sciences' Institute of Medicine (IOM) reports, whether particular illnesses warrant a presumption of service connection and, if so, to set compensation regulations that correlated with specific illnesses and levels of impairment that veterans experience.

In 1998, President Clinton signed into law the Rehabilitation Act of 1973 Amendments, which included Section 508, a segment which led to access to the federal government's electronic and information technology. This legislation covered all types of electronic and information technology in the federal sector and did not limit access to assistive technologies used by people with disabilities.

The *Olmstead v. L. C. and E. W.* decision by the Supreme Court (1999) led to integration beyond philosophical expectations. In this landmark decision, the Court ruled that individuals with mental disabilities must be offered services in the most integrated setting possible.

Industry/Technology and Social Landmarks

On the international front, in 1990, the world saw the collapse of the Soviet Union. Undoubtedly, the collapse of the Soviet Union moved Russia from being considered one of the world's superpowers to a struggling economic capitalistic nation. This also led the way for other Communist European nations to become capitalist. The Berlin Wall came down in 1990, reuniting Germany into one nation. Also in 1990, Iraq invaded Kuwait. In response, Operation Desert Storm, launched in 1991, successfully drove Iraqi forces out of Kuwait.

The ADA was signed into law in 1990 by President George H. W. Bush and, through its five titles, paved the way for inclusion of older adults into community life. Although intended for people with disabilities, nondisabled older adults were also benefactors of this legislation.

Changes in technology made worldwide communications more efficient through the development of the World Wide Web. Search engines such as Google and Yahoo would then extend the use of web-enabled home computers into virtual gateways of information. Libraries also benefited remarkably through the use of technology for database management.

In Michigan, the notion of assisted suicide was promoted by Dr. Jack Kevorkian. Although eventually arrested, disbarred from practicing medicine, and imprisoned, Dr. Kevorkian prescribed medication to chronically ill patients interested in assisted suicide as an option to care. Despite being illegal under federal law and in most states, the Kevorkian paradigm was adopted by the state of Oregon to develop state legislation in support of physician-assisted suicide as an option for patients with chronic health conditions. Physician-assisted suicide has since been replicated in other U.S. states, Canada, and several European countries.

Labor Front Landmarks

The NAFTA was approved by Congress in 1993, leading to changes in the labor-market pool within the United States and shifting jobs and industries to Mexico. While NAFTA was used to stimulate business across North American countries, business was stimulated within the United States through Empowerment/Enterprise zones during the Clinton administration (1993).

Racial, Ethnic, and Gender Landmarks

The 1990s also witnessed a growing ethnic diversity in the United States, and women challenged the "glass ceiling." In 1992, Carol Moseley-Braun became the first African American woman to be elected to the United States Senate.

During this decade, the United States Supreme Court rulings in two landmark cases, *Bush v. Vera* and *Shaw v. Hunt,* demonstrated that the use of race as a factor when creating congressional districts was unconstitutional. In the case of *Bush v. Vera,* the court ruled that gerrymandered districts to address effects of past discrimination was a violation of the Voting Rights Act. In *Shaw v. Hunt*, the Court reversed a decision by the Eastern District of North Carolina, noting relieving past discrimination was not a compelling state interest and the gerrymandered district was therefore a violation of the Equal Protection Clause.

Poverty Landmarks

Welfare reform and changes in AFDC impacted people in poverty. New legislation known as Temporary Aid to Needy Families (TANF) led to a ceiling in the number of years one could collect funds (5 years). TANF, spearheaded by the then Secretary of Health and Human Services, Tommy Thompson, was modeled after Thompson's Wisconsin welfare initiative, which had been successfully implemented while he was governor.

The Dawning of a New Century: 2000–2009

Aging Policy Landmarks

A number of advances within the aging policy arena have already occurred during the 21st century. In 2000, Social Security earnings tests were eliminated for full retirement age. In 2003, the Medicare Part D prescription drug benefit was passed, opening up options for people seeking financial assistance for pharmaceutical medications.

The fifth White House Conference on Aging took place in 2005, in Washington, DC. This conference was, according to many professionals within the field, mired in politics, and devoid of meaningful constituent input. Fifty priorities were developed as a result of the conference, and these priorities helped shape the 2006 amendments to the Older Americans Act.

These amendments laid the groundwork for some significant changes in community services, which can address prevention services as well as services for existing conditions. The concept of Centers for Prevention to address mental health and healthcare are welcome additions to the act. Dealing with self-neglect is also introduced in the Older Americans Act.

Disability Policy Landmarks

The Help America Vote Act (HAVA) became law in 2002, and it required voting "systems" to be accessible for all those with disabilities. This legislation made it easier people with mobility impairments, the visually impaired, and those requiring special assistance to be able to exercise their civil rights.

In 2004, President George W. Bush signed into law the "Special Olympics Sport and Empowerment Act," Pub. L. No. 108–406. The bill authorized funding for its Healthy Athletes, Education, and Worldwide Expansion programs.

The Genetic Information Nondiscrimination Act (Pub. L. No. 110–233; 2008) prohibits group health plans and health insurers from denying coverage to a healthy individual or charging that person higher premiums based solely on a genetic predisposition to develop a disease in the future. The legislation also bars employers from using individuals' genetic information when making hiring, firing, job placement, or promotion decisions.

The ADA Amendments Act of 2008 broadened the scope of who is considered disabled under the law passed in 1990.

The American Recovery and Reinvestment Act (ARRA; Pub. L. No. 111–5, 2009) included billions of dollars to protect and expand disability services and benefits. Most critical were the funding increases to Medicaid, special education, early intervention, and vocational rehabilitation.

The Paul Wellstone and Pete Domenici Mental Health Parity and Addiction Equity Act (contained in Pub. L. No. 110–343, 2008) mandated that commercial insurers set mental health insurance copayments and treatment limits equal to those for coverage of physical conditions. It also banned cost-sharing requirements that apply only to mental health or substance abuse disorder benefits.

The Higher Education Opportunity Act (Pub. L. No. 110–315, 2008) enacted significant federal efforts to assist students with disabilities to access and succeed in postsecondary education programs. It included groundbreaking provisions regarding inclusion, enrichment, socialization, independent living, and person-centered planning in the development of the course of study. The law also had provisions for teacher training in special education.

The SSI Extension for Elderly and Disabled Refugees Act (Pub. L. No. 110–328, 2008) extends SSI eligibility for elderly and disabled refugees, those who have sought asylum, and other humanitarian immigrants from 7 to 9 years. In addition, a provision of the bill covers those who have already lost their SSI benefits. These individuals fled persecution or torture in countries such as Iran, Russia, Iraq, Vietnam, and Somalia and now meet the criteria for SSI eligibility based on disability or age.

The Improving Long-Term Care Choices Act (contained in Pub. L. No. 109–171, the Deficit Reduction Act, 2006) gives states the option of creating home- and community-based services and supports within the state Medicaid plan without obtaining a waiver. States were permitted to allow individuals to choose to self-direct services. States must establish a more stringent eligibility standard for placement of individuals in institutions than for services in a home- and community-based setting.

The Money Follows the Person Act (contained in Pub. L. No. 109–171, the Deficit Reduction Act, 2006) provides demonstration grants to states to help individuals transition from institutions to community settings. The program provides financial incentives for states to rebalance their long-term care systems and provide more cost-effective choices between institutions and the community.

The Individuals with Disabilities Education Improvement Act (2004) makes changes in IEP requirements, transition services, and the way in which school districts identify students as having disabilities with special attention to the issue of over-identification of members of ethnic and racial minority groups. The law also encourages more early intervention referrals, makes changes in the way disciplinary actions are handled, and adopts portions of the No Child Left Behind (NCLB) Act. The Act also adopts the NCLB definition of "Highly Qualified Teacher," provides for "risk pool" programs to address high needs children with disabilities, makes changes in procedural safeguards and dispute resolution, and encourages "universal design" as defined in the Assistive Technology

Act. It also has provisions for assessments of special education students under NCLB for paperwork reduction activities and for monitoring and technical assistance to school districts and states.

Industry/Technology and Social Landmarks

A number of events have taken place in the 21st century, including terrorist attacks, the toppling of dictatorships (e.g., Saddam Hussein in Iraq), and natural disasters (e.g., Hurricane Katrina).

On September 11, 2001, the United States witnessed a number of terrorist attacks on American soil. These began with two planes crashing into the Twin Towers of the World Trade Center in New York City and were followed by one crashing into the Pentagon in Washington, DC. A fourth plane, which was perhaps intended to crash into the Capitol building in Washington, DC, was forced into a field in Pennsylvania. These attacks spurred President George W. Bush's "War on Terror."

In 2002, the world witnessed the toppling of a major dictatorship, that of Saddam Hussein in Iraq. The United States sought to topple this dictatorship as one of its strategies to address the war on terror. By 2006, United States military forces remained in Iraq as an attempt to bring about a democracy within the country.

In the spring of 2005, the world bid farewell to Pope John Paul II, who passed away in Rome. The pontiff was known for his vision to bring about world peace, and he impacted religious leadership well beyond the Roman Catholic faith, to include Islam, Judaism, Buddhism, and other world religions. His successor, elected by papal conclave, was Pope Benedict XVI.

In 2008, the first African American president, Barack Obama, was elected.

Hurricane Katrina, in 2005, stormed through New Orleans and other parts of Louisiana, Mississippi, and the Gulf areas in the United States leaving many people homeless, particularly the marginalized and poor. This devastating natural disaster led to the displacement of many people.

In 2007, the most devastating massacre in the history of postsecondary institutions took place in Virginia. More than 35 victims (students and faculty) were shot by a troubled student one warm day on a college campus, just weeks before the end of the spring semester.

Racial, Ethnic, and Gender Landmarks

A major issue was same-sex marriages. Canada legalized same sex marriages, with at least five states in the United States, by 2006. However, legalization of nontraditional marriage continued to lead to major challenges to the paradigm of the family and controversy about the contract of marriage. This issue continued to be contentious into the next decade, even after it was legally resolved.

The Age of Individualism (2010 and Beyond)

Aging Policy Landmarks

Attempts to reauthorize the Older Americans Act took place in 2010; however, the amendments were not reauthorized until 2016. The reauthorization led to an expansion of services into the disability arena to help address the new needs presented through the merged Administration on Aging and Administration on Disability sectors, known as the Administration of Community Living. Older adults benefit from this merge because the face of aging services become more person-centered as opposed to services driven by a medical model.

Disability Policy Landmarks

The Patient Protection and Affordable Care Act (informally known as the ACA or Obamacare) became law in 2010, but was met with opposition following the change of Administration in 2016. As a result of this legislation, effective 2012, employers' health insurance policies cannot drop or deny coverage when a person falls ill or put a lifetime cap on how much care the policy will pay if a person gets sick. Effective 2014, companies cannot deny coverage based on preexisting conditions or put an annual cap on how much care the policy will pay for if a person becomes ill. During President Trump's administration (effective 2018) some of the original components of the ACA have been repealed.

On March 15, 2011, the new ADA came into effect. Its provisions expanded accessibility requirements for recreational facilities such as swimming pools, golf courses, exercise clubs, and boating facilities. They also set standards for the use of wheelchairs and other mobility devices in public spaces and changed the standards for things such as selling tickets to events (which account for accessibility needs) and reserving accessible hotel rooms.

Industry, Technology, and Social Landmarks

Businessman and reality television star, Donald Trump was elected to lead the country in 2016. His term, which began in 2017 brought forward many conservative approaches to social policy. This tough presidential election was fought against the first major-party female candidate for president, Hillary Rodham Clinton.

Rights of marginalized people saw an upswing during this era. In a 2013 Supreme Court case, people living in same sex relationships won the right to formal marriage in all 50 states in the United States.

Technology moved forward in many ways including advances in technology for communication, social media, robotics, and transportation. The first automatic cars appeared in this era, and the first licenses are granted for some cars. The first 3D printer is used during this era to aid in reconstructive surgery. In addition to these technological advances, this era also witnessed the final NASA shuttle flight which ended the NASA space program as it was known.

Gun violence rises to an all-time high during this era, and becomes a major public health issue as identified by the Centers for Disease Control and Prevention (CDC) and the American Public Health Association (APHA). Incidents ranged from Congresswoman Gabby Gifford shot during a community rally, to a mass shooting in Las Vegas killing about 50 people and injuring nearly 500 to school shootings such as Sandy Hook, Charleston, and Parkland. The Sandy Hook shooting took place at an elementary school on December 14, 2012 in Newtown, Connecticut, leaving 28 fatalities and two nonfatal injuries. The Charleston church shooting took place in South Carolina by a white supremacist Dylann Roof. Parkland, Florida was the site of a major shooting in Marjory Stoneman Douglas High School.

On the international front, diplomatic relations with Cuba were reinstated by President Barack Obama, but when Donald Trump succeeded him, restrictions on commercial and personal interaction between the two countries remained restricted. ISIS becomes a strong force and terrorist attacks are seen in public spaces not only in the on the international arena within the Middle East and Europe and include sites such as Ankara, Istanbul, Brussels, and Nice. This extremist group of Islamic fundamentalists appear to focus their attacks on more mainstream Muslims than on non-Muslims.

Labor Landmarks

During this era, labor unions lost traction, and some states became "right to work" states, leaving workers to feel more vulnerable and less secure. Several states enacted legislation intended to erode the power of unions within their workplaces.

Racial and Ethnic Landmarks

The death of Freddie Gray, an unarmed Black man, while in police custody in Baltimore, and deaths of other African Americans in Florida, St. Louis, Minnesota, and elsewhere, led to the "Black Lives Matter" movement, which took place in major cities across the United States. Although initiated as a result of perceived unjust treatment to the victims, the movement has led to extreme upheaval and recognition of the differences in treatment between ethnic minorities, specifically African Americans, by the judicial system.

Poverty Landmarks

During this era, the Occupy Wall Street protests became a major vehicle to protest financial interests of Wall Street businesses. In addition, the protest also fought against the relationship between Wall Street Financiers and the recession not only experienced within the United States, but also within the world economy.

SUMMARY

A number of changes have occurred within the fields of aging and disabilities over the last century. These changes, however, do not come close to the changes we have witnessed within the social, technological, and political arenas in the United States or worldwide. This relative dearth in changes can also be attributed to the fact that economic climate plays a tremendous role in social programs. Philosophical perspectives also play a major role in the development of our social fabric and the social welfare of domestic policies and programs. The next chapter lays out a range of philosophical paradigms that play a part in the development of social policies and programs and ultimately influence the aging and disability arenas. See Table 2.1.

Erica and Theresa sat back and examined the history lesson that they had just unfolded. The two women found the overview of events illuminating and the public laws and legislation fascinating. The information gave them a strong background to help them build their blueprint for programs and services within the aging and disability arenas of the communities that they will be assessing.

DISCUSSION QUESTIONS

1. Compare and contrast the different changes that have evolved between aging and disability legislation over the decades. Why do you think that there have been more input and advances in the disability arena than in aging-related legislation?
2. Is there a difference in the kind of expectations that one would have across the lifespan for people with disabilities and for people who are growing older? How do these expectations play a role in the development of public policy and legislation?
3. Can you compare and contrast advances made in social conditions, science, and technology versus advances in aging and disability policy/legislation. What do you think accounts for these differences?
4. How does the ageing arena benefit from advances in disability legislation and vice versa?

Table 2.1 Historical Landmarks, Social and Political Trends, and Their Relationship With Aging and Disability Policies

Decade	Policy Landmarks in the Aging and Disability Arenas	Social Landmarks	Political Influences and Landmarks
1920–1929	1920: The Civil Service Retirement Act: provides a retirement system for many government employees. Includes members of Congress, uniformed and civil servants.	Widespread availability of petroleum and electricity. The advent of new products: refrigerators, vacuum cleaners, wristwatches, foam rubber, disposable tissues, frozen foods. 1919: Prohibition is enacted. 1920: League of Nations begins. 1924: Immigration Act seeks to control immigration, to maintain the "racial preponderance of the basic strain of our people." 1925: Scopes trial takes place. 1927: Charles Lindbergh makes his first transatlantic flight. 1927: The first sound movie, *The Jazz Singer,* is released. Dancing of the "Charleston." This is an era of social experimentation. 1929: The Great Stock Market crash occurs.	*Labor*: Labor tries to organize but meets with major resistance, 1926: Senate passes law to allow unions to organize. An era of trickle-down economics and company unions. *Racial/ethnic*: Blacks, Hispanics, Native Americans, and Asian Americans are systematically discriminated against, often by laws. Quotas are set based on national origin. Immigration Act sets immigration quotas to restrict people of African descent. *Gender*: Women are realizing that getting the vote does not improve their economic position or lead to improved social policies. New sexual freedom, characterized by the flappers and encouraged by popularity of Freud. *Poverty*: It is assumed that all will share in prosperity as the economy grows, with this era.

(*continued*)

Table 2.1 Historical Landmarks, Social and Political Trends, and Their Relationship With Aging and Disability Policies (*continued*)

Decade	Policy Landmarks in the Aging and Disability Arenas	Social Landmarks	Political Influences and Landmarks
1930–1939	1935: The Social Security Act becomes law. 1937: The Railroad Retirement Act is enacted to provide annuities (pensions) for retired railroad employees and spouses. 1939: Social Security Administration adds survivor's insurance.	1933: Hitler assumes leadership in Germany. 1936: Roosevelt elected President of the United States. Indian Reorganization Act passes (1934). World War II (1939–1945) begins.	*Labor*: 1938: National Labor Relations Act (Wagner Act) are legalizes and empowers unions. Coalition forms between unions and the Democratic party. New York Association of Social Workers organizes social workers into unions. *Racial/ethnic*: The Social Security Act effectively excludes Blacks and some other minority groups from coverage. Syphilis study recruits African Americans, then leaves them untreated. Mary McLeod Bethune founds the National Council of Negro Women. Roosevelt appoints "Black cabinet." *Gender*: Women mostly excluded from Social Security, except as widows. *Poverty*: Rampant poverty is rampant. New Deal programs are assumed to be temporary, until the economy rights itself. 1933: Roosevelt drafts "grand design" to include FERA NIRA PWA CWA. Frances Perkins appointed first female Secretary of Labor.

(*continued*)

Table 2.1 Historical Landmarks, Social and Political Trends, and Their Relationship With Aging and Disability Policies (*continued*)

Decade	Policy Landmarks in the Aging and Disability Arenas	Social Landmarks	Political Influences and Landmarks
1940–1949	1945: Connecticut is first to establish a state agency on aging through its designation of a State Commission on the Care and Treatment of Chronically Ill, Aged, and Infirm.	1941: Japan attacks Pearl Harbor. 1943: Soviet victory at Stalingrad. 1945: United Nations established. 1947: UN splits Palestine into two nations, Palestine and Israel. India gains independence from Britain through the efforts of Gandhi. 1948: Israel becomes independent country. The declaration of Human Rights is ratified by the United Nations General Assembly.	*Labor:* Unions consolidate economic and political power. The post–World War II compromise allows wages and prices to grow. *Racial/ethnic:* Discrimination against returning Black soldiers. Growing dissatisfaction; civil rights groups beginning to become active. Blacks migrate north. 1948: President Truman orders the military desegregated. *Gender:* Women enter the workforce in large numbers during the war, but are driven out after the war. Marketers begin targeting women as consumers. 1946: Baby Boom generation begins. *Poverty:* Poverty is ignored. Social work is in Freudian stage.

(*continued*)

Table 2.1 Historical Landmarks, Social and Political Trends, and Their Relationship With Aging and Disability Policies (*continued*)

Decade	Policy Landmarks in the Aging and Disability Arenas	Social Landmarks	Political Influences and Landmarks
1950–1959	1950: First National Conference on Aging in DC, sponsored by Federal Security Agency. 1956: Special staff on aging is assigned coordinative responsibilities for aging within the Office of the Secretary of Department of Health, Education and Welfare. 1958: Representative John E. Fogarty introduces bill in Congress calling for White House Conference on Aging. 1959: The Housing Act is enacted, authorizing a direct loan program of nonprofit rental projects for the elderly at low interest rates. Also the U.S. Senate Special Committee on Aging is created.	People move from farms into suburbs. Development of psychotropic medications unleashes potential for people with mental illness. Most homes are furnished with televisions. Birth of rock and roll. 1950: Korean War begins. 1952: *MAD Magazine* appears. Sugar-free soft drinks appear Puerto Rico becomes an independent commonwealth of the United States. 1954: *Brown v. Board of Education.* Geneva Accord splits Vietnam into two parts, one Communist, one noncommunist. 1955: Rosa Parks refuses to move from the front of a bus to the segregated section; The 1954 Polio vaccine becomes widely available 1959: Barbie doll debuts.	*Labor:* Unions consolidate their power both economically and politically. The post–World War II compromise allows wages and prices to grow. 1952: Truman seizes the steel mill industry to avert strike. 1954: Jim Crow laws struck down. 1955: The American Federation of Labor and Congress of Industrial Nations (AFL-CIO) merger creates organized superpower. *Racial/ethnic:* Blacks migrate north. 1955: “Family of Man” exhibition at Museum of Modern Art *Gender:* Women enter the workforce in large numbers during the war, but are driven out after the war. Marketers begin targeting women as consumers. 1955: Ann Landers revolutionizes women’s expectations in advice column. *Poverty:* AFDC population increased dramatically along with Baby Boom. Accessibility to public assistance did not encourage productivity or employability, and over the decade public aid expenditures rose from \$2.30 to \$3.30 million.

(*continued*)

Table 2.1 Historical Landmarks, Social and Political Trends, and Their Relationship With Aging and Disability Policies (*continued*)

Decade	Policy Landmarks in the Aging and Disability Arenas	Social Landmarks	Political Influences and Landmarks
1960–1969	1960: Social Security amendments eliminated age 50 as a minimum to qualify for disability benefits and liberalized retirement test and requirement for fully insured status. 1961: First White House Conference on Aging. 1962: More than 160 bills introduced in Congress related to the aged and aging; eight are enacted. 1965: Medicare health insurance program for the elderly is legislated. Older Americans Act becomes law 1967: Amendments to the Older Americans Act extend its provisions for 2 years and directed the Administration on Aging to undertake a study of personnel needs in the aging field. Age Discrimination Act becomes law. Administration on Aging is placed in a newly created Social and Rehabilitation Service Agency (SRS) within the Department of Aging. 1969: Amendments to Older Americans Act extend its provisions for 3 years and authorize use of Title III funds to support area-wide model projects.	1960: Kennedy elected president 1962: Cuban missile crisis. 1963: Kennedy assassinated . United States enters as advisors to the Vietnam War. 1964: Civil Rights Act passes. Martin Luther King Jr.'s "I Have a Dream" speech. 1967: Haight-Ashbury sit-in in San Francisco. 1968: Martin Luther King, Jr. and Robert Kennedy assassinated. 1969: U.S. astronauts land on moon.	*Labor:* Farm workers begin to organize. *Racial/ethnic:* Civil rights movement catches the popular eye. Several civil rights acts are passed. *Gender:* Opponents of civil rights legislation include gender in acts. Gender later becomes basis of several lawsuits. Birth control pill and sexual revolution in full swing. *Poverty:* 1963: Community Mental Health Act passed. This and the Great Society legislation change social work. 1964: War on Poverty declared. In a year, 1,000 community action centers open.

(*continued*)

Table 2.1 Historical Landmarks, Social and Political Trends, and Their Relationship With Aging and Disability Policies (*continued*)

Decade	Policy Landmarks in the Aging and Disability Arenas	Social Landmarks	Political Influences and Landmarks
1970–1979	1971: Second White House Conference on Aging convened in Washington, DC. 1972: SSI programs created 1973: Older American Comprehensive Service Amendments establish areas agencies on aging and authorize model projects for senior centers. The Domestic Volunteer Service Act provides for Foster Grandparent programs. The CETA provides job training for those facing barriers to employment commonly experienced by older workers. 1975: Age Discrimination Act passed.	Rise of technology improves age of mechanization through computers. President Reagan's fiscal policies (Reaganomics) affect nations worldwide. 1972: End of Vietnam War.	*Labor:* 1970: Occupational Safety Health Administration (OSHA) is created. *Racial/ethnic:* A time of consolidating gains. *Gender:* Women's movement grows. 1973: *Roe v. Wade. Poverty:* Food stamp program is nationalized and national eligibility standards are established. Nixon takes away the ability of Legal Aid to file class action suits against government agencies.
1980–1989	1981: Amendments to the Older American Act extended the program for 3 years. 1984: Amendments to the Older Americans Act clarified the roles of state and area agencies on aging in coordinating community-based services and in maintaining accountability for the funding of national priority services.	1987: Reagan and Gorbachev sign historic arms treaty. 1980: John Lennon is murdered. End to era of rock revival	*Labor:* 1980: OSHA amendments. *Racial/ethnic:* Increased recognition for affirmative action and hiring goals. *Gender:* Women increase presence in labor market and nontraditional sectors. *Poverty:* Increased poverty, particularly among people with disabilities and people with severe persistent mental illness.

(*continued*)

Table 2.1 Historical Landmarks, Social and Political Trends, and Their Relationship With Aging and Disability Policies (*continued*)

Decade	Policy Landmarks in the Aging and Disability Arenas	Social Landmarks	Political Influences and Landmarks
	1985: *A Compendium of Papers Honoring the 20th Anniversary of the Older Americans Act* is compiled by the U.S. House of Representatives Select Committee on Aging. 1987: Amendments to the Older Americans Act authorized new initiatives on mental health, elder abuse, home healthcare for the frail elderly, and outreach to eligible SSI recipients.		Decreased support to social programs through the impact of "Reaganomics" on poverty—impacts those with fewest resources and creates a narrowing of middle-class income.
1990–1999	1992: Amendments to the Older Americans Act include the addition of Title VII, the Vulnerable Elders Rights Protection Title and fund efforts to increase education on healthy lifestyles. 1995—The fourth White House Conference on Aging convenes in Washington, DC. 1997—The Older Americans Act is up for reauthorization.	Changes in technology make worldwide communications more efficient. Assisted suicide movement begins under leadership of Dr. Jack Kevorkian in MI. 1990: Iraq invades Kuwait. The Americans with Disabilities Act signed. Nelson Mandela released from prison in South Africa. Clean Air Act passed. 1991. Operation Desert Storm. Collapse of the Soviet Union.	1990: Stewart B. McKinney Assistance Act for the Homeless reauthorized 1993: NAFTA approved by Congress. *Racial/ethnic:* Growing ethnic diversity changes the face of America (23.9% white) *Gender*: Women challenge the "glass ceiling." *Poverty:* Welfare reform and changes in AFDC impact people in poverty. 1996: TANF replaces AFDC and subsumes other assistance programs.

(*continued*)

Table 2.1 Historical Landmarks, Social and Political Trends, and Their Relationship With Aging and Disability Policies (*continued*)

Decade	Policy Landmarks in the Aging and Disability Arenas	Social Landmarks	Political Influences and Landmarks
2000–2009	2000: Social Security earnings test eliminated for full retirement age. 2003: Medicare Part D Prescription drug benefit passed.	2001: 9/11 Terrorist attack. 2002: Overthrow of Saddam. Hussein in Iraq. 2004: Death of Ronald Reagan. 2005: Hurricane Katrina. Death of Pope John Paul II. Same sex marriage passed as a constitutional right in Canada, several states in the United States follow suite. 2006: Execution of Saddam Hussein. 2007: Massacre of 39 victims on Virginia Technology University campus. 2008: Election of the first African American president, Barack H. Obama. 2011: Final NASA space flight. 2011: Shooting of Rep. Gabby Giffords in Tucson, AZ. 2012: Self-driving cars granted first licenses.	*Gender*: Same sex marriage is legalized in Canada and several U.S. states.

(*continued*)

Table 2.1 Historical Landmarks, Social and Political Trends, and Their Relationship With Aging and Disability Policies (*continued*)

Decade	Policy Landmarks in the Aging and Disability Arenas	Social Landmarks	Political Influences and Landmarks
2010 onward	2016: Reauthorization of Older Americans Act Amendments addresses both disability and aging arenas.	2013: 3D printer used for innovations in surgery. 2014: ISIS becomes a strong force, launching terrorist attacks.	*Racial/Ethnic:* 2015: Black Lives Matter movement develops.
	2015: Administration on Aging and Administration on Disability merge to form the Administration on Community Living. 2013: Patient Protection and Affordable Care Act becomes Law, enables many who have disabilities and people without health insurance access.	2015: Full diplomatic relations reinstated in Cuba. 2016: Donald Trump elected 45th president. 2017: Mass shooting at a country music festival in Las Vegas, NV.	*Gender:* 2015: Legalization of same sex marriages in all 50 states. Hillary Clinton is first major-party female candidate for presidency.

AFDC, Aid to Families with Dependent Children; AFL CIO, American Federation of Labor and Congress of Industrial Organizations; CETA, Comprehensive Employment and Training Act; CWA, Civil Works Administration; FERA, Federal Emergency Relief Act; NAFTA, North American Free Trade Agreement; NIRA, National Industrial Recovery Act; OSHA, Occupational Safety and Health Administration; PWA, Public Works Administration; SRS, Social and Rehabilitation Service Agency; SSI, Supplemental Security Income; TANF, Temporary Aid to Needy Families.

REFERENCES

Blatt, B., & Kaplan, F. M. (1966). *Christmas in purgatory: A photographic essay on mental retardation*. Boston, MA: Allyn and Bacon.

Compton, B. R. (1980). *Introduction to social welfare and social work: Structure, function, and process*. Homewood, IL: The Dorsey Press.

Day, P. J. (2006). *A new history of social welfare*. Boston, MA: Allyn & Bacon.

Glennon, L. (1995). *Our times: The illustrated history of the 20th century*. Atlanta, GA: Turner Publishing.

Wolfensberger, W. (1969). *The origin and nature of our institutional models*. Washington, DC: President's Committee on Mental Retardation.

Woolley, J., & Peter, G. (2018). Dwight D. Eisenhower remarks at opening session of the White House Conference on Aging, January 9, 1961. *The American presidency project*. Retrieved from http://www.presidency.ucsb.edu/ws/index.php?pid=12059

3

Philosophical Paradigms and Policy Frameworks Impacting Aging and Disability Policy

LEARNING OBJECTIVES

At the end of this chapter, readers will:

1. *Be familiar with philosophical paradigms that impact aging and disability-related policies.*
2. *Understand theories of implementation that impact public policies for people advancing in age or with disabilities.*
3. *Be familiar with a model for needs assessment and public policy analysis.*

> *Erica and Theresa put their heads together to attempt to understand the steps and forces that played a role in policy development as they proceeded to decide how to build agency policy and programmatic supports. They began by trying to understand the philosophical paradigms that play a role in policy development. In the process, the two quickly realized that they also needed to build an understanding of implementation strategies. Through their search, they uncovered many of the nuggets of wisdom that follow in this chapter.*

Public policy is a fabric woven from threads of numerous sources and through various influences. In the first two chapters, we see that aging policy is shaped by a variety of demographic, social, and economic factors. However, these factors are not the only influences on the development of public policy or aging/disability policies. Philosophical paradigms and theoretical frameworks also influence the actual development of policy and play a strong implicit role in how public policy is drafted.

PHILOSOPHICAL PARADIGMS AND THE RELATIONSHIP TO AGING POLICY AND POLICY ANALYSIS

Having a working knowledge of the social welfare and policy arena, including how to analyze public policy offers a number of benefits. All too often, policy decisions have been made on the basis of economic and political considerations, while the experiences

 DOI:10.1891/9780826128393.0003

of those who are directly affected, such as the constituents, and sometimes stakeholders, have been given little attention. Human service specialists are often called upon to provide insight into programs and policies, and within this context often have a vision for what policy or programs they would like to see implemented. However, the reality is that there is often a mismatch between what planners and public health/human service professionals have in mind for aging policy and what is either signed into legislation or becomes a program or service. This lack of agreement is often the result of competing philosophical paradigms or the implementation process. An explanation of these issues and concepts as a part of the policy analysis process helps facilitate an understanding of these competing philosophical paradigms.

WHAT IS POLICY ANALYSIS?

Policy analysis can be explained as an investigation and inquiry into the causes and consequences of public policies. *Public policy* is the general term for decisions, laws, and regulations put forth by governing bodies. Policy analysis also considers the political process and stakeholders and can interpret issues using a political lens (i.e., the interests and goals of elected officials) and tries to explain the role and influence of stakeholders within the policy process (Jimenez, Mayers-Pasztor, Chambers, & Pearlman Fujii, 2015). Information gained through the analysis of public policies can be used to develop policy alternatives for the future, to assess existing or previous policies, or to explain public problems and social phenomena (Dobelstein, 1996). Within this framework of policy analysis, various philosophical paradigms play a role in the development of healthy public policy, and various implementation strategies play a role in the process of moving policy from a legislative effort to programs and services. In the next sections these factors, such as philosophical paradigms and implementation strategies, will be explored, within the context of policy development and implementation.

PHILOSOPHICAL PARADIGMS

Public policy is never shaped in a vacuum, and it is strongly influenced by a variety of philosophical perspectives, which may run the range from very conservative to very liberal. These perspectives are essential to understanding the prevailing views that influence or shape current social policy. Understanding these various views can help build strategies to promote new perspectives, directions, or amendments to existing policy/legislation. In this chapter, a variety of philosophical paradigms are presented.

Individual values and ideology greatly influence the content and structure of public policy, and theories explain how social problems receive recognition and then become the objects of the policy debate. One's individual values color how public policy can be developed and how public policy may either be introduced as a bill or eventually be signed into legislation. In fact, a close examination of public hearings and personal testimonies and legislative proceedings can reveal some very significant value-laden perspectives. These values can be categorized into paradigms, which can help serve as a framework to understand social policy or the values that underpin social policy. Although no one paradigm stands clearly as the best explanation of why and how certain public policies came to be, paradigms do help to provide a framework for the analysis of the current welfare system and aging system. Some specific paradigms include blaming the victim, elitism, social welfare as a right, econometric perspectives, cause versus function, cronyism, egocentrism, and feminism. An exploration of each of these paradigms will help shape our understanding of how public policy can be developed.

Blaming the Victim

The philosophical paradigm of blaming the victim embraces the notion that individuals are at fault for their shortcomings or their status in society, rather than considering the systemic or universal issues (Ryan, 1976). This concept helps explain inequity in our society by suggesting that there are individuals who are inherently in a cycle of poverty, culturally deprived, or career criminals because of their choice, rather than because of an inherent problem in society or with the social care system. Ryan characterizes these cycles of victimization due to three dimensions: (a) perceived differences versus similarities, (b) individual behaviors versus collective action, and (c) internal factors versus external forces. The exclusion of specific groups of people from legislative efforts incorporates this blaming the victim perspective. For example, people with addictions and substance abuse histories are excluded from policies like the Americans with Disabilities Act. This also explains why self-neglect has only recently been added to the Older Americans Act. Both of these social issues are perceived to be attributed to behaviors that are not similar to the majority of older adults and people with disabilities, but rather to those who exhibit some form of deviance. Second, they are as a result of individual behaviors, and last, often perceived as due to inherent individual weaknesses. Hence, legislative efforts for programs and services do not address the needs of these specific groups of people, since these individuals are perceived to be responsible for their own problematic behaviors and thus responsible for their own solutions, rather than requiring solutions as a result of collective efforts or broad social and public responses through public policy. Unfortunately, historically speaking, many legislative efforts have not been as comprehensive as they could have been in meeting human needs because of this paradigm of blaming the victim and placing the responsibility squarely on the individual and his or her behavior.

This concept can be further articulated if we examine a basic premise in American culture—the belief that all older Americans have access to adequate food, clothing, and shelter. For the most part, we would assume that this is true, and the majority of our educated program planners and policy makers would subscribe to this perspective. Hence, if an older adult is at risk of being homeless because of an inadequate pension, we often perceive this as an individual difference, and a problem for the individual, not the collective; thus, we blame the victim. Similarly, if disability benefits do not meet the cost of living standards for one's basic subsistence, blame is placed on the individual rather than on the program providing financial support. Often individuals may be blamed for not managing their resources rather than looking at what resources are available.

Elitism

In the paradigm of elitism, policy development is in the hands of a few stakeholders. This group of stakeholders tends to dictate the rules and influence public policy based on their own values, preferences, and interests rather than the needs of the public or desire to serve the greater good (Bruggerman, 2013; Domhoff, 1956, 1974; Dye, 1975). Individuals with financial resources tend to play a more critical role in policy making, than those who do not have access to such resources (Galbraith, 1973). Corporate giants or their executives have been thought to utilize government as a resource in efforts to influence public policy in their favor (Wright-Mills, 1956). Recent examples of the use of elitism can be traced to the passage of the Affordable Care Act (ACA) through the support of the pharmaceutical industry and the American Medical Association, or the 2016 election of Donald Trump.

John Kenneth Galbraith argues that the "public bureaucracy . . . can be effectively and durably influenced by another organization. And between public and private organizations there can be a deeply symbiotic relationship" (Galbraith, 1973, p. 46). Hence, the elite have access to opportunities that other groups may not be privy to, which enhance their ability to influence public policy. To illustrate: "the president of General Motors, has a prescriptive right, on visiting Washington, to see the president of the United States. The president of General Electric has a right to see the Secretary of Defense" (Galbraith, 1973, p. 46). These examples illustrate how corporate elites use their opportunities to shape the legislative fabric of our state through their values (Galbraith, 1973).

In addition, many of these same individuals may have been appointed to high-level policy-making positions within government as a result of their circle of relationships or stakeholders. Since many may have a track record of running effective corporations, they are often appointed to run massive federal bureaucracies. Through these positions, they can often wield tremendous influence on public policy by imposing their own policy and value preferences within the federal agencies they direct. A recent example of this practice is the Trump administrative appointees into cabinet positions.

"The power," argues Galbraith, of this elite system "rests on its access to belief." What is good for the specific elite group in question is believed to be good for the general public. People in "elite power" believe that a model of public policy making is best because "the masses are largely passive, apathetic, and ill-informed." Public policy results in "not reflecting the demands of the people in so much as it does the interests and values of the elites" (Dye, 1975, p. 25).

Aging and disability policy arenas have been influenced by elitism through entities such as the American Medical Association, long-term care associations such as the American Health Quality Association and the American Association of Homes and Services for the Aging, the American Dental Association, and investment houses. Disability policy has also been influenced by elites opposing proactive policies such as the health insurance industry and transportation industry. When the Americans with Disabilities Act was up for passage, the transportation industry lobbied for the negative impact this would have and financial burden to the transportation industry if passed.

Social Welfare as a Right

The paradigm of social welfare as a right dates back to the Elizabethan Poor Laws of 1654, in which the deserving poor were perceived to have a right to services and support. Under this philosophical paradigm, a group in society—such as widows or those with congenital disabilities—is perceived to have a right to services. It is seen that these individuals are widowed or disabled, not through their doing, but through some negative or adverse event. The original Aid to Families and Dependent Children (AFDC) program, a title that was a component of the Social Security Act, was drafted to care for mothers who had been widowed or affected by the loss of their husbands through honorable service. This program was intended as a right for women and children whose spouses were assuming responsibility for their country. As civil rights expanded in the United States for people who were minorities, and particularly African Americans, the inclusion of minority groups into social welfare policies was seen as a right, rather than a privilege. Similarly, the rise of gay rights movements forced the inclusion of people who aligned with lesbian, gay, bisexual, and transgender (LGBT) principles (aging, disabled, or otherwise) the right to many benefits of social welfare programs.

Econometric Perspectives

Within an econometric paradigm, costs and the economic impact are always considered when developing programs and drafting policy. The Government Accounting Office is mandated to conduct evaluations on policy initiatives with cost in mind. Unfortunately, the costs of programs and of implementation are often a major deterrent to building incremental changes to current public policy. Support for public policy is weighed through the lens of costs to society and a quantitative view of how many people will benefit from such investment (Kemp & Denton, 2003). An example of how the econometric paradigm plays a role in the development of public policy can be seen with some of the amendments to the retirement ages that must be attained for the receipt of Social Security benefits.

When Social Security was originally conceptualized in 1935, the life expectancy was about 62 years, a few years shy of the age required to collect Social Security benefits. Thus, from a financial or economic perspective, it made good financial sense to have legislation that would provide a social safety net for people and their families as they advanced in age. If we fast forward 80 to 85 years, we see people living long past the retirement age originally established for Social Security, and we no longer see the same widespread support for the legislation due to the increased cost.

Currently, we see many valuable policies and programs either vetoed or introduced into the legislature without becoming law or not being implemented because of the costs associated with implementation. Cost benefit analysis plays a critical role in the policy process and is a crucial component of the econometric component of policy's philosophical paradigm.

Cause Versus Function

Through the cause versus function paradigm, policy and programs are drafted in an attempt to placate the cause, rather than have any utilitarian or functional value or impact (Karger & Stoesz, 1990; Piven & Cloward, 1979; Wilensky & Lebeaux, 1965). Hence, with this approach, the very purpose of the drafted policy or legislation is to create the impression to the general public that some effort has been taken to care for a specific social problem or issue. However, in reality, the program or legislative effort really plays a limited role or function for the individual or group. An example of this paradigm at play occurred after Hurricane Katrina in Louisiana, in 2005. As a result of the Homeland Security Act, all skilled nursing care and nursing home facilities were to have an emergency response evacuation plan in the event of a community-wide emergency. The "cause" was to be responsive in time of public emergency; however, in reality, these plans failed because of other systemic features within the larger community. Hence, the actual results of these plans were minimal, even if as a result of the legislative efforts the expectation was that a complete emergency response plan was in effect.

Often, policies, programs, and services are available but address a specific cause without fully addressing the problem or needs of the older adult or person with disabilities. However, when criticized, government officials can brag about the enactment of legislation to address the issues. Sometimes this approach can be referred to as "window dressing." Access and availability may still be issues for the constituent groups that the policies or programs are intended to impact. Another example, more widespread than the response to Katrina, is the availability of respite services to families or caregivers caring for a person with dementia or Alzheimer's disease or a parent of a child with autism. Although respite services are available through programs flowing via the Older Americans' Act, in reality they may amount to only 5 or 10 hours per month in rural communities—hardly adequate to provide a caregiver needed respite. Hence, the cause—burnout—is addressed by legislative efforts, but the functionality of the programs available is lacking.

Cronyism

Cronyism as a public policy paradigm was coined by the author of this text. The term refers to the use of one's inner circle of acquaintances and business collaborators not to develop public policy based on what is best for the community or stakeholders, but rather to benefit the stakeholders most closely connected as either business affiliates or family to those in the policy-making position. Throughout history influential families have been involved in politics and the policy-making process. One may argue that these connections benefitted from a relative or close ally in political power rather than what may have been advantageous to the broader community. In the last half century families such Kennedy family, the Bush family, and the Clinton family may be perceived in this light.

One may question what the difference is between elitism and cronyism. While it is likely that those in a position of influence in an example of cronyism could be a part of the elite, the difference is that elitism also includes the interest groups that wield political power. Examples include the American Medical Association and the American Dental Association. Cronyism refers to the process of policy-making resulting from a network of close friends or allies, with the end result having some impact on this network's business profit or outcomes.

Feminism

The feminist perspective is increasingly playing a role in the policy-making process, given that increasing numbers of women are entering state and local legislatures and Congress. Feminism refers to the ideology that pursues the goal to advance political, economic, individual, and social rights for women (Beasley, 1999; Hawkesworth, 2006). This perspective includes the goal of establishing policies to advance opportunities for women that are consistent with those of their male counterparts. Policies within the realm of aging and disability arenas have pushed toward helping people marginalized as well as women have the same status as their male counterparts (Hooks, 2000; Roberts, 2017). In some countries within the developing world, where educational and rehabilitation resources are limited, disparities between males and females still exist in terms of who receives interventions. A feminist paradigm strives toward equality regardless of gender and uses the approach of inclusivity as a guiding principle (Roberts, 2017).

Public Policy Advocates' Understanding of the Paradigms

In summary, various paradigms are at play when legislation is drafted or programs or services developed. Insight into these various philosophical perspectives can help enable public policy advocates to become better prepared with responses or rebuttals to support their own perspective and to help equip them with responses to assure that some of the gaps within legislation or programs are addressed. A working knowledge of these philosophical paradigms and how they influence policy makers is helpful to novice advocates as they attempt to build arguments to address these perspectives in the policy analysis and advocacy process. The next segment of this chapter addresses specific policy implementation strategies.

IMPLEMENTATION STRATEGIES

Social policy is developed and implemented within the context of both philosophical paradigms and specific implementation strategies. These implementation strategies help one to understand why specific policies and programs are implemented and others are not, and once understood, enable the reader to develop strategies to use to more effectively recognize the implementation of public policy. Values and ideology greatly influence the content and structure of public policy, although theories explain how social problems receive recognition and then become the objects of the policy debate. Although no one theory stands clearly as the best explanation of why and how certain public policies came to be, theories do help to provide a framework for the analysis of the current welfare system and aging system. Implementation strategies include window of opportunity, implementation, incrementalism, rationalism, and street-level bureaucrats.

Window of Opportunity

The timing of a public decision has been characterized by Kingdon (1984) as the opening of a policy window of opportunity, and an essential consideration in the implementation of public policy. Three elements need to be present for the success of the window of opportunity, which include (a) a compelling public problem, (b) a solution, and (c) broad political support for the solution. When these three elements come together, there is a strong likelihood that public policy will be developed. The events of the 1930s demonstrate the three streams coming together to develop the Social Security Act. Timing was right, depression brought about economic hardship, and a solution had been debated by political leaders and advocates for years. The Homeland Security Act is another example of the window of opportunity implementation theory. At the time of its passing, the social problem was impending attacks from terrorist sources, the solution was controls imposed through the Homeland Security Act, and since this was a compelling social issue, broad bipartisan political support ensued. Another example is the ACA, which was signed into legislation during the Obama presidency. The window of opportunity included the need for medical coverage for a wide sector of uninsured Americans (compelling public problem). The ACA provided a solution to these health insurance coverage needs (along with various other concerns such as an unskilled workforce prepared to support older adults and people with disabilities). In addition, President Obama was able to secure enough support from both sides of the political aisle (Republicans and Democrats) for this piece of legislation.

Implementation

It is no surprise that what develops as a policy and what actually gets implemented as a program or service frequently differ. This reality is often considered the implementation theory of policy development. Pressman and Wildavsky (1979) suggest that the implementation of public policy is an evolutionary process and the actual legislated policy changes when it is implemented. Although policy makers develop policy, the initial perception of what had been written in the legislation, or even what had been initially envisioned, is seldom what is implemented. Unfortunately, these differences may be accounted for by the reality that those who devise the policy are not the same people who are responsible for actually putting the ideas into practice. There is room for interpretation and values, especially for social welfare programs. What might make sense politically, when passed in the legislature, may make no sense once this same policy is implemented at a local level or in rural communities, for example. An illustration of this theory is the implementation of Medicare Part D. While seniors are required to apply on a computer, using a URL and through a specific Medicare Part D website, a vast number of older adults and people with disabilities, particularly, those living in rural communities, are in serious need of technology support in order to apply for Medicare Part D. This problem can be compounded in rural communities with limited band access to the Internet or limited resources and supports available to help them apply for Medicare Part D benefits. People may have access to the computer but the process is very intimidating for older adults, and may limit access to those who could qualify. Ironically, Barbara Bush, President George W. Bush's mother, also cited problems with attempting to apply.

Incrementalism

Charles Lindblom (1959), in "The Science of Muddling Through," articulates that public policy is developed through small changes to existing policies. In the implementation process, Lindblom suggests, there is never enough time to consider all information, that information on all possible choices is not possible, that choices are not readily available, and that it is easier to make small changes to existing policies than to create something entirely new. The Social Security Act and The Older Americans Act are good examples of how policy development occurred through incrementalism, since amendments over time have shaped both pieces of legislation to include important updates that enable the policies to address programs and services needed by the general population.

If you trace the history of these pieces of legislation, it is no surprise that may components have been added over time and have provided for a range of options for the constituent group to be served. If one would try to pass legislation to meet all stakeholder/constituent needs upfront, the legislation may never see fruition, due to cost. Thus, incrementalism may also be seen as a mechanism to initiate legislative action, with additional amendments to follow.

Rationalism

Rational policy making requires knowledge of the values of all segments of society, all possible policy alternatives, the consequences of those alternatives, and the costs and benefits. This knowledge is often hard to come by because it is not necessarily realistic, but rather, the ideal. Numerous factors affect this rational process, such as values, attitudes, interest groups with varying resources, lack of time to weigh all possibilities, and lack of adequate information. Unfortunately, within the policy-making process, there is often not the time or the resources to really examine all possible alternatives, such as short-term and long-term implications, costs, and benefits to a particular proposal. Although a number of interest groups may present themselves to the legislature, it may not be possible to hear from all groups that may be affected by a specific legislative effort, because of time and resources. Consequently, interest groups that have the resources and person power to be heard are often those whose perspectives are considered, rather than the perspectives of all who will be affected, and the end result is that a rational policy-making approach is not carried out.

Street-Level Bureaucrats

The implementation theory known as street-level bureaucrats is best characterized by Lipsky (1980), who suggests that the implementation process should focus on what happens after policy is implemented. He calls the power to shape social policy exercised by public services workers the power of street-level bureaucrats, since the administrative and human service workforces play a tremendous role in the actual implementation of the intended public policy. Street-level bureaucrats have significant power and control over people's lives, making decisions that affect who gets what, how quickly, and under what circumstances (Moore, 1987, 1990). Actions affecting policy can be as simple as how quickly applications are processed or whether phone calls are returned. These resources and their implementation are further controlled by administrative structures that may include severe personnel shortages, thus leading to additional constraints upon a public care system (Jewell & Glasser, 2006; Smith, Novak, & Frank, 2001; Vinzant & Crothers, 1996).

Public Policy Advocates' Understanding of the Implementation Strategies

An understanding of specific implementation strategies is an initial step to the development of effective public policies. Developing an awareness of specific strategies such as rationalism, implementation, incrementalism, window of opportunity, and street-level bureaucrats can help the policy advocate better understand the system and why specific policies may be limited in their impact, or why specific policies do not meet the intended goals. The next step in this process is to conceptualize a model for social welfare policy analysis.

A MODEL FOR SOCIAL WELFARE POLICY ANALYSIS

Within the context of philosophical paradigms and implementation strategies, one must consider how to pull these together to best understand the implementation of social welfare policy analysis. Although public policies such as aging policy are developed for a purpose (that is, to meet a specific community need) within this purpose, one can examine what values or philosophical paradigms were at play in the development and intention of the policy, and second, what specific strategies are or can be used to help address the intended and actual impact. Hence, within this framework, one must consider several key concepts that will help build a model for social welfare policy analysis. These concepts include the social problem/social issue, the goal, the policy or legislation, the implementation of legislation, the affected population, the intended impact, and the actual impact. Let us review each of these considerations to help build an understanding of how they develop an overall framework or model for policy analysis.

Social Problem/Social Issue

The first step in this process is to understand what the social problem or social issue is. How is this social issue shaped by demographic, social, technological, or economic factors? How prevalent is it within the community of concern? Is this a universal issue, or is it localized within a specific region? What data are available to support that this is indeed an issue of concern? Within this phase, a community needs assessment can be very useful in articulating the incidence and prevalence of a specific social issue.

Goal

The second step in this process is to articulate a goal. This goal can be developed to meet the need or social problem. The goal may thus help identify the purpose of the specific legislation—what is the intended purpose and how this will be designed to meet the social problem or need. An important question to consider is, how does this help us address the issue of the social problem? What values and philosophical paradigms underlie this goal? How are these values used to meet the goal or address the social problem?

Policy or Legislation

In the policy or legislation step within the framework of public policy analysis, one must consider the actual policy or piece of legislation. What is it? What does it attempt to do in terms of meeting the social needs or social problem? What are the specific features of the legislation? What programs or services does the legislation mandate?

Implementation of Policy or Legislation

What are the actual features of the policy or legislation? How has the implementation process altered the original intention of the policy or legislation? Who are the affected populations? What was the intended impact of the policy or legislation? What is the actual impact? How does this impact mirror or come close to meeting the original goal and addressing the social problem that was initially cited?

Affected Population

In this stage of the policy analysis, consider who the affected population is. What role do these people play, and who, in fact, are impacted by the legislative efforts described? It is important to note that many times the affected population may not necessarily be the same population as those intended to be addressed, especially if a policy or legislation is developed to meet the needs of a specific group. For example, the Social Security Act was intended to provide a safety net for people in their retirement. Since African Americans were originally excluded from this legislation, the affected population in the original legislation became White civil servants. Thus the affected population may not necessarily have included all those identified within the original social problem or issue.

Intended Impact

An important step within the analysis framework is to ask what was the intended impact of the legislation? How was it developed to meet the needs of the social problem identified initially? What goals did the policy or legislation have in mind?

Actual Impact

Finally, within this framework, it is essential to identify the actual impact. Who was affected and to what degree? What role did the policy play, and to what extent was the social issue/social problem addressed?

Figure 3.1 provides an overview of this policy analysis framework. Using this framework and the questions addressed within this text helps one to more effectively analyze a social problem or issue and how it has been addressed within the context of social policy/legislation. Lastly, it enables one to examine how both philosophical paradigms and implementation strategies play a role in meeting the intended goal of the legislation and/or to address a gap in social policy or legislation. It also enables one to address a specific social issue or problem.

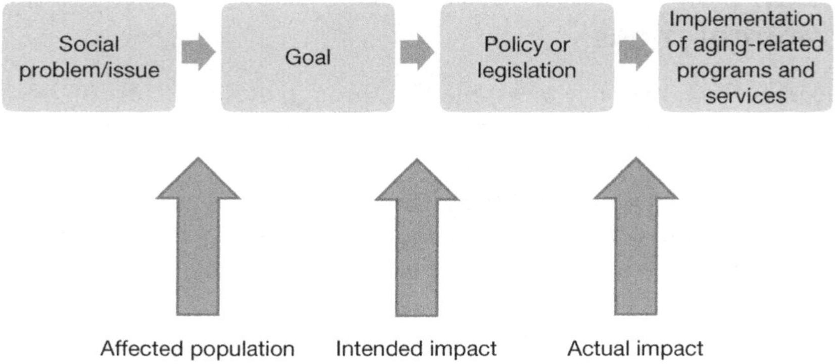

Figure 3.1 A framework for public policy analysis.

THE USE OF NEEDS ASSESSMENTS FOR POLICY DEVELOPMENT AND COMMUNITY PLANNING

Community-based needs assessments can be very useful in the process of identifying specific community needs and specific issues or problems to be addressed. In fact, community needs assessments can be vital tools in the process of policy development and community planning and are addressed in Part III of this text, as a specific tool in the process of policy development. What is important at this juncture, however, is to understand how these needs assessments fit with the overall model for policy analysis. It is also important to keep in mind that within the policy development process, needs assessments can be objective and provide some measure of evidence to support an objective view of a problem. Philosophical paradigms, however, will color this process, as well as, the implementation strategies. Hence it is important to consider how paradigms impact the social issue at hand. A needs assessment can help one to be able to utilize objective evidence to better address how the philosophical paradigms and the implementation strategies discussed within this chapter play a critical role in this process. The needs assessment process is outlined in more detail within Chapter 18. The following chapter will address the use of evidence in policy development and will revisit the concept of using evidence as part of a needs assessment.

SUMMARY

Public policy, especially aging and disability policy, is not created in a vacuum, nor is it value free. Values and philosophies guide the development of specific philosophical paradigms and shape how aging and disability policy is developed and implemented. This chapter explores how these realities play a role in the development and implementation of public policy and aging/disability policy. Although advocates for aging/disability policy may have a vision for policies and programs that address issues in a more utopian manner, this chapter showcases some of the realities that may prevent the implementation of the policy or program as envisioned. As a safeguard against a subjectively devised policy and program base, objective evidence and empirically driven initiatives can be developed by aging and disability policy advocates. The next chapter facilitates these skills within the policy development process.

DISCUSSION QUESTIONS

1. Consider a current policy that is moving through the legislature (either at a local, state, or federal level), and identify what philosophical paradigms are at play within the congressional testimony or presenting arguments.
2. Consider a current policy at either your local/regional level or at the federal level that interests you. What implementation strategies have been implicit within the policy as you track it from its first appearance as a public law and at the current time?
3. Using the framework presented in this chapter and Figure 3.1, identify a social policy of interest and analyze it through the framework presented.

REFERENCES

Beasley, C. (1999). Feminism's critique of traditional social and political thought. In C. Beasley (Ed.), *What is feminism? An introduction to feminist theory* (pp. 3–11). London, UK: Sage.

Bruggerman, W. G. (2013). *The practice of macro social work*. San Francisco, CA: Cengage.

Dobelstein, A. W. (1996). *Social welfare policy and analysis* (2nd ed.). Chicago, IL: Nelson-Hall.

Domhoff, G. W. (1956). *Who rules America?* Englewood Cliffs, NJ: Prentice-Hall.

Domhoff, G. W. (1974). *The powers that be*. New York, NY: Random House.

Dye, T. (1975). *Understanding public policy*. Englewood Cliffs, NJ: Prentice-Hall.

Galbraith, J. K. (1973). *Economics and the public purpose*. Boston, MA: Houghton-Mifflin.

Hawkesworth, M. E. (2006). *Globalization and feminist activism* (pp. 25–27). New York, NY: Rowman & Littlefield.

Hooks, B. (2000). *Feminism is for everybody: Passionate politics*. Cambridge, MA: South End Press.

Jewell, C. J., & Glasser, B. E. (2006). Toward a general analytic framework. Organizational settings, policy goals, and street-level behavior. *Administration & Society, 38*(3), 335–364. doi:10.1177/0095399706288581

Jimenez, J., Mayers-Pasztor, E., Chambers, R. M, & Pearlman Fujii, C. (2015). *Social policy and social change: Toward the creation of social and economic justice* (2nd ed., pp. 25–28). Thousand Oaks, CA: Sage.

Karger, H. J., & Stoesz, D. (1990). *American social welfare policy: A structural approach*. New York, NY: Longman.

Kemp, C. L., & Denton, M. (2003). The allocation of responsibility for later life: Canadian reflections on the roles of individuals, government, employers and families. *Aging and Society, 23*(6), 737–760.

Kingdon, J. W. (1984). *Agendas, alternatives and public policies*. Boston, MA: Little, Brown.

Lindblom, C. E. (1959). The science of muddling through. *Public Administration Review, 19*, 79–88. doi:10.2307/973677

Lipsky, M. (1980). *Street level bureaucrats*. Thousand Oaks, CA: Sage.

Moore, S. T. (1987). The theory of street-level bureaucracy. A positive critique. *Administration & Society, 19*(1), 74–94.

Moore, S. T. (1990). Street-level policymaking: Characteristics of decision and policy in public welfare. *The American Review of Public Administration, 20*(3), 191–209.

Piven, F. F., & Cloward, R. A. (1979). *Poor people's movements: How they succeed and how they fail*. New York, NY: Random House.

Pressman, J. L., & Wildavsky, A. (1979). *Implementation*. Los Angeles, CA: University of California Press.

Roberts, J. (2017). Women's work. *Distillations*. 3 (1): 6–11.

Ryan, W. (1976). *Blaming the victim*. New York, NY: Random House.

Smith, B. W., Novak, K. J., & Frank, J. (2001). Community policing and the work routines of street-level officers. *Criminal Justice Review, 26*(1), 17–37.

Vinzant, J., & Crothers, L. (1996). Street-level leadership: Rethinking the role of public servants in contemporary governance. *The American Review of Public Administration, 26*(4), 457–476.

Wilensky, H. L., & Lebeaux, C. N. (1965). *Industrial society & social welfare*. New York, NY: The Free Press.

Wright-Mills, C. (1956). *The power elite*. New York, NY: Oxford University Press.

4

Evidence-Based Policy Development: Tools for Public Policy Development and Analysis

LEARNING OBJECTIVES

At the end of this chapter, readers will:

1. *Be familiar with how evidence and an evidence base guide policy development.*
2. *Be familiar with various sources of public and private data sources that can guide the policy development process.*
3. *Be aware of Healthy People 2020 benchmarks used to guide program planning and policy development.*

> *After running a series of focus groups with care providers, Erica thought that many of the issues presented could be supported with data and documentation. Her concern was that she had a series of case-specific issues that were identified but was not certain that these could be backed up with specific numbers. Further, she also was concerned that many of the issues presented to her may not appear to be priorities in any specific government documents. She turned to her colleague Theresa for some help in this matter. Thus, the two of them began to wade their way through government documents to identify which documents may be of use; they summarized documents available for community planning in the materials identified in this chapter. Let us begin to examine how some of these sources were put together.*

WHAT IS AN EVIDENCE BASE?

Evidence seems to be the buzz word that is used repeatedly; however, what does it really imply and how can it be used in the process of program planning and policy development? Witkin and Harrison (2001) define *evidence based* as using the "best available" evidence, or empirically based/research-driven "knowledge" about specific issues or concerns. Evidence is defined as "something that furnishes proof" (*Merriam-Webster* 2018). In Chapter 3, the case is made that philosophical paradigms play a major role in the development of public policy, and within the context of many philosophical paradigms, a rational, data-driven evidence base is often negated. Hence, an evidence base provides some research-based theory and/or empirically driven background/rationale to support the need for specific directions for policy development or program planning. Historically, we have been acclimated to the idea of needs assessment and have been familiarized with this concept in order to identify issues that require redress, and in essence, the process of a needs assessment provides an evidence base for decision making and planning efforts.

WHAT IS EVIDENCE-BASED PROGRAM AND POLICY DEVELOPMENT?

Evidence-based needs assessment and program development is the use of data and benchmarks to inform one's decision making and the development of resource allocation.

Professional judgments and policy development should be guided by two principles:

- Policy should be grounded upon prior findings, likely to produce predictable and effective results.
- Client systems over time should be evaluated to determine the efficacy of the intervention (i.e., policy decision; Howard, McMillen, & Pollio, 2003).

Thus, at the core of policy development and program-planning initiatives should be the best evidence, which would include integrating knowledge that one gleans from practice, clinical trials, and practical experience (Institute of Medicine, 2003; Johnson & Austin, 2006; Proctor, 2003; Rosen, 2003). An evidence base to policy development envisions a scientifically based approach that uses the best available evidence to guide policy and practice decisions. It also strives to move beyond one's cultural perspective for decision making and bridges the cultural perspective about what power relations tell us is real (Witkin & Harrison, 2001), and what data showcase as real (Jurkowski, 2005) when developing policy or building programs for older adults (OA).

WHY AN EVIDENCE BASE?

The first question to ask when examining evidence-based policy development is to ask, what is evidence and how does it provide the basis for decision making. An evidence base provides several advantages. First, it strives toward policy development from a rational philosophical paradigm perspective. An evidence base also minimizes values that may be political as opposed to objective reasons for policy development. In addition, it provides a measure of accountability and solicits data for the basis of policy and program-related decisions (McNeill, 2006). The field of public health is steeped in epidemiologic data, much of which is used for decision making, program planning, and policy development. Other allied health professions, such as social work, have been lagging in their use of epidemiologic data and available data sources to assist in building a case for program planning and policy development (Morago, 2006; Plath, 2006). In fact, some professions such as social work have been considered "authority based" and have relied upon this authority basis for the development of programs, policies, and services until the last decade or so. The heart of this authority may be the need to identify what constitutes an evidence base, and how empirical knowledge and evidence are really defined (Gibbs & Gambrill, 2002; Rubin & Parrish, 2007).

Erica reviewed what she had found on evidence-based policy development above, and once again tried to identify these issues with Theresa, an MSW graduate. She wondered how the social work profession viewed this idea of an evidence base, since Erica was trained to use "authority," evidence, and professional expertise for decision-making. Theresa provided her with the following explanations.

SOCIAL WORK AND PROGRAM PLANNING FOR OLDER ADULTS AND PEOPLE WITH DISABILITIES: AN AUTHORITY-BASED OR EVIDENCE-BASED PROFESSION?

Traditionally, our profession has been seen as "authority-based practice (ABP)" (Gambrill, 1999), which means we utilized our expertise to make the best possible clinical judgments, as opposed to driving our decisions. Although a move has been popularized to address the dearth of evidence, through the integration of practice wisdom and evidence-based approaches, this section addresses some of the dilemmas of an authority-based approach and the need for an evidence-based approach (Gambrill, 2001). Based upon this notion, several dilemmas of social work as an authority-based profession have been identified, including the following:

- Clients may not be adequately informed of the range of options available to them.
- Social workers may lack adequate information and evidence to support programs or policies that have been developed to guide practice.
- Decisions may not be informed by empirical or realistic outcomes and findings.

While social work is being critiqued here for not being an evidence-based profession, other allied health professions may also follow with some of the same limitations when evidence supporting the authority is concerned. Thus, the debate around what evidence-based practice is and how it plays into program planning and policy development also emerges. What strategies can be used to create an evidence-based approach to program planning and policy development for OA? Do clinical trials alone provide adequate evidence to develop an implementation framework for policy development, or do we need to consider alternative sources of evidence to support program and policy decisions, while waiting for our clinical trials to gestate data?

Such alternative approaches provide for substance, while assuring that some of the objections to evidence-based practice, such as value-driven approaches to discipline specific practice, are negated (Gibbs & Gambrill, 2002). The profession of social work has struggled with the concept of evidence-based approaches to practice (EBP), since the concept of an evidence base is dependent upon clinical trials in the broadest sense of the definition of EBP. In addition, the profession, and documentation of outcome measures, is still in its childhood; thus some alternative ways to consider sources of evidence at this time, while building policy and program initiatives within the aging arena, will be necessary.

Erica, now convinced that she should utilize data sources to help her build her rationale for work-force development, decided to build along with Theresa, a series of approaches that could be used for evidence-based policy development. Together they cultivated a repository of specific sources.

APPROACHES TO EVIDENCE-BASED POLICY DEVELOPMENT

A number of approaches guide the process to assure evidence-based policy development. These approaches include efficiency, effectiveness, cost, cost-benefit studies, and cost-effectiveness. In terms of efficiency, one must consider the question: does the policy/intervention work? In terms of effectiveness: does the policy meet the stated objectives under normal conditions? In addition, do the service outcomes associated with a policy differ across consumer subpopulations? In terms of cost, how much does it cost to deliver an intervention per unit of service? And finally, one must consider the cost-benefit of the process or policy in question. From this perspective, do the dollar benefits exceed the dollar costs of the policy/programs? If in fact policies lead to programs that are cost-effective, how do these policies compare with regard to the resources required to implement them? Thus, each of these questions leads to a different approach that can be used in the process of gathering evidence to build an evidence base for policy development.

The National Association of Social Workers (NASW) code of ethics challenges social workers to develop policies and programs that draw from practice-related research. Through this challenge, one makes use of data, evaluation, and outcomes measures to evaluate practice (and policy) decisions. This process enables one to monitor progress and trends over time and can also be translated into impact assessment.

Public health, on the other hand, can be considered an empirically based profession, which utilizes a variety of tools that incorporate the use of counts, incidence, and prevalence. These epidemiologic sources of data are useful for building a case to showcase the impact of specific public policy or the need for revision of social policy and should be borrowed by other professions within the multidisciplinary relationship.

SOURCES OF EVIDENCE

A number of sources that can provide evidence and support policy directions or programmatic choices are available to practitioners and advocates within the health and human service (HHS) arenas. Some of these include Congressional Universe, Congressional Record, *Congress.gov*, Government Printing Office (GPO), Government Accountability Office (GAO), and databases from secondary data sources. This section provides an overview of these evidence-based sources and summarizes some of the content of these databases. These databases provide the best available data that currently exists within secondary data sources to help us understand policies or the impact of policy and program initiatives.

Congressional Universe

A comprehensive online resource known as "Congressional Universe" enables the researcher/policy advocate search for Congressional hearings, public issues, legislation, history, and legal research. This tool also provides the ability to research using an in-depth approach to access the full text of congressional information, dating back for at least 200 years. This resource provides detailed information about Congress, including member biographies, committee assignments, voting records, financial data, and the full text of key regulatory and statutory resources. Specifically, Congressional Universe can enable some of the following:

- Pinpoint expert testimony on the leading issues of the day.
- Tap authoritative sources of statistics, projections, and analyses.

- Discover a law's intent by tracing its legislative history.
- Gauge Congressional attitudes toward current topics.
- Find out how members of Congress voted on legislation.
- Investigate the finances of members of Congress.
- Monitor legislation and public policy on almost any topic.
- Review the federal regulations that implement legislation.
- Learn the makeup and mission of Congressional committees.
- Access "hot bills" and topics of Congress.

This tool can provide the background necessary to enable a policy advocate to identify the philosophical paradigms behind either a proposed bill or current legislative efforts. Congressional Universe provides an up-to-date holding of the federal *Congressional Record*.

Congress.gov Database

The Congress.gov database (formerly known as THOMAS.gov) is a publicly funded resource that makes United States federal policy-related materials available to the general public through a variety of links to current federal legislative information. This resource was first launched in January 1995, at the inception of the 104th Congress, and it resulted from leadership in this Congress directing the Library of Congress to assure that federal information was easily available to the general public. Since 1995, Congress.gov has been expanded to include a range of resources of interest to the policy advocate. These include bills and resolutions, activity in Congress, Congressional Record, schedules and calendars, committee information (House and Senate), presidential nominations, treaties, government resources, and a segment for teachers.

Bill resolutions can be found through the Congress.gov home page, which provides the text of legislation for the current Congress. In addition, one can search a bill summary and the status of a particular bill. The summary and status information includes: sponsor(s); cosponsor(s); official, short, and popular titles; floor/executive actions; detailed legislative history; Congressional Record page references; bill summary; committees of referral; reporting and origin; subcommittees of referral; links to other committee information provided by the House of Representatives; amendment descriptions (and text, when available); subjects (indexing terms assigned to each bill); a link to the full text versions; and if the bill has been enacted into law, a link to the full text of the law on the GPO website.

Bill summary and status information is searchable by word/phrase, subject (index) term, bill/amendment number, stage in the legislative process, dates of introduction, sponsor/cosponsor, and committee. Lists of all legislation, public laws, private laws, vetoed bills, and bills/amendments sponsored/cosponsored by each member during each Congress are also available.

Search Bill Text or Bill Summary and Status for Previous Congresses

The Bill Text and Bill Summary and Status features both contain the ability to search previous Congresses. Users can select a Congress from the menu on the search pages.

Public Laws by Law Number

This feature contains Bill Summary and Status records for each bill that became public law. Laws are listed both by law number order and in bill number sequence (House Joint Resolutions, House Bills, Senate Joint Resolutions, and Senate Bills).

House and Senate Roll Call Votes

Roll call votes are recorded votes from the House of Representatives and the Senate. Votes are listed in reverse chronological order by roll call vote number. The vote summary page lists roll call vote number, vote date, the issue (bill/amendment number being voted on, quorum call, or Journal approval), the question (description of the vote), the result (passed, failed, or agreed to), and the title/description of the legislation. Detailed vote pages show individual members' votes and vote totals by party.

Legislation by Sponsor

Legislation can be browsed by sponsor (senator or representative) for the current Congress. Legislation sponsored by a particular member or members can also be found for previous Congresses.

Search Committee Reports

Committee Reports include the full text of House and Senate committee reports (including conference reports and joint committee reports) printed by the GPO. Most committee reports are printed by the GPO. Reports can be searched by word/phrase, report number, bill number, and committee. Searches can be limited by type of report (House, Senate, Conference, or Joint). Reports can be browsed sequentially by House/Senate committee report number, conference report, and joint committee report.

Treaties

Information provided about treaties includes treaty number, the date the treaty was transmitted, short title, formal title, treaty type, legislative actions, and index terms. New information is added throughout the day by the executive clerk of the Senate. It becomes available early the next morning. This feature does not contain the actual text of the treaty itself. The full text of treaties can be searched at GPO Access.

Government Resources

Congress.gov contains a list of legislative and other government resources. Congress.gov also provides resources for learning about the legislative process and resources for legislative researchers. Congress.gov also provides resources for teachers, including classroom activities, lesson plans, guides to congressional information, and more.

Government Printing Office

The GPO is the federal government's primary centralized resource for gathering, cataloging, producing, providing, authenticating, and preserving published information in all its forms. GPO is responsible for the production and distribution of information products and services for all three branches of the federal government. GPO's main mission is to ensure the American public has access to government information.

The U.S. GPO's core mission, which is stated as "Keeping America Informed," dates to 1813, when Congress determined the need to make information regarding the work of the three branches of government available to all Americans. This is the inherent function of government, which GPO carries out for federal agencies on behalf of the public.

Many of the United States' most important information products, such as the Congressional Record and Federal Register, are produced at the GPO's main plant in Washington, DC, a 1.5 million square-foot complex that is the largest information processing, printing, and distribution facility in the world, located just five blocks from the Capitol. In addition to the agency's production facilities, GPO procures between 600 and 1,000 print-related projects a day through private-sector vendors across the country. The majority of the government's printing needs are met through a long-standing partnership with America's printing industry. GPO competitively buys products and services from thousands of private sector companies in all 50 States. It is one of the government's most successful procurement programs, assuring the most cost-effective use of the taxpayers' printing dollars. The GPO also publishes reports drafted through GAO and makes these available to the general public and Federal Book Depositories. Thus, the materials are easily available to the general public, public HHS policy advocates, and lobbyists interested in building evidence-based cases for aging-related causes.

Government Accountability Office

The GAO is an agency that works for Congress and the American people. Congress asks GAO to study the programs and expenditures of the federal government. GAO, commonly called the investigative arm of Congress or the congressional watchdog, is independent and nonpartisan. In the recent past, the GAO was known as the Government Accounting Office. This entity studies the impact of how the federal government spends taxpayer dollars. GAO advises Congress and the heads of executive agencies (such as Administration on Community Living [ACL], Environmental Protection Agency [EPA], Department of Defense [DOD], and HHS) about ways to make government more effective and responsive to current social, economic, and political issues. GAO evaluates federal programs, audits federal expenditures, and issues legal opinions. When GAO reports its findings to Congress, it recommends actions. GAO's work leads to laws and acts that improve government operations and hopefully save dollars for the public. An example of how the GAO interfaces with policy developments in the aging arena can be found with evaluation reports, which advise legislative amendments to the Older Americans Act or Social Security amendments.

The GAO is not subject to the Freedom of Information Act (FOIA; 5 USC 552). However, GAO's disclosure policy follows the spirit of the act consistent with GAO's duties and functions as an agency with primary responsibility to the Congress.

Secondary Data Sources Useful in an Evidence-Based Approach

A number of data sources are also available from state-based and federal agency sources, which can also be used to advise policy and program developments in the aging and disability arenas. Although a comprehensive listing of databases is available from the Federal Interagency Forum on Aging-Related Statistics (2016) in its report *Older Americans 2016: Key Indicators of Well-Being* and on its website (agingstats.gov), this segment provides a short overview of some of the publicly available data sources. Table 4.1 also provides an overview of data sources that can provide empirical data that are helpful to program planners and policy advocates interested in advancing policies and legislation that will impact the segment of our population growing older and/or living with disabilities.

State Departments of Public Health (Data for Community Assessment)

Every state-based health department currently has a data system available that provides a composite picture of the health of communities. Although the actual variables within

Table 4.1 Secondary Data Sources That Can Provide Empirical Data on Aging and Disability Measures

Source	Website
Census Bureau	www.census.gov
Current Population Survey	www.bls.gov/cps/home.htm
Centers for Disease Control and Prevention	www.cdc.gov/index.htm
Behavioral Risk Factor Surveillance System	www.cdc.gov/brfss/index.html
Longitudinal Studies on Aging	www.cdc.gov/nchs/lsoa/index.htm
National Ambulatory Medical Care Survey	www.cdc.gov/nchs/ahcd/index.htm
National Death Index	www.cdc.gov/nchs/ndi/index.htm
National Health and Nutrition Examination Survey	www.cdc.gov/nchs/nhanes/index.htm
National Health Interview Survey	www.cdc.gov/nchs/nhis/index.htm
National Home and Hospice Care Survey	www.cdc.gov/nchs/nhhcs/index.htm
National Hospital Ambulatory Medical Care Survey	www.cdc.gov/nchs/ahcd/index.htm
National Hospital Discharge Survey	www.cdc.gov/nchs/nhds/index.htm
National Mortality Followback Survey	www.cdc.gov/nchs/nvss/nmfs.htm
National Nursing Home Survey	www.cdc.gov/nchs/nnhs/index.htm
National Study of Long-Term Care Providers	www.cdc.gov/nchs/nsltcp/index.htm
National Vital Statistics System (Vital Statistics)	www.cdc.gov/nchs/nvss/index.htm
Centers for Medicare and Medicaid Services	www.cms.gov/index.html
Health and Retirement Study	hrsonline.isr.umich.edu/index.html
National Long Term Care Survey	www.icpsr.umich.edu/icpsrweb/NACDA/studies/9681
New Immigrant Survey	nis.princeton.edu/index.html
Panel Study of Income Dynamics	psidonline.isr.umich.edu/default.aspx
Drug Abuse Warning Network	www.datafiles.samhsa.gov/study-series/drug-abuse-warning-network-dawn-nid13516

(*continued*)

Table 4.1 Secondary Data Sources That Can Provide Empirical Data on Aging and Disability Measures (*continued*)

Source	Website
National Survey on Drug Use and Health	www.samhsa.gov/data/data-we-collect/nsduh-national-survey-drug-use-and-health
The Survey of Mental Health Organizations	wwwdasis.samhsa.gov/webt/NewMapv1.htm
American Time Use Survey	www.bls.gov/tus/home.htm
Uniform Reporting System	wwwdasis.samhsa.gov/dasis2/urs.htm
Consumer Expenditure Surveys	www.bls.gov/cex/home.htm
Current Population Survey	www.census.gov/programs-surveys/cps.html
National Longitudinal Surveys	www.bls.gov/nls/home.htm
National Survey of Veterans	www.bls.gov/nls/home.htm
FedStats/Federal Committee on Statistical Methodology	nces.ed.gov/FCSM/index.asp
Institute for Community Inclusion	www.communityinclusion.org/project.php?project_id=16

each data set may differ from state to state based upon health priorities, essentially all states collect data on acute and chronic conditions across the life span; thus, policy and program advocates can secure data related to health conditions of OA. These data have been collected in a standardized manner based upon the Assessment Protocol for Excellence in Public Health (APEX-PH) model for public health practice and are readily available to constituents through the state-based departments of public health. Many state-based departments of public health also have these data available through state-based websites. State-based data are also compared to the benchmarks identified in the *Healthy People 2020's Health Objectives for the Nation*. (Note: Appendix A and B include a listing of these objectives related to OA and people with disabilities.)

U.S. Census Bureau

The U.S. Census Bureau collects data on its residents on a decennial basis for two specific purposes. The first is to apportion the 435 seats in the U.S. House of Representatives among the 50 states. According to the U.S. Constitution (Article 1, Section 2), apportionment of representatives among the states must take place every 10 years (decennially). The second reason to carry out the census is to enumerate the resident population. The census can provide data on sex, race, Hispanic origin, and age for 100% of the enumerated population, and data on income, education, housing, occupation, and industry from a representative sample. Data are enumerated from a short form with seven basic questions, and a long form, which includes the same seven questions and an additional set of questions. Although all residences are enumerated, only one in every six households receives the long form. Data are available from the census through the census bureau at www.census.gov.

Department of Health and Human Services

The Department of Health and Human Services offers resources to fund a variety of products that provide data related to OA and conditions of aging and across the life span. These resources are available through the Centers for Disease Control and Prevention (CDC), the National Center for Chronic Disease Prevention and Health Promotion, the National Center for Health Statistics (NCHS), and the Centers for Medicare and Medicaid Services. This section describes each of the secondary data sets available through these entities, which can be useful in the process of building a vision for developing an evidence base for program planning or policy development.

Centers for Disease Control and Prevention

Within the CDC, the National Center for Chronic Disease Prevention and Health Promotion is responsible for the Behavioral Risk Factor Surveillance System (BRFSS). The BRFSS is designed to collect state-specific data on behaviors that can relate to leading causes of morbidity and mortality. Since comparable methods are used from year to year, states can compare risk factors and the prevalence of specific behaviors across states and over time. Thus, it becomes possible to track the impact of health interventions over time as well. The questionnaire used within the BRFSS has four components: a fixed core, a rotating core of questions, standardized optional modules, and some specific state-devised questions. State and local health departments take advantage of the data provided from the BRFSS to do the following:

- Identify priority health needs and populations most at risk for illness and disability.
- Develop strategic plans and target prevention programs and activities.
- Examine trends in behaviors over time and monitor the effectiveness of interventions vis-à-vis Healthy People 2020 objectives.
- Support community policies and programs that promote health and prevent disease.

The data from the BRFSS can be exceedingly helpful for program planners interested in examining the impact of specific programs and policies that will impact OA within state-based initiatives. The data are available from the BRFSS website at www.cdc.gov/brfss. Surveillance summaries and reports relevant to the BRFSS are also available through the website.

National Center for Health Statistics

The NCHS, in collaboration with the National Institute on Aging (NIA), sponsors a data site with a Longitudinal Study on Aging (LSOA), and the Supplement on Aging (SOA). These surveys provide data to measure changes in health, health-related behaviors, healthcare, and causes/consequences of such changes across two cohorts of elderly Americans. Variables covered within the questionnaires include housing characteristics, family structure and living arrangements, relationships and social contacts, use of community services, occupation and retirement (income sources), health conditions and impairments, functional status and assistance with basic activities, utilization of health services and nursing home stays, and health opinions. The sample includes adults 55 years of age or older. Table 4.1 provides the website to find these data.

Other secondary database products available through the NCHS include some of the following databases:

- National Ambulatory Medical Care Survey (NAMCS)
- National Death Index (NDI)
- National Health and Nutrition Examination Survey (NHANES)
- National Health Interview Survey (NHIS)
- National Home and Hospice Care Survey (NHHCS)
- National Hospital Ambulatory Medical Care Survey (NHAMCS)
- National Hospital Discharge Survey (NHDS)
- National Mortality Followback Survey (NMFS)
- National Nursing Home Survey (NNHS)
- National Study of Long-Term Care Providers (NSLTCP)
- National Vital Statistics System (NVSS)

All of these surveys can be accessed through the CDC and NCHS websites.

Centers for Medicare and Medicaid Services

The purpose of collecting data sources through the Centers for Medicare and Medicaid Services is assessment of the Medicare and Medicaid programs. These secondary data sets include the following:

- Consumer Assessment of Healthcare Providers and Systems (CAHPS)
- Medicaid (Claims and Enrollment) data
- Medicare (Claims and Enrollment) data
- Medicare Current Beneficiary Survey (MCBS)
- Medicare Health Outcomes Survey (HOS)
- Minimum Data Set (MDS)
- Outcome and Assessment Information Set (OASIS)
- Chronic Conditions Data Warehouse (CCW)

National Institutes of Health

The National Institutes of Health include two institutes that house data relevant to aging. These are the National Cancer Institute (NCI) and the NIA. NIA provides a database on surveillance epidemiology and end results (SEER), while NIA supports four specific data sets of interest to aging policy advocates: the Health and Retirement study (HRS), the National Long-Term Care Survey (NLTCS), the New Immigrant Survey (NIS), and the Panel Study on Income Dynamics (PSID).

Office of the Assistant Secretary for Planning and Evaluation

The office of Disability, Aging, and Long-Term Care Policy (DALTCP) is a division within the Office of the Assistant Secretary for Planning and Evaluation. In particular, the Division of Disability and Aging Policy evaluates programs authorized by the Older Americans Act. Furthermore, the National Alzheimer's Project Act (NAPA) was passed in 2010, establishing the groundwork for DALTCP and other agencies to create a National Plan focused on Alzheimer's disease and related dementias (AD/ADRD).

Substance Abuse and Mental Health Services Administration

The Substance Abuse and Mental Health Services Administration (SAMHSA) program provides oversight to mental health and substance abuse programs nationwide in the

United States. In efforts to develop programs and services that are meaningful to the aging population, several databases are available that provide data on the usage and attitudes of OA and substance use or mental health service provision. These include the following:

- Drug Abuse Warning Network (DAWN)
- National Survey on Drug Use and Health (NSDUH)
- National Survey of Substance Abuse Treatment Services (N-SSATS)
- Treatment Episode Data Set (TEDS)
- Uniform Reporting System (URS)

The DAWN was developed as an ongoing, national public health surveillance system that collected data related to adverse health consequences resulting from drug misuse and abuse. Data were collected from hospital emergency room visits drawn from a national probability sample of hospitals. Although the system ended in 2011, DAWN still provides valuable data to showcase emerging drug-related trends and provides these data to communities, member facilities, local public health authorities, federal agencies, and policy makers.

The N-SSATS collects information from all facilities in the United States, both public and private, that provide substance abuse treatment. Some of the objectives of collecting this information include the following: to assist SAMHSA and state/local governments to assess the nature and extent of services provided in state-supported and other treatment facilities; to analyze treatment service trends and provide a comparative analysis for the nation, regions, and states; and to provide a national directory of drug abuse treatment facilities.

The TEDS was compiled annually until 2005 and provided demographic data on the characteristics and substance abuse problems of people admitted for substance abuse treatment. The records are not compiled per individual, but rather per admission, and agencies included within this data set are receiving funds for alcohol or drug services or Federal Block Grant money. The TEDS system included both an Admissions Data Set and a Discharge Data Set.

The URS is an annual survey that provides state-level data regarding the impact and usage rate of state-run community mental health programs and psychiatric facilities.

Department of Housing and Urban Development

The Department of Housing and Urban Development, through the Office of Policy Development and Research, disseminates the American Housing Survey (AHS), which addresses the nation's housing situation. The AHS provides data on the characteristics; conditions; financing; and costs of housing, nationally and in selected metropolitan areas; on neighborhood conditions and amenities; and on households. Specifically, the AHS conducts a national survey every 2 years and a metropolitan areas survey once every 6 years. Public use data files are available through www.huduser.org/portal/datasets/ahs.html.

Department of Labor

The Department of Labor, through the Bureau of Labor Statistics, provides for four specific surveys with relevance to aging adults: the American Time Use Survey (ATUS), The Consumer Expenditure Survey (CEX), Current Population Survey (CPS), and the National Longitudinal Surveys (NLS).

Department of Veterans Affairs

The Department of Veterans Affairs (VA) collects data on their veterans through the National Survey of Veterans (NSV). The intent of this survey is to describe characteristics of the veteran population and of users and nonusers of Department of VA benefit programs. The survey topics include sociodemographic and economic characteristics, military background, health status measures, and VA and non-VA benefits usage. The sample is based upon a population of veterans 65 years of age and older.

Federal Committee on Statistical Methodology

The Federal Committee on Statistical Methodology (FCSM), created by the Office of Management and Budget, administers a website entitled FedStats, which is an interagency effort that provides access to a full range of official statistical information available to the public through the federal government. Users can access official statistics, which are collected and published by more than 13 federal agencies.

Social Security Administration

The Social Security Administration compiles a system of data on its new beneficiaries known as the New Beneficiary Data System (NBDS). The NBDS provides important data on the changing circumstances of aged and disabled beneficiaries. The data system includes two studies, the New Beneficiary Survey (NBS) and the New Beneficiary Follow-Up (NBF). A wide range of topics are covered, including demographic characteristics, marital and childbearing history, employment history, current income and assets, and health status. Some data are also gathered from spouses and added to the administrative records. Data are available from www.ssa.gov/policy/.

Administration on Community Living

The Administration on Community Living (ACL) provides databases related to functioning and ability across the lifespan. The ACL provides data and statistics on OA as well as persons with physical and intellectual and developmental disabilities. In addition, the ACL has developed a strong focus on measurement of program results, including the following: implementation and strengthening of program information reporting from the states, development of targeted performance measures, and national surveys. Data can be found at the following website: www.acl.gov/programs/program-evaluations-and-reports

The Centers for Disease Control and Prevention

The Disability and Health (DH) branch of the Centers for Disease Control and Prevention conducts studies and collects data through community-based panel surveys on disability-related topics. Disability and Health Data System (DHDS) is an online source of state-level data on adults with disabilities. Users can access information on five functional disability types: cognition (serious difficulty concentrating, remembering, or making decisions), mobility (serious difficulty walking or climbing stairs), vision (serious difficulty seeing), self-care (difficulty dressing or bathing), and independent living (difficulty doing errands alone). Information on limitation status (use of special equipment or activity limitation because of physical, mental, or emotional problems) is also available.

Data on more than 30 health topics among adults with or without disabilities can be explored in DHDS, including smoking, physical activity, obesity, hypertension, heart disease, and diabetes. Data can be accessed through www.cdc.gov/features/disability-health-data/index.html.

The World Health Organization

The World Health Organization, an agency of the United Nations, provides databases on health-related data, disability, and aging. Its databases also provide a user with the opportunity to compare the data between countries. With assessment tools utilizing the *International Classification of Functioning, Disability, and Health* (*ICF*) and *International Statistical Classification of Diseases and Related Health Problems, 10th Revision* (*ICD-10*), the end user can examine functional status and mobility limitations with common assessment tools and compare data between the United States and other countries around the world. The website for the World Health Organization is www.who.org (See Appendix E for more information about ICD10).

Theresa and Erica have now developed an arsenal of data sources to begin to address workforce-related issues. In their discussions with each other, they realized that they needed to prioritize some issues for the workforce specific to the aging and disability fields. Theresa suggested that they explore what the health outcomes and goals for the nation actually are through a review of Healthy People 2020's goals and benchmarks.

BENCHMARKS USED IN THE HEALTHCARE ARENA FOR PROGRAM PLANNING AND POLICY DEVELOPMENT

A blueprint for the health of the United States has been developed through the use of a document entitled *Healthy People 2020: Health Objectives for the Nation*. The Department of Health and Human Services has undertaken this initiative, which provides benchmarks for the progress of the health of Americans for the next 10 years, with supporting objectives in disease prevention and health promotion. The two main goals of the health objectives are (a) to increase quality and years of healthy life and (b) to eliminate health disparities. The Future of Public Health (Institute of Medicine, 1988) called for a national system of benchmarks to articulate the health objectives of the nation, and these have been revised for 1990, 2000, 2010, and 2020. Benchmarks currently have been established in order to identify where health goals for the nation and individual states should be, and the program is evaluated routinely by local and state health departments. Healthy People 2020 is also used to gauge the impact of health policy. Within the objectives, benchmarks are listed for a variety of health issues that impact OA, including mental health, access to care, physical activity, oral healthcare, and disability. The data sources cited within this chapter are used in the process of identifying how closely benchmarks have been met. Healthy People Objectives have been in force since HP1990, and by the year 2020 we will see a version of Healthy People 2030.

Specific topical areas have been identified within Healthy People 2020, and health objectives with accompanying data for the nation and the specific state-related data are available within the HP2020 website www.healthypeople.gov.

These benchmarks can be used as a part of rationale for proposing legislation to provide resources or address specific policy/program needs by policy advocates. Public health officials consistently make use of this resources as an opportunity for understanding and building rationale for policy and program development. Healthy People 2020 benchmarks for people growing older are available in the Older Adult (OA) objectives, while benchmarks for people growing older are available in the Disability and Health (DH) objectives (CDC, 2018, Office of Disease Prevention and Health Promotion [ODPHP], 2018a, 2018b). Appendices A and B expound on these objectives.

EVIDENCE AND ITS ROLE IN POLICY DEVELOPMENT AND COMMUNITY PLANNING

Thus far this chapter has focused on sources of evidence for evidence-based policy development. Now we need to ask the question, "What role does evidence play in the development of policy and community resources for aging services?" How can this information be put to use in the development of revised policies to benefit OAs and programs or services to improve the health and well-being of OAs? The first step in this process is to use the information for needs assessments.

What Is a Needs Assessment?

Needs assessments take on a variety of different meanings and definitions; however, Witkin & Altschuld (1995) sum this up in their definition, which suggests that a needs assessment is "a systematic set of procedures undertaken for the purpose of setting priorities and making decisions about program or organizational improvement and allocation of resources. These priorities are based upon identified needs" (p. 4).

Several strategies can be used in the process of developing this inventory of community resources and gaps in the resources. Kirst-Ashman and Hall (2002) identifies five specific strategies that can be used: social indicators, key informants, community forums, surveys, and agency-related data. Each is important and can make a significant contribution in part or in combination with other methods in order to create a composite sketch of a community's needs. Although presented cursively here, these approaches are revisited as a tool for policy and program development in Chapter 18 and will be elaborated upon. These needs are based upon evidence or data, much of which can also be obtained from the sources cited earlier in this chapter.

SUMMARY

The struggle to reach a vision of rational policy development based upon evidence is paramount at this stage in our journey to build aging policies and services. This chapter explores some of the dilemmas with developing an evidence base and provides a range of empirical sources within the aging and disabilities arenas that can be used in building an evidence-based approach to policy development. The journey, however, will not be without struggle—since philosophical paradigms, and social and economic factors will interface and play a role in the development of evidence-based policy. Policy advocates, however can help with this cause through the use of data-driven and evidence-based approaches to building public policy and program planning for OAs and people with disabilities.

ADDITIONAL RESOURCES

Websites

Centers for Disease Control and Prevention: www.cdc.gov

The official site for the Centers for Disease Control and Prevention, which provides links to the host of national data sets, collected through the NCHS.

Congressional Record: www.congress.gov

Cornell ILR: A Guide to Disability Statistics from the CPS—Annual Social and Economic Supplement (March CPS): digitalcommons.ilr.cornell.edu/edicollect/1233

This website provides a useful manual and step-by-step instructions on how to access and utilize data on people with disabilities among various community- and employment-oriented statuses. All data are derived from state and federal data repositories.

GAO: www.gao.gov

This portal provides access to governmental evaluation and assessment reports on a variety of topics. The topics range from evaluations of existing legislation to issues that may require legislative intervention.

GPO: www.gpo.gov

There are approximately a quarter of a million titles available to the public via the Internet on the GPO Access website at www.gpoaccess.gov. Through GPO's partner websites, an additional half a million titles are accessible to the public. Printed copies of more than 5,500 of those documents ranging from Supreme Court opinions to reports from the Bureau of Labor Statistics may also be purchased from the GPO Sales Program in person, online, via phone, fax, email, or postal mail.

Healthy People 2020: www.healthypeople.gov

The official website for Healthy People 2020 containing the health objectives for the year 2020, as well as midcourse progress reports.

IRIS Data Repository: iris.wpro.who.int

This site serves as The WHO Regional Institutional Repository for Information Sharing (WPRO IRIS) and is the digital library of WPRO's published material and technical information in full text produced since 1951. The material and available content is freely accessible and searchable in English; however, content in Chinese and French are currently digitized and are available if requested.

Local Disability Data for Planners: www.infouse.com/disabilitydata/organizations/index.php

This website provides useful data for state and locally based disability planning entities and links the consumer with a range of websites that provide disability statistics.

PubMed: www.ncbi.nlm.nih.gov/entrez/query.fcgi?otool=ilusiclib

An online index to articles in medical and life science journals, many available in full text without charge. Also available are other online subject specific indices, NLM and NIH resources for consumers and professionals, and the TOXNET database on toxicology and related subjects, for example, you can search "healthcare reform and statistics."

Congress, Library of Congress: congress.gov

Congress.gov provides full text legislative information on the Internet beginning with the 104th Congress (1995/1996). It includes congressional bills, public laws, roll call votes, the Congressional Record, committee reports, and information on the legislative process. Searching is by word or phrase, bill number, stage of legislative process, or public law number. Years of Coverage: 104th Congress (1995/1996) to present with some accessibility to earlier years.

World Health Organization: www.who.org

This site provides links to the World Health Organization. Data collected for countries worldwide in the areas of health, disability, and social indicators.

DISCUSSION QUESTIONS

1. If you wanted to identify the need for a specific policy in your community, how would you go about identifying the need, and what data sources could you utilize to document the population and need from the resources identified in this chapter?
2. How can you use the *Healthy People 2020* benchmarks to build a baseline and goals for specific policy and program initiatives you want to address in your community/county or state?
3. What uses can the Government Accountability Office (GPO) documents be for building advice on specific program or policy issues that you would like to draw attention to either within your county/community/state or at the federal level?
4. How can you and your colleagues or classmates build a needs assessment intervention strategy that would address a specific policy/program need using the secondary data sources outlined within this chapter?
5. Consider the data sources in this chapter and identify how you can use some specific aspects of quantitative data to go along with anecdotal data or case-specific examples in efforts to address a specific aging/disability-related gap that exists.

REFERENCES

Administration for Community Living. (2016). *Data and research*. Retrieved from http://www.acl.gov/aging-and-disability-in-america/data-and-research

Centers for Disease Control and Prevention. (2018a). *Disability and health: data system (DHDS)*. Retrieved from http://www.cdc.gov/ncbddd/disabilityandhealth/dhds/index.html

Centers for Disease Control and Prevention. (2018b). *Healthy People 2020: Objectives*. Retrieved from http://www.cdc.gov/nchs/healthy_people/hp2020.htm

Federal Interagency Forum on Aging-Related Statistics. (2016). *Older Americans 2016: Key indicators of well-being*. Washington, DC: U.S. Government Printing Office.

Gambrill, E. (1999). Evidence-based practice: An alternative to authority-based practice. *Families in Society, 80*(4), 341–350. doi:10.1177/1044389418786699

Gambrill, E. (2001). Social work: An authority-based profession. *Research on Social Work Practice, 11*, 166–175. doi:10.1177/104973150101100203

Gibbs, L., & Gambrill, E. (2002). Evidence-based practice: Counterarguments to objections. *Research on Social Work Practice, 12*(3), 452–476. doi:10.1177/1049731502012003007

Howard, M., McMillen, C., & Pollio, D. (2003). Teaching evidence-based practice: Toward a new paradigm for social work education. *Research on Social Work Practice, 13*(2), 234–259. doi:10.1177/1049731502250404

Institute of Medicine. (1988). *The future of public health*. Washington, DC: National Academies Press.

Institute of Medicine. (2003). *The future of the public's health in the 21st century*. Washington, DC: National Academies Press.

Johnson, M., & Austin, M. J. (2006). Evidence-based practice in the social services: Implications for organizational change. *Administration in Social Work, 30*(3), 75–104. doi:10.1300/J147v30n03_06

Jurkowski, E. (2005, December 14). *Evidence based policy development.* A paper presented to the American Public Health Association, Philadelphia, PA.

Kirst-Ashman, K., & Hall, G. H. (2002). *Understanding generalist practice*. Belmont, CA: Brooks Cole.

McNeill, T. (2006). Evidence-based practice in an age of relativism: Toward a model for practice. *Social Work, 51*(2), 147–156. doi:10.1093/sw/51.2.147

Merriam-Webster online dictionary. (2018). *Evidence*. Retrieved from http://www.merriam-webster.com/dictionary/evidence

Morago, P. (2006). Evidence-based practice: From medicine to social work. *European Journal of Social Work, 9*(4), 461–477. doi:10.1080/00981389.2013.834029

Office of Disease Prevention and Health Promotion. (2018a). *Healthy People 2020 topics and objectives: Older adults.* Retrieved from http://www.healthypeople.gov/2020/topics-objectives/topic/older-adults/objectives

Office of Disease Prevention and Health Promotion. (2018b). *Healthy People 2020 topics and objectives: Disability and health.* Retrieved from http://www.healthypeople.gov/2020/topics-objectives/topic/disability-and-health/objectives

Plath, D. (2006). Evidence-based practice: Current issues and future directions. *Australian Social Work, 59*(1), 56–72. doi:10.1080/03124070500449788

Proctor, E. K. (2003). Evidence for practice: Challenges, opportunities, and access. *Social Work Research, 27*(4), 195–196. doi:10.1093/swr/27.4.195

Rosen, A. (2003). Evidence-based social work practice: Challenges and promise. *Social Work Research, 27*(4), 197–208. doi:10.1093/swr/27.4.197

United States Department of Health and Human Services. (2016). *Healthy People 2020: Health objectives for the nation*. Washington, DC: Government Printing Office.

Witkin, R. W., & Altschuld, J. W. (1995). *Planning and conducting needs assessments: A practical guide*. Thousand Oaks, CA: Sage.

Witkin, S., & Harrison, D. (2001). Whose evidence and for what purpose? *Social Work, 46*(4), 293–296. doi:10.1093/sw/46.4.293

Part II

The Legislative Basis for Programs and Services Affecting Older Adults and/or People With Disabilities

Part II of this text provides an overview of major federal policies and programs that impact older adults and people with disabilities in the various aspects of their lives. Some historical developments leading up to the actual development and implementation of the policies are also explored and discussed. This section begins to address the dynamics of social welfare in Chapter 5, which explores Social Security. Healthcare issues related to Medicare are examined in Chapter 6. Chapter 7 examines the Older Americans Act, while Chapter 8 introduces and explores the Americans with Disabilities Act. Chapter 9 elaborates on mental health policy and practice through the Community Mental Health Centers Act and other legislation impacting older adults and people with disabilities. Chapter 10 provides an overview of the Patient Protection and Affordable Care Act and implications for older adults and people with disabilities. Chapter 11 provides an overview of the Elder Justice Act. The Caregiver Support Act is addressed in Chapter 12. Housing and long-term care is examined in Chapter 13, and substance use/misuse is addressed in Chapter 14. The chapters within this section of the book articulate key components of the legislation and unfold some of the programs and services that emanate from the legislation.

5

The Social Security Act

LEARNING OBJECTIVES

At the end of this chapter, readers will:

1. *Understand the history of the Social Security Act (SSA).*
2. *Understand specific components of the SSA.*
3. *Understand how Social Security provides resources to older adults and people with disabilities.*

Can you imagine a system within our current industrialized and technological society with no safety net for one's economic and medical resources upon retirement or disability? In agrarian societies, people bore many children as insurance for themselves when they were into their old age—thus, they would have person power to provide for them in their golden years. In today's society, with families opting to have one or two children, it hardly seems realistic that one would rely upon their children to care for them in their old age. In fact, these were some of the dilemmas that Franklin D. Roosevelt faced when he considered the passage of the Social Security Act (SSA).

This chapter provides a backdrop to our current Social Security Program and an overview of some models for Social Security programs in Europe and Canada; it explores the genesis of the Social Security program in the United States. The contents of the original SSA is explored and compared to the titles and programs mandated through the current SSA. The chapter also offers some guidelines for the current administration of the program, examines the debate around current proposals for revision, and reviews why these proposals are current issues for consideration. The chapter concludes with an overview of useful websites that can provide up-to-date information.

BACKDROP TO OUR CURRENT SOCIAL SECURITY PROGRAM

Social Security in the United States is a program that by worldwide standards was a relative latecomer to this country. Although the original Social Security program was signed into law by President Franklin D. Roosevelt in 1935 to provide for the welfare and financial

© Springer Publishing Company DOI:10.1891/9780826128393.0005

security of older Americans without means testing. Programs from other corners of the world have been more comprehensive in nature than what we began with in the United States. The early social insurance schemes were designed in Western Europe to address three fears of industrial workers:

- Poverty in old age
- Illness
- Unemployment

The German Chancellor Otto Von Bismarck established and designed Europe's first social insurance program in 1880; however, the program was not officially adopted until 1889, thus leading the campaign for an old-age social security program. The idea was first put forward, at Bismarck's behest, in 1881 by Germany's emperor, William I (more commonly known as Kaiser Wilhelm), in a groundbreaking letter to the German Parliament. William wrote: "those who are disabled from work by age and invalidity have a well-grounded claim to care from the state" (Mann, 1970, p. 269).

Two specific motivations can be credited for Bismarck's introduction of a social security program in Germany. The first was to encourage the health and well-being of workers as an effort to promote and maximize the efficiency of the German economy; the second was to thwart any more radical "socialist alternatives." Despite Bismarck's right-wing perspective and commitment to commerce and trade, Bismarck would be coined a socialist for introducing these programs, as was President Roosevelt 70 years later.

The German system provided contributory retirement benefits and disability benefits as well. Participation was mandatory, and contributions were taken from the employee, the employer, and the government. Coupled with the workers' compensation program established in 1884 and the "sickness" insurance enacted the year before, these features gave the Germans a comprehensive system of income security based on social insurance principles.

An interesting myth has prevailed throughout history, to suggest that Bismarck chose an arbitrary retirement age of 65, since he himself was said to have been 65 years of age at the time. In reality, however, Germany initially set their retirement age at 70 years, while Bismarck himself was 74 at the time. The retirement age was lowered to 65 in 1916, although Bismarck had been deceased since 1898. The myth is significant, however, because the United States examined the German model and utilized its features as a blueprint when designing its own Social Security program, including a retirement age of 65.

Social Security in Europe

In England, the first vestiges of a SSA were seen in the early 1900s through England's Pension Act of 1908. France was a latecomer to the development of a social security system and did not evolve its program until 1930.

European models for a social security system were based upon investment schemes as opposed to a "pay as you go" system. Essentially, this approach meant that systems invested the taxation revenues and used the proceeds to finance a social security or disbursement plan. In contrast, the "pay as you go" approach has revenue coming into a system and paid out at the same time, with no or limited investment of the resources.

Social security programs enhanced workers' loyalty to the state by giving laborers a stake in the government, especially if they were not landowners. In some cases, labor unions revolted.

The Genesis of Social Security in the United States

In the United States, the Great Depression was a major economic upheaval. Hence, reform proposals suggested taking taxes to fund guaranteed incomes in old age. The 1932 presidential election brought Franklin D. Roosevelt into office with a clear mandate to "do something." Roosevelt established a cabinet-level Committee on Economic Security (CES). The mandate of CES was to draft a proposal for a New Deal program in collaboration with Frances Perkins (a trained social worker with a master's degree in social work) appointed to serve as the Secretary of Labor (the first female member of a presidential cabinet). In 1935 the SSA was passed, which provided programs to address the unemployed, women, children, and the elderly within one single piece of legislation.

Initially, Social Security paid benefits in the form of a single, lump sum payment (1937–1940). These onetime payments were designed to give some payback to those people who contributed to the program but would not participate long enough to be vested for monthly benefits. Under the 1935 law, monthly benefits were to begin in 1942; however, the time span between 1937 and 1942 was designed to be a period of time to build up the trust funds and to provide a minimum period for participation in order to qualify for monthly benefits.

It should also be noted that a hallmark of the Social Security System in the United States is that it is known as a "pay as you go" system. In this model, funding to pay benefits comes from contributions from employers and employees, so that the funds available for retirees and other beneficiaries is directly related to the number of people that have been and are paying into the system. This model, unlike many retirement programs worldwide, does not invest a portion of the funds so that the revenue from these funds can be used to pay for benefits to future retirees.

The original Social Security legislation provided only retirement benefits, and only to the worker. In 1939, amendments made a fundamental change in the Social Security program. The amendments added two new categories of benefits: payments to the spouse and minor children of a retired worker (so-called dependents benefits) and survivors benefits paid to the family in the event of the premature death of a covered worker. This change transformed Social Security from a retirement program for workers into a *family-based* economic security program.

Amendments made to the Social Security program in 1954 initiated a disability insurance program that lent support to the public with additional coverage against economic insecurity. Although the disability program did not offer any cash benefits, it did prevent disability from reducing or wiping out one's retirement and survivor benefits. In 1956, the SSA was again amended, this time to provide benefits to disabled workers 50 to 64 years of age and disabled adult children of recipients, and to enable women to retire at 62 years of age with benefits actuarially reduced. Additional amendments to the Social Security program made under President Dwight D. Eisenhower in September 1960 changed the disability rules to permit payment of benefits to disabled workers regardless of their age as well as to their dependents.

On June 30, 1961, President John Kennedy signed amendments that permitted workers to elect a reduced retirement age, enabling men to retire at 62 with benefits actuarially reduced.

Medicare

The Medicare bill was signed on July 30, 1965, by President Lyndon B. Johnson. This bill provided health coverage to all Americans who were 65 years of age and older. Amendments to the original legislation enabled people with disabilities who had worked during

Table 5.1 Contents of the Social Security Act of 1935

Preamble: An act to provide for the general welfare by establishing a system of Federal old-age benefits, and by enabling the several states to make more adequate provision for aged persons, blind persons, dependent and crippled children, maternal and child welfare, public health, and the administration of their unemployment compensation laws; to establish a Social Security Board, to raise revenue; and for other purposes.

Title I: Grants to States for Old-Age Assistance
Title II: Federal Old-Age Benefits
Title III: Grants to States for Unemployment Compensation Administration
Title IV: Grants to States for Aid to Dependent Children
Title V: Grants to States for Maternal and Child Welfare
Title VI: Public Health Work
Title VII: Social Security Board
Title VIII: Taxes with Respect to Employment
Title IX: Tax on Employers of Eight or More
Title X: Grants to States for Aid to the Blind
Title XI: General Provisions

Source: Social Security Act of 1935 [H.R. 7260 ; Pub. L. No. 74–271, 49 Stat. 620]. Retrieved from https://www.ssa.gov/history/35act.html

their adult life as well as children with disabilities to be eligible for Medicare. Chapter 6 provides more information about Medicare and its administration.

Contents of the Original Social Security Act

The original SSA of 1935 comprised 11 titles, listed in Table 5.1. These titles reflect the thinking and philosophy at the time, when women, children, and those disabled by blindness were seen as the groups who should be cared for by the state.

It is also interesting to note that the original SSA was not exclusively designed to provide retirement or old-age benefits, but rather to provide for the public's health and the well-being of the vulnerable within the community, such as dependent children, mothers and children, the visually impaired, and the unemployed. It is noteworthy that in 1935, during the "Great Depression," these vulnerable groups were considered most at risk.

THE CURRENT SOCIAL SECURITY ACT

Over time, the original 11 titles of the SSA have expanded to now cover 21 titles; however, two have been repealed (Barusch, 2002). Within these titles, there is now a provision that includes special benefits for certain World War II veterans. SSA also includes block grants for social services and the state-based Children's Health Insurance Program (CHIP). Health insurance for the aged and disabled are also included through the Medicare program (which was enacted in 1965). Chapter 6 elaborates on the Medicare program. The titles of the current Social Security program are summarized in Table 5.2.

TABLE 5.2 Compiled Titles of the Social Security Act, 1935 to Present

Title I: Grants to states for Old-Age Assistance (Supplemental Security Income)
Title II: Old Age, Survivors and Disability Insurance Benefits
Title III: Grants to States for Unemployment Compensation
Title IV: Grants to States for Aid and Services to Needy Families with Children and for Child Welfare Services
Title V: Maternal and Child Health Services Block Grant
Title VII: Administration
Title VIII: Special Benefits for Certain WWII Veterans
Title IX: Miscellaneous Provisions Relating to Employment Security
Title X: Grants to States for Aid to the Blind—Supplemental Security Income
Title XI: General Provisions
Title XII: Advances to State Unemployment Funds
Title XIII: Reconversion Unemployment Benefits for Seamen
Title XIV: Supplemental Security Income (Grants to States for Aid to the Permanently and Totally Disabled)
Title XVI: Supplemental Security Income (Grants to States for the Aged, Blind, and Disabled)
Title XVII: Grants for Planning Comprehensive Action to Combat Mental Retardation
Title XVIII: Health Insurance for the Aged and Disabled
Title XIX: Grants to States for Medical Assistance Programs
Title XX: Block Grants to States for Social Services
Title XXI: State Children's Insurance Program

Note: Titles VI and XV have been repealed. Title XIIIi was repealed but the eligibility for seamen remained.

Source: Social Security Administration. (2018a). *Social Security Act table of contents*. Retrieved from http://www.ssa.gov/OP_Home/ssact/ssact-toc.htm.

Some Guidelines for Social Security Programs

The SSA and related laws establish a number of programs that have the following basic purposes:

- To provide for the material needs of individuals and families.
- To protect aged and disabled persons against the expenses of illnesses that may otherwise use up their savings.
- To keep families together.
- To give children the chance to grow up healthy and secure.

Although we tend to think that Social Security is specifically retirement benefits, a number of current social welfare programs designed for families, women, and children are also a part of this initiative.

The following programs are included within the Social Security program:

- Retirement insurance
- Survivors insurance
- Disability insurance

- Hospital and medical insurance for the aged, the disabled, and those with end-stage renal disease
- Prescription drug benefit
- Extra help with Medicare prescription drug costs
- Supplemental security income (SSI)
- Special veterans benefits
- Unemployment insurance
- Public assistance and welfare services, including:
  - Temporary assistance for needy families
  - Medical assistance
  - Maternal and child health services
  - Child support enforcement
  - Family and child welfare services
  - Food stamps
  - Energy assistance

Individuals are eligible for Social Security Benefits if they fall into the following categories:

- A disabled insured worker who has not reached full retirement age.
- A retired insured worker age 62 or over.
- The spouse of a retired or disabled worker entitled to benefits who:
  - Is age 62 or over
  - Has in care a child who is either under age 16, or over age 16 and disabled, who is entitled to benefits on the worker's Social Security record.
- The divorced spouse of a retired or disabled worker entitled to benefits if at least 62 and married to the worker for at least 10 years.
- The divorced spouse of a fully insured worker who:
  - Has not yet filed a claim for benefits if both the worker and his or her ex-spouse are at least 62 years of age.
  - Was married for at least 10 years.
  - Has been finally divorced for at least 2 years in a row.
- The dependent, who is an unmarried child of a wage earner who is retired, disabled, or a deceased insured worker is entitled to benefits if he or she is:
  - Under age 18.
  - Under age 19 and a full-time elementary or secondary school student.
  - Age 18 or older but under a disability which began before age 22.
- The surviving spouse (including a surviving divorced spouse) of a deceased insured worker age 60 or older.
- The disabled surviving spouse (including a surviving divorced spouse in some cases) of a deceased insured worker if they are age 50 to 59 and become disabled within the period specified.
- The surviving spouse (including a surviving divorced spouse) of a deceased insured worker, regardless of age, if caring for an entitled child of the deceased who is either under age 16 or was disabled before age 22.
- The dependent parents of a deceased insured worker age 62 or over.

Note: In addition to monthly survivors' benefits, a lump sum death payment is payable upon the death of an insured worker.

SSI is a federal program administered by SSA.

The SSI program was established to provide cash assistance to individuals who:

- Have limited income and resources
- Are age 65 or older
- Are blind
- Are disabled

Disabled and blind children are also included in the SSI program. Details on the eligibility and process of securing coverage are addressed in the next section.

> *Although Mary has been on Social Security for a few years, since she has just recently celebrated her 70th birthday, she has also had the Power of Attorney for her four older sisters. She has thus had the opportunity for many dealings with Social Security and its representatives. Mary initially had questions about when payments would begin and how one received Social Security Disability benefits, especially since two of her sisters became medically disabled in their early 50s. In the case of one sister, originally denied coverage, Mary questioned the decision and wanted to have the case reexamined. Mary also wanted to assist her second sister in returning to work, but she was fearful that doing so would result in benefits being discontinued or denied. Many of Mary's concerns and questions are captured in the next section of this chapter.*

Basic Information When One Is Receiving Social Security Disability Benefits

About Benefits

When do Payments Begin?

An individual's disability payments typically begin on the 6th month of the disability because of the law that does not allow disability payments to start being paid until the individual has been disabled for a minimum of five full months.

How Long do Payments Continue?

It is the responsibility for individuals receiving Social Security Disability Income (SSDI) to notify the Social Security Administration if there is any change in their ability to work, if they return to work, or if their medical condition improves.

What Happens If One Disagrees With a Decision Made by the Social Security Administration?

If there is any disagreement about a decision made by the SSA, the individual has the right to appeal the decision, and a request must be submitted in writing and delivered to any office of the SSA no later than 60 days after receiving the SSA's letter containing its decision. Additional steps can be taken if the individual is still not satisfied at this point. In addition, it is important to remember that all individuals have the right to hire an attorney, other representative, or anyone else to represent them. This does not indicate that an attorney or other representative must be hired on behalf of the individual seeking SSDI (SSA, 2018b).

When and How Are Benefits Are Paid?

Social Security benefits are paid to the beneficiaries each month. Typically, the day that the individual receives a benefit payment depends on the birthdate of the individual on whose work record benefits are received. The SSA has been attempting to discontinue all disability payments received through the mail by check every month, and instead, have the benefit payment deposited into a checking or savings account, or onto a prepaid debit card.

How do Electronic Payments Work?

If an individual applied for benefits after May 1, 2011, payments must be received electronically. Individuals were strongly advised to sign up for electronic payments by March 1, 2013 because if not, the United States Treasury Department may send the payments via the Direct Express card program to avoid an interruption in payment. The majority of individuals have three options to receive their benefits:

1. Individuals may choose to receive their benefits by direct deposit to their bank account and can accomplish this by contacting their bank or Social Security Office.
2. The Direct Express card program is the second option; it allows for deposits from federal payments to be made directly to the card account.
3. The third option is an "Electronic Transfer Account," which is known as a low-cost federally insured account; it allows individuals to enjoy the safety, security, and convenience of automatic payments.

What Happens If One Receives Checks by Mail and the Check Is Not Delivered

For those beneficiaries who are still eligible to receive their monthly check by mail, and it is not delivered on the due date, they should wait three workdays before reporting the missing check to the SSA. Not reporting a change of address is the most common reason that checks are late. These beneficiaries should contact the SSA immediately if their check is ever lost or stolen, and the check can be replaced. As a precaution, beneficiaries should cash or deposit their checks immediately after receiving them. A government check must be cashed within 12 months after the date of the check or it will be void.

How Does One Return Benefits not Due?

At times, electronic payments may be made when in fact these are not due to those receiving them, such as an executor for a deceased enrollee who is settling the affairs of the estate. If an individual receives a check from the Social Security Administration that is knowingly not due, the check can be returned to a Social Security office or to the United States Department of Treasury at the address provided on the check envelope. The individual should write VOID on the front of the check and enclose a note stating the reason for sending the check back. An individual who knowingly accepts payments from the Social Security office that is not due is at risk for facing criminal charges.

Who Must Pay Taxes on Benefits?

Some individuals who receive Social Security must pay taxes on their benefits. SSA reported that approximately 1/3 of the nation's current beneficiaries pay taxes on their benefits. The beneficiary is affected only if he or she is receiving Social Security benefits along with an income that is considered "substantial." If an individual files a federal tax return as an "individual" and has an income of more than $25,000, that individual will have to pay taxes on a portion of that income. If a couple files a joint return, taxes may have to be paid if the couple has a combined income that is more than $32,000 (these figures are current as of 2018). Married individuals who file a separate tax return will most likely have to pay taxes on their benefits.

How Does the SSA Contact a Recipient?

When the SSA needs to contact an individual, they will typically call the individual on the phone or through the postal service, however, in particular matters, a Social Security Representative may arrive at the individual's home. The SSA acknowledged that it is a good idea to call the Social Security office to determine whether a representative was sent to see the individual before letting the representative into the home.

What Special Accommodation Does SSA Offer Individuals Who Are Blind?

Individuals who are blind can chose to receive notices from the SSA in one of the following ways: standard print notice by first-class mail; standard print notice by certified mail; standard print notice by first-class mail and a follow-up telephone call; braille notice and a standard print notice by first-class mail; Microsoft Word file on a data compact disc (CD) and a standard print notice by first-class mail; audio CD and a standard print notice by first-class mail; or large print (18-point size) notice and a standard print notice by first-class mail.

What Are Cost-Of-Living Adjustments?

Each January, benefits increase automatically if the cost of living has gone up. For example, if the cost of living has increased by 2%, benefits also will increase by 2%. People who receive benefits are notified in advance by mail of the cost-of-living adjustment (COLA).

What Happens When One Reaches Full Retirement Age?

If an individual is receiving Social Security disability benefits and reaches full retirement age, the disability benefits will automatically convert to retirement benefits, and the amount received will remain unchanged. An individual who is receiving a reduced widow's benefit and reaches full retirement age is responsible for notifying Social Security when full retirement age is reached.

Other Benefits One May Be Eligible For

Supplemental Security Income

An individual with limited income and resources may be eligible to receive SSI. SSI is a federal program that provides monthly payments to people age 65 or older and to people who are blind or disabled. An individual who receives SSI may also be eligible for additional benefits such as Medicaid and Supplemental Nutrition Assistance Program (SNAP), formerly known as food stamps.

Medicare

After an individual has been receiving disability benefits for 24 months, he or she becomes eligible for Medicare on month 25. The individual will receive information about Medicare several months before coverage starts. An individual who is living with a permanent kidney failure requiring regular dialysis or a transplant or has amyotrophic lateral sclerosis (Lou Gehrig's disease) may qualify for Medicare almost immediately.

Help for Low-Income Medicare Beneficiaries

If an individual receives Medicare and has low income and few resources, the state may pay the Medicare premiums and, in some cases, other "out-of-pocket" medical expenses such as deductibles and coinsurance. This coverage is known as Medicaid, and because

Medicaid is a state program, only the state can decide whether an individual qualifies by a state's own rules on qualification. To find out, an individual must contact his or her state or local welfare office or Medicaid agency.

Supplemental Nutrition Assistance Program (Food Stamps)

One may be able to get help through the SNAP, formerly known as food stamps. This program, originally designed to provide supplemental nutritious food for individuals and their families (including people with disabilities and older adults), originally provided coupons for specific food items of nutritional value. Currently, the program is an electronic deposit into one's Food Stamp account, and a debit card is presented to a vendor to pay for items. The program, originally designed for retailer use, has been expanded to include Farmer's Market vendors in many states.

What Must Be Reported to SSA?

Whenever a change occurs that could affect an individual's benefits, it must be reported to the SSA immediately by phone, mail, or in person. Family members receiving benefits based on that person's work also should report events that might affect their payments. Information given to another government agency may be provided to Social Security by the other agency, but one also must report the change directly to the SSA.

The following circumstances must be reported to the SSA:

- One is working while receiving disability payments.
- One is receiving other disability benefits in addition to Social Security benefits.
- One is offered services under the Ticket to Work Program.
- One moves to a different location or changes direct deposit accounts.
- One is unable to manage his or her benefits.
- One is receiving a pension from work not covered by Social Security.
- One gets married or divorced.
- One changes his or her name.
- One cares for a child who receives benefits.
- One becomes a parent after entitlement.
- A child receiving benefits is adopted.
- An individual has an outstanding warrant for arrest.
- One is convicted of a crime or has violated a condition of parole or probation.
- One leaves the United States, or one's citizenship status changes.
- A beneficiary dies.
- One is receiving Social Security and Railroad Retirement benefits

Gerry was born with cerebral palsy and hydrocephalus, and was hospitalized for several months following his birth. His parents were encouraged to apply for Social Security Disability Insurance for him, as a child. At the outset, his parents had many questions, many of their questions were not easily addressed by family and friends. As Gerry was nearing his 18th birthday, new challenges for funding options came into play. His parents' concerns included many of the points addressed in the next section of this chapter.

SOCIAL SECURITY DISABILITY INSURANCE FOR CHILDREN

There are some important things to know about a child's benefits if an adult is receiving benefits on behalf of that child.

When a Child Reaches Age 18

A child's benefits stop with the month before the child reaches age 18 unless the child is disabled or is a full-time elementary or secondary school student and unmarried. About 3 months before the child's 18th birthday, he or she will get a letter explaining how benefits can continue. The SSA will send the child a student form along with the letter. If the child's benefits stopped at age 18, they can start again if he or she becomes disabled before reaching age 22 or becomes a full-time elementary or secondary school student before reaching age 19. The student must contact the SSA to reapply for benefits.

If an 18-Year-Old Child Is Still in School

A child can receive benefits until age 19 if he or she continues to be a full-time elementary or secondary school student. When the child's 19th birthday occurs during a school term, benefits usually can continue until completion of the term, or for 2 months following the 19th birthday, whichever comes first. The parent of the child receiving benefits should tell the SSA immediately if the child marries, is convicted of a crime, drops out of school, changes from full-time to part-time attendance, is expelled or suspended, or changes schools. The parent must notify the SSA if the child has an employer who is paying for the child to attend school. In general, a student can keep receiving benefits during a vacation period of 4 months or less if he or she plans to go back to school full time at the end of the vacation.

If a Child Is Disabled

A child can continue to receive benefits after age 18 if he or she has a disability that begins before age 22. The child also may qualify for SSI disability benefits.

If One Has a Stepchild and Gets Divorced

If an individual has a stepchild who is receiving benefits based on the stepparent's work and the stepparent divorces the child's parent, the SSA must be informed as soon as the divorce becomes final. The stepchild's benefit will stop the month after the divorce becomes final.

Reviewing One's Medical Condition

All people receiving disability benefits must have their medical conditions reviewed from time to time. An individual's benefits will continue unless there is strong proof that the condition has improved medically and that the individual is able to return to work.

Frequency of Reviews

How often an individual's medical condition is reviewed depends on how severe it is and the likelihood it will improve. The award notice tells the individual when to expect the first review.

Medical improvement expected—If the condition is expected to improve within a specific time, the first review will be 6 to 18 months after the start of disability benefits.

Improvement possible—If improvement in the medical condition is possible, the case will be reviewed about every 3 years.

Improvement not expected—If the medical condition is unlikely to improve, the case will be reviewed only about once every 5 to 7 years.

What Happens During a Review?

To start the review process, the Social Security office will send a letter stating that it is conducting a review. Soon after that, someone from the local Social Security office will contact the individual to explain the review process and appeal rights. The Social Security representative will ask the individual to provide information about his or her medical treatment and any work that he or she may have done. A team consisting of a disability examiner and a doctor will review the file and request personal medical reports. The individual may be asked to have a special examination. SSA will pay for the examination and some of the transportation costs.

When a decision is made, SSA will send a letter to the individual. If a decision is made that the individual is still disabled, the benefits will continue. An individual who disagrees with a decision that he or she is no longer disabled can file an appeal. If the individual decides not to appeal the decision, benefits will terminate 3 months after the SSA decides that the individual's disability has ended.

Helping One Return to Work

An individual who begins receiving disability benefits may want to try working again. There are special rules called "work incentives" that can help individuals keep their cash benefits and Medicare while they test their ability to work.

Protection of One's Personal Information

Social Security keeps personal and confidential information for millions of individuals including, names, Social Security numbers, earnings records, ages, and beneficiary addresses. Generally, the SSA will discuss personal information only with the individual. The Social Security office asks several questions to assist in verifying a caller or visitor's identity before discussing personal information.

Erica and Theresa have been working on building training and information sessions related to older adults and people with disabilities. They have noted the information in the previous sections of this text about demographic changes within the nation and wondered what impact this may have on reforms to the Social Security System. As they dug deeper into these issues and met with researchers, they were able to better understand some of the political perspective on the Social Security program and programs and political will which has had an interest in the overall benefit program.

SOME REFORMS WORTH NOTING

The notion of revising or reforming the Social Security system is definitely not a new concern or issue and has been a subject of discussion in several administrations since the inception of the program. In 1981, President Ronald Reagan appointed the National Commission on Social Security Reform, headed by Alan Greenspan, who Regan would later appoint as chair of the Federal Reserve Bank in the United States. The four areas of recommendations included:

1. Revisions in the cost of living adjustment.
2. Taxation of benefits.
3. Increased retirement ages.
4. Work incentives.

Table 5.3 Retirement Ages at Which One Can Collect Social Security Benefits

Year of Birth	Full Retirement Age	Number of months of reduction
1937 or earlier	65 years	36
1938	65 years and 2 months	38
1939	65 years and 4 months	40
1940	65 years and 6 months	42
1941	65 years and 8months	44
1942	65 years and 10 months	46
1943–1954	66 years	48
1955	66 years and 2 months	50
1956	66 years and 4 months	52
1957	66 years and 6 months	54
1958	66 years and 8 months	56
1959	66 years and 10 months	58
1960 and later	67 years of age	60

The end result has included revisions particularly in increased retirement ages. Although many of the recommendations that Greenspan identified did not take place during the Reagan administration, some of these revisions did come to pass, and particularly full retirement ages have increased and continue to increase to age 67, based upon one's year of birth (Ball, 1996). One may begin to collect retirement benefits at age 62; however, there will be a reduction in benefits, depending upon one's year of birth. Table 5.3 provides a listing of eligible retirement year according to one's birth year (USDHHS, 2018). See Table 5.3.

PROPOSALS FOR REVISION AND WHY

During President Bill Clinton's administration, an effort was made to privatize Old Age Survivors and Disability Insurance (OASDI). President Clinton had appointed Jose Obera (the former labor minister of Chile) to head up a task force through the Social Security Advisory Council. President Clinton's Social Security Advisory Council developed three proposals, based upon a successful model used in Chile to privatize Social Security benefits. The three proposals included:

1. Maintenance of benefits plan.
2. Individual accounts.
3. Personal savings accounts (PSAs).

These three proposals, although different, all had similarities, and most importantly, they were all in support of maintaining a mandatory, universal, public social insurance program, and within this program retirement, survivor, and disability benefits were paramount (Quinn & Mitchell, 1996). None of the proposals called for a revision of the Social Security system into a welfare-oriented system that would be means tested.

The Maintenance of Benefits Plan proposed to raise the revenues to preserve the system's solvency. A proportion of this increase could be accomplished through an investment of up to 40% of the trust fund reserves within private capital markets. This plan would also result in a 2% increase in payroll taxes, which would begin in 2050.

The Individual Accounts proposal would end up reducing benefits paid by states or the current Social Security program and increasing the establishment of individual contribution accounts that would ultimately be funded through increasing payroll taxes. Individual participants would have some discretion (not completely) in how their accounts were invested.

The PSAs would completely replace the Social Security System, into a two-tier system. This was the most radical of all the proposals. The first tier would provide a low flat rate of benefits for people with at least 10 years of contributed benefits, regardless of their earning history. Individuals with 35 years of contributions would have their benefits prorated. At a maximum, this approach could provide benefits to about two-thirds of the poverty levels for older adults. The second tier would provide for a mandatory PSA, which would be directed and held by the individual. After age 62, these accounts could be withdrawn as lump sum payments.

One must also consider why these proposals came to the forefront and what hidden agendas were at play in this process as a 16-member bipartisan Commission on Social Security was appointed in 2001. Its task was to modernize and ensure financial soundness to Social Security. The end result of this commission has been a task force report offering three possible scenarios that are fairly similar for how the long-range financing for Social Security should be addressed. Bear in mind that these ideas had been initiated under a Republican administration and have continued to be on the radar of succeeding Republican administrations. In recent years (2013), Senator Rand Paul used privatization of Social Security as one of his campaign priorities.

According to Veghte and Schreur (2016), the concept of modernizing the Social Security system has not made much progress, although the issues and concern are still active. Their 2016 Trustees Report updates projections about the future finances of Social Security's two trust funds, the Old-Age and Survivors (OASI) Trust Fund and the Disability Insurance (DI) Trust Fund.

Of the 6.2% of earnings that workers and employers each pay into Social Security, 5.015% goes into the OASI trust fund and 1.185% goes into the DI trust fund. The Bipartisan Budget Act of 2015 set these rates effective for the period January 1, 2016 through December 31, 2018. After 2018, the allocation of Social Security payroll contributions reverts to what it had been since 2000: 0.9% to the DI trust fund, and the remaining 5.3% to OASI. The DI fund is projected to cover scheduled benefits until 2023, and the OASI fund until 2035. On a combined OASDI basis, Social Security is fully funded until 2034, but faces a projected shortfall thereafter.

In 2015, Social Security income from payroll contributions, tax revenues, and interest on reserves exceeded outgo by $23 billion, leaving a surplus. Reserves, now at $2.8 trillion, are projected to grow to $2.9 trillion by the end of 2019. If Congress takes no action before then, reserves would be drawn down to pay benefits.

Implications of a Privatized System

Several implications accompany a privatized Social Security system and leave this proposal in great debate. One of these implications includes the loss of bond treasury.

Funds are used to invest in the bond treasury and thus are paid out in benefits. As a result of the inability for many working-class people to save and/or invest for their older age, we can predict that there would be an upsurge of the elderly poor (two-thirds of our older adult population), which is dramatic, especially in a country that is known to be one of the most affluent in the world.

A second implication of a privatized system is an increase in stock market investments. While this could prove to be an advantage and lucrative, it may benefit only about 10% of the population. Hence, the remaining 90% may be left to struggle on their own. Another consideration is that while investments may benefit a narrow segment of the population, one cannot guarantee how long this benefit may last. There could be disaster if there were a crash in the stock market such as occurred in 1929. It is also interesting to note in testimony presented by Alan Greenspan, the former chair of the Federal Reserve Board, in 1999. His testimony argued that it would be impossible to keep politics out of the stock market if major public funds were invested there by the Social Security system.

The most important implication of major revisions to the program would be the loss of a safety net program that benefits millions of older adults within the United States. The outcome and implication of this initiative could potentially leave huge pockets of people in poverty. This may also have some serious impacts for a nation that has people growing older and living longer as well as for those living in rural communities.

DILEMMAS FOR THE FUTURE

A number of issues discussed within this chapter also lead to dilemmas for the future. Specifically, poverty and the threat of a dismantled Social Security system are two major factors that would lead to some profound impacts on the safety net system that was originally envisioned for older adults. A central question asks how these specific issues affect our current Social Security system as well as its future.

A Culture of Impoverished Older Adults

The dilemma of a potential culture with impoverished older adults could become a reality if corporate pension plans continue to erode, and are replaced with private 401(k) accounts. This so-called erosion could potentially place more pressure on the current Social Security system and lead to more older adults with fewer resources and thus a subculture of poverty. These factors, coupled with smaller families and more fragmented families and social networks, could potentially lead to more people who, in their old age, could become impoverished. The Government Accountability Office has studied this issue, with projections for 2030 and 2050, only to raise alarming concerns about a growing culture of poverty.

Older Women and Poverty

Women who survive to age 65 can plan to outlive men of the same age by at least 7 years. They face far more challenges today and will continue to face challenges into the future. One of the most important of these challenges is that of poverty. A significant proportion of women who reach retirement age today may not have worked at their capacity during their lifetime and may not have accumulated a comfortable pension, resulting in women living at or far beneath the poverty level during their retirement years. Three additional factors that lead to older women living in poverty include the reality of women outliving their male counterparts, earning less than their male counterparts, and the changing family structure. Far more frequently, women have lost secure marriages because of divorce or death and have become victims of a limited safety net. Pension splitting, as a result of divorce, often does not provide ample funds for a divorced spouse to live comfortably, or even to live substantially above the poverty level. Thus, a dilemma for the future is the significant increase in the number of women living in poverty.

An Empty Pot at the End of the Rainbow

A dilemma for the future is the reality that the "pot," or resources available to retirees through the Social Security Fund, may not exist. Thus, the "pot" that people looked toward as income to support them in retirement may no longer exist or may be either depleted and empty or close to empty by the time an individual reaches his or her retirement. Depending upon the types of reforms that are instituted, current reports (Social Security Trustee Report, 2016) suggest that without revision, by the 100th anniversary of the SSA of 1935, funds may not be available to fully fund retirees.

SUMMARY

This chapter has presented the current Social Security system, which provides for older adults, but has also grown to cover dependent women and children. The historical background behind the program and its evolution have also been discussed. Although many people have argued for their vision to privatize the system, the reality is that there is much more political support to maintain the program as a safety net program rather than a means-tested program and a desire to maintain this universal retirement program.

DISCUSSION QUESTIONS

1. The SSA responds to needs other than retirement income and income for people with disabilities. Why do you think this has happened? What implementation strategy (see Chapter 3) has had an impact here and why?
2. The retirement age continues to increase depending upon the age of the worker. Is this a positive or negative strategy and why?
3. What proposals or strategies do you think are going to be useful to help keep Social Security solvent in the future?

ADDITIONAL RESOURCES

Websites

The official web site of Social Security: www.ssa.gov

This Website provides a comprehensive array of materials to address every possible question regarding Social Security and Disability benefits. This official governmental website provides the reader with background information on the Social Security and Disability programs, as well as current publications.

AARP's website related to Social Security: www.aarp.org/work/social-security

This website provides an overview of how Social Security works and some of the current issues that the Social Security program faces. Debates about privatization of the Social Security program are also discussed on this website.

National Committee to Preserve Social Security and Medicare: www.ncpssm.org

This website provides the reader with the opportunity to participate as a consumer in the preservation of the Social Security movement. It serves as a portal to a number of essays that address strategies to preserve the Social Security program and Social Security trust funds.

The Urban Institute Tool Kit on Social Security: apps.urban.org/features/social-security-data-tool

This website provides a wide array of materials that address issues for and against the Social Security program. A variety of educational materials are also available.

YouTube Resources Related to Social Security

Social Security and What is new for 2018: www.youtube.com/watch?v=2ClhXq4TeNc

This YouTube video provides an overview of Social Security benefits and what is new for 2018 as well as benefits to the program.

Social Security and Supplemental Disability Income: www.youtube.com/watch?v=ncTu2jmBfeM

This YouTube video provides the viewer with information about Social Security Disability benefits.

REFERENCES

Ball, R. M. (1996). Medicare's roots: What Medicare's architects had in mind. *Generations*, *20*(2), 13–18.

Barusch, A. S. (2002). *Foundations of social policy: Social justice, public programs, and the social work profession.* Itasca, IL: Peacock.

Mann, G. (1970). *The history of Germany since 1789.* New York, NY: Praeger.

Quinn, J. F., & Mitchell, O. S. (1996). Social security on the table. *American Prospect*, *26*, 6–81.

Social Security Act of 1935 [H.R. 7260]. Retrieved from https://www.ssa.gov/history/35act.html

Social Security Administration. (2018a). *Social Security Act table of contents.* Retrieved from http://www.ssa.gov/OP_Home/ssact/ssact-toc.htm

Social Security Administration. (2018b). *What you need to know when you get Social Security Disability Benefits.* Retrieved from http://www.ssa.gov/pubs/EN-05-10153.pdf

United States Department of Health and Human Services. (2018). *Retirement planner: Social Security online.* Retrieved from http://www.ssa.gov/retirechartred.htm

Veghte, B., & Schreur, E. (2016, June). *Social security finances: Findings of the 2016 trustees report* (Social Security Brief No. 46). National Academy of Social Insurance. Retrieved from https://www.nasi.org

6

Medicare

LEARNING OBJECTIVES

At the end of this chapter, readers will:

1. *Understand the history of the Medicare in the United States.*
2. *Understand specific components of Medicare Parts A, B, C, and D.*
3. *Understand how Medicare provides healthcare resources to older adults and people with disabilities.*

Now that Erica and Theresa have reviewed income through Social Security, they realized they had not addressed another component of the Social Security Act which addressed healthcare needs through Medicare. Both women decided that it would be helpful initially to identify programs and services through Medicare and then review these through the lens of service utilization based upon real case approaches. Their pair decided to examine this approach through cases from both an urban and rural perspective and through cases, which represent both aging and disability perspectives. The cases they decided to view Medicare policy through included the following.

INTRODUCTION

In a country as prosperous as the United States, one would expect all people to be healthy and prosperous. The inception of Medicare in 1965 gave many people the illusion that there would be a "pot" at the end of the rainbow to take care of their healthcare concerns once they reached the magic age of 64 and were ready to move into their retirement or if they became disabled before reaching that age. In 2016, 93% of people 65 years of age and older were covered by Medicare for their health insurance. While the Medicare managed care programs have expanded the healthcare market, there are still many people without healthcare insurance who are struggling for coverage.

Despite these limitations, Medicare serves as a guaranteed source of insurance coverage; hence contributing to billable services in situations where research and development with older adults or people with disabilities will take place (Ball, 1996). The Centers for Medicare and Medicaid Services (CMS) administer Medicare, the nation's largest health insurance program, which covers nearly 60 million Americans (Alliance for Retired Americans, 2018). Medicare is a health insurance program for people 65 years of age

 DOI:10.1891/9780826128393.0006

and older, some disabled people under 65 years of age, and people with end-stage renal disease (ESRD; permanent kidney failure treated with dialysis or a transplant). Recipients included 49.3 million people 65 years of age and older and 9.1 million people with disabilities (Alliance for Retired Americans, 2018).

HISTORICAL PERSPECTIVE

Congress enacted Medicare and Medicaid in 1965 as Titles XVIII and XIX of the Social Security Act. Medicare is a social insurance program available to all citizens of the United States if they have worked and contributed into the program. While this is not a means-tested program, and all who have contributed can benefit, an additional benefit is available known as Medicaid, which is a means-tested public assistance program. Although Medicare (conceived originally as universal healthcare by President Franklin Delano Roosevelt) had been conceptualized along with Social Security in 1935, it was dropped from the original proposal in 1935 because of fear that the healthcare program would not receive bipartisan support (DiNitto & Johnson, 2016). Thus, it took an additional 30 years for this program to reach approval into a public law.

Robert Ball, the architect for the program, argued that Medicare was the first step toward a universal healthcare coverage program (Ball, 1996). Ball, who had served as commissioner of Social Security under Presidents Kennedy, Johnson, and Nixon, also suggested that when the initial thoughts of a universal healthcare program came into play in 1916, the American Medical Association was in support of the plan. In actual fact, a prior version of the Medicare program had been developed in the 1930s, along with the Social Security Act, with the intention of serving as universal healthcare coverage. This began with a Committee on Economic Security created by President Roosevelt (June 1934), which subsequently filed a report regarding the feasibility of a Social Security and health insurance program. This Report of the Committee on Economic Security was sent to Congress (January 1935) without any health insurance recommendations but spelling out principles and promising further efforts to evolve a plan.

The first government health insurance bill introduced in Congress, the "Epstein bill" (S. 3253) drafted by Abraham Epstein (lobbyist and founder of the American Association for Social Security) and sponsored by Senator Arthur Capper of Kansas, was introduced in July 1935. The goal of this bill was to provide healthcare coverage along with Social Security to provide economic and medical safety nets for Americans. Although it was struck down, President Franklin D. Roosevelt continued his campaign to develop a healthcare coverage plan, appointed a National Health Survey to be conducted, and in 1938, a *Report of the Technical Committee on Medical Care, A National Health Program*, was published. As a direct result of this survey, in 1939 Senator Robert F. Wagner of New York introduced a "National Health Bill" (S. 1620) incorporating recommendations of the National Health Conference. This was struck down and died in committee. However, after several attempts to introduce versions of a universal health coverage plan for older adults and the poor by Presidents Truman, Eisenhower, and Kennedy, a version of a healthcare coverage program known as Medicare was developed, debated, and eventually signed into legislation, by President Johnson in 1965.

Unfortunately, business groups, especially those associated with the insurance industry, opposed a universal healthcare program; thus, Medicare was a compromise with bipartisan support. Leaders of the labor movement sought to develop Medicare coverage as early as 1957; however, this legislation was not successfully passed until Johnson's expansion of the Great Society programs, in the mid-1960s. Thus, the labor movement used a window of opportunity to see these programs come to passage.

Medicare, in 1965, initially did not include coverage for people with disabilities. This target group was given Medicare coverage as a result of the 1972 Social Security amendments, which added coverage for the disabled and people with ESRD. The amendments also included a venue for quality control through the Professional Standards Review Organizations (PSRO). This oversight, however, was replaced with Peer Review Organizations (PRO) through the 1982 Social Security amendments. These amendments also included benefit expansion that added coverage for hospice care to Medicare enrollees.

The freedom of choice waivers and home- and community-based care waivers were established for Medicaid through 1981 legislative amendments. In 1987, the Omnibus Budget Reconciliation Act (OBRA) strengthened the protection for residents of nursing homes.

In 2003, the Medicare Prescription Drug Improvement and Modernization Act (MMA) probably impacted the Medicare program the most since its inception in 1965. MMA created a drug prescription card, valid until 2006, which then rolled over into a new voluntary program known as Medicare Part D. This outpatient prescription drug program makes prescription drugs available to beneficiaries from private drug plans, as well as Medicare Advantage plans (CMS, n.d.; DiNitto & Johnson, 2016).

HOW DOES MEDICARE WORK?

Currently four components of Medicare insurance are available—specifically Part A, Part B, Part C, and Part D. In a nutshell, each of these programs offers specific coverage.

Medicare Part A (Hospital Insurance) helps cover the following:

- Home healthcare
- Inpatient care in hospitals
- Hospice care
- Skilled nursing facility care (SNFC)

Medicare Part B (Medical/Physician Insurance) helps cover the following:

- Durable medical equipment
- Home healthcare
- Outpatient care
- Services from doctors and other healthcare providers
- Some preventative services

Medicare Part C (Medicare Advantage) has the following features:

- It includes all benefits and services covered under Part A and Part B.
- It is run by Medicare-approved private insurance companies.
- Advantage plans are offered with and without prescription drug coverage.
- It may include extra benefits (such as coverage for hearing, vision, and dental) and services for an additional cost such as ambulance coverage and preventative screening services.

Medicare Part D

- It is run by Medicare-approved private insurance companies.
- It helps cover the cost of prescription drugs.
- It may help lower prescription drug costs and help protect against higher costs in the future.

Hospital Insurance (Part A)

Medicare Part A is a hospital insurance, which is funded through mandatory contributions through employment and payroll taxes (1.45% each or 2.9% if self-employed). These funds are held in the Hospital Insurance Trust Fund. Some of the specific services and provisions that are covered through Medicare Part A include care in hospitals as an inpatient, critical access hospitals (small facilities that give limited outpatient and inpatient services to people in rural areas), skilled nursing facilities, hospice care, and some home healthcare. Services covered under Medicare Part A are those considered "medically necessary."

More specifically, some of the medically necessary services fall under the categories of blood, home health services, hospice care, hospital stays, and SNFC. Blood that one receives through a hospital or skilled nursing facility during a covered stay, although perceived as a minute detail, is one item covered under Medicare Part A. Enrollees pay all costs for the first three pints of blood received as an inpatient, then 20% of the Medicare-approved amount for the additional pints of blood.

A second area covered under medically necessary services is home health services. These services must be ordered by one's physician and be provided for by a Medicare-certified home health agency. Home health services are limited to intermittent skilled nursing care and home health aide services, physical therapy, occupational therapy (OT), and speech-language pathology. Medically necessary services also include medical social services; other services; durable medical equipment such as wheelchairs, hospital beds, oxygen, walkers, and medical supplies that can be used in one's home. Under Medicare coverage, individuals pay nothing for home healthcare services and 20% of the Medicare-approved amount for durable medical equipment.

A third area of services under Medicare Part A includes hospital stays. Medicare enrollees are eligible for semiprivate rooms, meals, general nursing care, and other hospital services and supplies. Inpatient care that one receives through critical access hospitals and mental healthcare are also covered. Private rooms are not considered an eligible hospital stay unless such a stay is considered medically necessary. Other areas within this category of hospital stays that are not included as Medicare benefits are private-duty nursing services and a television or telephone in one's room. Inpatient mental healthcare within psychiatric hospitals is limited to 190 days within one's lifetime. As of 2018 one pays $952 for the first 60 days of each benefit period. Following this first 60-day period, individuals are levied at least $335 per day for days 61 to 90 of the benefit period (note: $335.00 is a 2018 rate). From days 91 to 150, individuals pay $670 per day for care. Individuals also may take advantage of "lifetime reserve days" or 60 extra days of coverage that can be used during their lifetime. As of 2016, one pays $476 per day during the 60 days of coverage. Beyond these lifetime reserve days, all costs for each day of care beyond the 150 days are the responsibility of the individual.

A fourth area of services covered under Medicare Part A is SNFC. Although Medicare does not cover long-term care, one can take advantage of 100 days in a benefit period of SNFC. SNFC includes a semiprivate room, meals, skilled nursing and rehabilitative services, and other services and supplies. This period of 100 days per benefit period kicks in after a 3-day inpatient hospital stay for a related illness or injury. The costs of SNFC as of 2018 is nothing for the first 20 days of each benefit period, then $167.50 per day for days 21 to 100 of each benefit period, and then 100% for each day after day 100 in the benefit period.

One additional area covered within Medicare Part A is hospice care. Hospice care is available to individuals receiving Medicare if in fact they are deemed to have only 6 months or less to live. Services one can utilize include drugs for symptom control and pain relief, medical and support services from a Medicare-approved hospice, and other services not otherwise covered by Medicare, such as grief counseling. Hospice care is generally provided within one's home or in a nursing facility if that is considered one's home. Hospice also covers short-term hospital and inpatient respite care, which generally takes the form of care that is given to a hospice patient so that the usual caregiver can rest. Under hospice care benefits, an individual pays a copayment of up to $5.00 for outpatient prescription drugs and 5% of the Medicare-approved amounts for inpatient respite care (short-term care given by another caregiver so that the usual caregiver can rest). If a drug is not covered by the hospice benefit, it may be covered under Medicare Part D.

Medical Insurance (Part B)

Medicare Part B is an optional voluntary supplemental insurance that subscribers may opt into for coverage. This component of Medicare insurance can help pay for medical services such as physicians' services, outpatient care, and additional medical services that are not covered under Part A. Part B can be helpful in paying for items considered medically necessary, but not covered under part A, and it also covers preventative services. "Medically necessary" has been defined for the purposes of Medicare as "an item or service that is needed for the diagnosis or treatment of one's medical condition." It should be noted, however, that not all preventative services are covered under Medicare Part B. Services that are available and covered under Medicare Part B are listed and described in Table 6.1 include abdominal aortic aneurysm screening; alcohol misuse screening and counseling; ambulance services; ambulatory surgical centers; blood; bone mass measurement (bone density); breast cancer screening (mammograms); cardiac rehabilitation; cardiovascular disease (behavioral therapy); cardiovascular disease screening; cervical and vaginal cancer screening; chemotherapy; chiropractic services (limited coverage); clinical research studies; colorectal cancer screenings; concierge care; continuous positive airway pressure (CPAP) therapy; defibrillator (implantable automatic); depression screening; diabetes screenings; diabetes self-management training; diabetes supplies; doctor and other healthcare provider services; durable medical equipment (like walkers); durable medical equipment, prosthetics, orthotics, and supplies (DMEPOS) Competitive Bidding Program; EKG or ECG screening; ED services; eyeglasses (limited); Federally Qualified Health Center (FQHC) services; flu shots; foot exams and treatment; glaucoma tests; hearing and balance exams; travel services (healthcare required when traveling outside the United States in Canada); and urgently needed care.

Table 6.1 Services Covered Under Medicare Part B

Service	Overview of What Is Covered
Abdominal aortic aneurysm screening	Covers a onetime abdominal aortic aneurysm ultrasound. Must be referred by doctor. Eligible if family history of abdominal aortic aneurysms or one is a man age 65 to 75 and smoked at least 100 cigarettes in a lifetime.
Alcohol misuse screening and counseling	Adults with Part B including pregnant women who use alcohol, but do not meet medical criteria for alcohol dependency can get the screening. Offers four brief face-to-face counseling sessions per year.

(continued)

Table 6.1 Services Covered Under Medicare Part B (*continued*)

Service	Overview of What Is Covered
Ambulance services	Transportation to a hospital or skilled nursing facility, when transportation by any other means would be considered a danger to one's health.
Ambulatory surgery	Facility fees covered for approved services.
Blood	Pints of blood received during outpatient services for Part B-covered services.
Bone mass measurement	Covered once every 24 months for patients at risk for bone fractures. Certain medical conditions may qualify for assessments more frequently than once every 24 months.
Cardiovascular screenings	Cholesterol, lipid, and triglyceride levels tested once every 5 years for prevention of stroke or heart attack.
Cardiovascular disease (behavioral therapy)	Covered once every 12 months. Helps lower the risk for cardiovascular disease. During the visit, the doctor may discuss aspirin use (if appropriate), check blood pressure, and give tips to ensure healthful eating.
Cervical and vaginal cancer screenings	Covers Pap tests and pelvic exams to check for cervical and vaginal cancer. Covers a clinical breast exam to check for breast cancer. Once every 24 months for all women, or every 12 months for individuals at high risk for breast cancer.
Chiropractic services	Limited services for manipulation of the spine to correct for subluxation (one or more of the bones out of position within the spine).
Clinical laboratory services	Blood tests, urinalysis, and some screening tests.
Clinical trials	Routine costs associated with qualifying clinical trials to test new regimens of medical care. Costs for the drugs or devices being tested within the clinical trial may not be covered.
Colorectal cancer screenings	1. Fecal occult blood tests: Once every 12 months if 50 years of age or older. Although one does not pay for the test, a fee for the doctor's visit may be levied. 2. Flexible sigmoidoscopy: Once every 48 months if 50 years of age or older, or once every 120 months when used instead of a colonoscopy for those not at high risk.

(*continued*)

Table 6.1 Services Covered Under Medicare Part B (*continued*)

Service	Overview of What Is Covered
	3. Screening colonoscopy: Once every 120 months, or 48 hours after a previous flexible sigmoidoscopy (high risk every 24 months). No minimum age. 4. Barium enema: Once every 48 months if age 50 or older (high risk every 24 months) when used instead of a sigmoidoscopy or colonoscopy.
Depression screenings	Covers one depression screening per year. Must be done in a primary care setting that can provide follow-up treatment if needed.
Diabetes screenings	Screenings up to two times per year based upon specific eligibility criteria including hypertension, dyslipidemia (history of abnormal cholesterol and triglyceride levels), obesity, or a history of high blood sugar. Also covers if two or more apply: age 65 or older, overweight, family history of diabetes, history of gestational diabetes, or delivery of a baby weighing more than 9 pounds.
DSMT	Provided for people with diabetes with a written physician order. In a rural area, one may be eligible to get DSMT services from a practitioner, like a registered dietician, in a different location through telehealth.
Diabetic supplies	Supplies to include glucose testing monitors, blood glucose test strips, lancet devices and lancets, glucose control solutions, and in some cases, therapeutic shoes. Syringes and insulin are covered if used with an insulin pump or if one has Medicare prescription drug coverage.
Durable medical equipment	Oxygen, wheelchairs, walkers, and hospital beds needed for use in one's home.
Emergency room services	Coverage for visits when one's health is in serious danger, following a bad injury, sudden illness, or an illness that quickly causes physical deterioration.
Eyeglasses	Limited coverage for eyeglasses is available for one pair of eyeglasses with standard frames following cataract surgery that implants an intraocular lens.
Flu shots	Once per flu season.
Foot exams and treatment	For individuals with diabetes-related nerve damage.

(*continued*)

Table 6.1 Services Covered Under Medicare Part B (*continued*)

Service	Overview of What Is Covered
Glaucoma tests	Tests to detect eye disease glaucoma, once per 12-month period for people with high risk for glaucoma (i.e., with a preexisting condition of diabetes or family history of glaucoma, are African American and 50 or older, or are Hispanic American and 65 or older, or specific risk factors).
Hearing and balance exams	Coverage is based upon physicians' requests to determine if medical treatment is required for condition. Exams for the purpose of fitting hearing aids are not covered.
Hepatitis C screening test	Covers one Hepatitis C screening test, and yearly repeat screening for certain people at high risk. People must have one of the following conditions: a past or current history of illicit injection drug use, a blood transfusion before 1992, or being born between 1945 and 1965.
HIV screening	Covered up to three times during pregnancy. Covered every 12 months for the following individuals: younger than 15 and older than 65, and are at increased risk for the virus. Individuals between 15 and 65, and ask for the test, and are pregnant.
Home health services	Limited to reasonable and necessary services to include part-time or intermittent skilled nursing care, home health aide services, physical therapy, OT, and speech-language pathology ordered by a physician. These services must also be provided for through a Medicare-certified home health agency. Medical supplies for use within the home are also covered and include medical social services and durable medical equipment to include wheelchairs, hospital beds, oxygen, and walkers.
Kidney dialysis services	Covered within a facility setting or at home.
Kidney dialysis supplies	Covered within a facility setting or at home.
Lung cancer screenings	Covers a lung cancer screening with LDCT once per year. People with Part B are eligible if they are 55 to 77, asymptomatic, either a current smoker or have quit smoking in the past 15 years, have a tobacco smoking history of one pack per day for 30 years, and must get written order from physician or qualified practitioner.
Mammograms (screening)	For women 40 years of age or older, preventative (screening) mammograms are covered once every 12 months. Women with Part B between 35 and 39 can get one baseline mammogram.

(*continued*)

Table 6.1 Services Covered Under Medicare Part B (*continued*)

Service	Overview of What Is Covered
Medical nutrition therapy	Individuals with diabetes or renal disease (prior to dialysis services or transplant), or for people up to 3 years post-kidney transplant with a doctor's order. Includes an initial nutrition and lifestyle assessment, one-on-one nutritional counseling, and follow-up visits to monitor progress in managing your individual diet. Mental healthcare (outpatient). Some limits and conditions will apply.
Mental healthcare (inpatient)	Covered by Medicare Part A (hospital insurance). Covers mental health services in a hospital. Services available either in a general hospital or a psychiatric hospital; if placed in a psychiatric hospital, Part A pays for up to 190 days during a lifetime.
Mental healthcare (outpatient)	Covered by Medicare Part B which covers mental health services and visits with a psychiatrist or other doctor, clinical psychologist, clinical social worker, clinical nurse specialist, nurse practitioner, and physician assistant. Covers mental health services that are usually provided outside hospital and services received in a hospital's outpatient department; covers outpatient services for the treatment of inappropriate drug and alcohol use.
Mental healthcare (partial hospitalization)	Covered by Part B, and individuals are provided a structured program of outpatient psychiatric services as an alternative to inpatient psychiatric care. The program is more intense than care received in a doctor's or therapist's office.
Obesity screening and counseling	Covers behavioral counseling to help lose weight. Eligible if you have Part B and have a BMI of 30 or more.
OT	OT services to facilitate one's ability to resume activities of daily living following an illness episode.
Outpatient hospital services	Services provided as an outpatient, as part of a doctor's care.
Outpatient medical and surgical services and supplies	Based upon approved procedures.

(*continued*)

Table 6.1 Services Covered Under Medicare Part B (*continued*)

Service	Overview of What Is Covered
Pap test and pelvic exams	Women considered low risk are covered once every 24 months, while women considered high risk for cervical and vaginal cancer, and those past childbearing age who have had an exam that indicated cancer or other abnormalities in the past 3 years are covered once every 12 months.
Physical therapy	Treatment for injuries and disease through heat, light, exercise, and massage.
Pneumococcal shots	To aid in the prevention of pneumococcal infection. Currently shots last one's lifetime.
Practitioner services	Services provided for by clinical social workers, physician assistants, and nurse practitioners.
Prescription drugs	Limited at the current time to drug coverage through Medicare Part D.
Preventive visit and yearly wellness exams	Covers a "Welcome to Medicare" preventive visit offered within the first 12 months of having Part B. Yearly "wellness" visits are offered to those who have had Part B over 12 months.
Prostate cancer screening	Once every 12 months for all men over 50 years of age. Exam includes preventative digital rectal exam and PSA test. All men over 50 (beginning the day after 50th birthday) and have Part B are eligible.
Prosthetic/ orthotic items	Arm, leg, and neck braces; artificial eyes; artificial limbs and replacement parts; breast prostheses (following mastectomy); prosthetic devices needed to replace an internal body part or function (including ostomy supplies and parenteral and enteral nutrition therapy).
Second surgical opinions	If surgery is not an emergency, subscribers may seek second and third opinions for potential surgical options.
STI screening and counseling	Covers STI screenings for chlamydia, gonorrhea, syphilis and/ or Hepatitis B once every 12 months or at certain times during pregnancy. Covers up to two individual 20 to 30 minute, face-to-face, high-intensity behavioral counseling sessions each year for sexually active adolescents or adults at increased risk for STI's, if referred to by primary care physician or practitioner.

(*continued*)

Table 6.1 Services Covered Under Medicare Part B (*continued*)

Service	Overview of What Is Covered
Smoking cessation	Up to eight face-to-face visits during a 12-month period, if ordered by a physician, provided that one is diagnosed with a smoking-related illness or is using medications that may be affected by tobacco use.
Speech-language pathology services	Treatment to regain or strengthen speech skills.
Surgical dressings	Treatment of surgical or surgically treated wound.
Telemedicine	Services within some rural communities, provided within a practitioner's office, a hospital, or federally qualified health center.
Transplant services	Within a Medicare-certified facility, services for heart, lung, kidney, intestine, liver, bone marrow, and some cornea transplants. If transplant was paid for by Medicare Part A or an employer/union group, and one is entitled to Medicare Part B, immunosuppressive drugs can be covered.
Travel services	Medical services provided for in Canada when one travels the most direct route to Canada between Alaska and another state.
Urgently needed care	Treatment for a sudden illness or injury not identified as a medical emergency.

BMI, body mass index; DSMT, diabetic self-management training; LDCT, low dose computed tomography; OT, occupational therapy; PSA, prostate specific antigen; STI, Sexually transmitted infections

Despite coverage that appears to identify a wide range of items, there still remain a number of services that are considered preventive in nature that are not covered in Medicare Part A and B. Some of these services include acupuncture, cosmetic surgery, dental care and dentures, hearing tests not ordered by a physician, eye care, custodial care, and long-term care. Services not covered by Medicare Parts A and B include (see also Table 6.2):

- Acupuncture
- Chiropractic services (except those listed in Table 6.1)
- Cosmetic surgery
- Custodial care (help with activities of daily living—bathing, dressing, toileting, or eating) either at home or within a nursing home setting
- Dental care, oral health screenings, and dentures
- Eye care (routine eye exams), eye refractions, and most eyeglasses
- Foot care such as cutting corns or calluses
- Hearing aids and hearing exams related to fitting a hearing aid
- Hearing tests without physician's orders
- Laboratory tests for screening purposes outside those listed in Table 6.1

- Long-term care and custodial care in a nursing home
- Orthopedic shoes (with the exception of people who are diabetics, and under certain conditions)
- Physical exams (routine or annual) except wellness exams as listed in Table 6.1
- Preventative vaccinations (outside of those listed in Table 6.1)
- Screening tests (outside of those listed in Table 6.1)
- Travel (healthcare received outside of the United States, except Canada, under certain conditions)

Medicare insurance (Part B) is based upon voluntary contributions and is financed through general revenues. One voluntarily enrolls in the program. In 2018, subscribers paid for a Medicare Part B premium $134.00 per month as a minim um, and the premium amounts are based on income. Table 6.3 provides an overview of these amounts. If an individual did not choose part Medicare Part B when eligible at age 65, the cost of Part B may go up 10% for each 12-month period that one could have had Part B but did not sign up for it, except in special cases. This penalty of an additional 10% is a premium that follows an individual requiring payment for the rest of one's life. Enrolling in Part B is an individual choice, and one is eligible to sign up for Part B anytime during a 7-month period that begins 3 months prior to one's 65th birthday.

Table 6.2 Services Not Covered by Medicare Parts A and B

Acupuncture
Chiropractic services (except those listed in Table 6.1)
Cosmetic surgery
Custodial care (help with activities of daily living—bathing, dressing, toileting, or eating) either at home or within a nursing home setting
Dental care, oral health screenings, and dentures
Eye care (routine eye exams), eye refractions, and most eyeglasses
Foot care such as cutting corns or calluses
Hearing aids and hearing exams related to fitting a hearing aid
Hearing tests without physician's orders
Laboratory tests for screening purposes outside those listed in Table 6.1
Long-term care and custodial care in a nursing home
Orthopedic shoes (with the exception of people who are diabetics, and under certain conditions)
Physical exams (routine or annual) except wellness exams as listed in Table 6.1
Preventative vaccinations (outside of those listed in Table 6.1)
Screening tests (outside of those listed in Table 6.1)
Travel (healthcare received outside of the United States, except Canada, under certain conditions)

The four categories of items and services that are not covered under the Medicare Program are as follows

1. Services and supplies that are not medically reasonable and necessary.
2. Noncovered items and services.
3. Services and supplies denied as bundled or included in the basic allowance of another service.
4. Items and services reimbursable by other organizations or furnished without charge.

Services and Supplies That Are Not Medically Reasonable and Necessary

Supplies or services are considered medically necessary if they meet the standards of good medical practice and are proper and needed for the diagnosis or treatment of the beneficiary's medical condition; furnished for the diagnosis, direct care, and treatment of the beneficiary's medical condition; and not mainly for the convenience of the beneficiary, provider, or supplier.

Noncovered Items and Services

These are items and services furnished outside the United States; items and services required as a result of war; personal comfort items and services; routine physical checkups, certain eye examinations, eyeglasses and lenses, hearing aids and examinations, and certain immunizations; custodial care; cosmetic surgery; items and services furnished by the beneficiary's immediate relatives and members of the beneficiary's household; dental services; nonphysician services furnished to hospital and skilled nursing facility inpatients that are not provided directly under arrangement; certain foot care services and supportive devices for the feet; investigational devices; and services related to and required as a result of services that are not covered.

Services and Supplies Denied as Bundled or Included in the Basic Allowance of Another Service

The following services and supplies denied as bundled or included in the basic allowance of another service will not be paid: fragmented services included in the basic allowance of the initial service; prolonged care (indirect); physician standby services; case management services; and supplies included in the basic allowance of a procedure.

Items and Services Reimbursable by Other Organizations or Furnished Without Charge

Services reimbursable under automobile, no-fault, or liability insurance or workers' compensation (the Medicare Secondary Payer Program); items and services authorized or paid by a government entity; items and services for which the beneficiary, another individual, or an organization has no legal obligation to pay for or furnish; and defective equipment or medical devices covered under warranty are not covered by Part B.

Although subscribers may opt into Medicare Part B and receive the services that are not considered medically necessary in Part A, some copayments or costs are still assigned to particular services and items. For example, blood received as an outpatient, as previously noted. No additional fees are levied for clinical laboratory services utilized under Medicare Part B if the services are deemed medically necessary. Under home health services, one pays nothing for Medicare-approved services, and 20% of the Medicare-approved amount for durable medical equipment. Medical and other services require one to pay 20% of the Medicare-approved amount for most doctor services, outpatient therapy (note that in 2018 some limits to physical therapy, OT, and speech-language pathology services may exist), most preventative services, and durable medical equipment. Mental health services require subscribers to pay for 50% of the outpatient mental healthcare. Other services require the subscriber to pay for the copayment and coinsurance amounts, while outpatient hospital services require that the subscriber pay a coinsurance or copayment amount that varies by service. The subscriber initially pays the first $166 yearly for Part B-covered services or items.

There are a few exceptions to the earlier policies related to Medicare Parts A and B. Some individuals automatically get Part A and Part B under the following circumstances

- An individual who is already receiving benefits from Social Security or the Railroad Retirement Board (RRB) will receive Part A and Part B the first day of the month of his or her 65th birthday.
- If individuals have amyotrophic lateral sclerosis (ALS, also referred to as Lou Gehrig's Disease), they will receive Part A and Part B automatically the month their Social Security disability benefits begin.
- If an individual is automatically enrolled, he or she will receive a Medicare card in the mail 3 months before the 65th birthday or the 25th month of receiving Social Security disability benefits.
- An individual who chooses to do nothing after receiving a Medicare card automatically can keep Part B and will have to pay Part B premiums. An individual who chooses not to keep Part B may have to wait to enroll and pay a penalty as long as he or she has Part B.

Some individuals have to sign up for Part A and/or Part B. Those who are close to age 65 and not receiving Social Security or RRB benefits will need to sign up by contacting Social Security 3 months before turning age 65. The 3-1-3 Rule is used during this time. This means that an individual can sign up for Part A and/or Part B 3 months before turning 65, the month of the 65th birthday, and 3 months after the 65th birthday. Individuals may sign up for Part A and Part B at socialsecurity.gov/retirement.

- It is important to note that individuals who worked for the railroad must contact the RRB. In most cases, an individual who does not apply for Part B when first eligible may have to pay a late enrollment penalty for as long as he or she has Part B.
- For individuals with ESRD who wish to sign up for Medicare, Social Security must be contacted to find out when and how to sign up for Part A and Part B.
- If one lives in Puerto Rico and receives Social Security benefits or benefits from the RRB, that person will automatically get Part A the first day of the month of the 65th birthday, or after receiving disability benefits for 24 months.

Special Enrollment Period

If an individual (or one's spouse) is still working, that person may have a chance to sign up for Medicare during a Special Enrollment Period. If an individual did not sign up for Part B (or Part A if required to buy it) when first eligible because he or she was covered under a group health plan based on current employment (one's own, a spouse's, or if one is disabled, a family member's), signing up for Part A and/or Part B under two circumstances

1. Anytime one is still covered by the group health plan.
2. During the 8-month period that begins the month after the employment ends or the coverage ends, whichever happens first.

Costs of Medicare Part A Coverage

Most people do not pay a monthly premium for Part A. If Part A has to be purchased at full costs, an individual would have to pay $422 per month (as of 2018). If a person enrolled on the original Medicare program, costs would be as follows for some specific areas of services such as the following

1. *Home healthcare*: Costs are $0 for home healthcare services and 20% of the Medicare-approved amount for durable medical equipment.
2. *Hospice care*: Costs are $0 for hospice care. The individual may need to pay a copayment for no more than $5 for each prescription drug and other similar products for pain relief and symptom control while at home. In rare cases, the drug may not be covered by the hospice benefit, the hospice provider must contact the individual's Medicare Prescription Drug Plan to see if the medication is covered under Part D. For inpatient respite care, the individual may need to pay 5% of the Medicare-approved amount. Medicare does not cover room and board when receiving hospice care in the home or another facility such as a nursing home.
3. *Hospital inpatient stay*: Costs are $1,340 deductible for each benefit period. *Days 1–60:* $0 coinsurance for each benefit period.
4. *Days 61–90*: $335 coinsurance per day of each benefit period.
5. *Days 91 and beyond*: $670 coinsurance per each "lifetime reserve day" after day 90 for each benefit period, up to 60 days over one's lifetime (CMS, 2018).
6. *Mental health inpatient stay:* Costs are $1,340 deductible for each benefit period. *Days 1–60:* $0 coinsurance per day of each benefit period. *Days 61–90:* $335 coinsurance per day of each benefit period. *Days 91 and beyond:* $670 coinsurance for each "lifetime reserve day" after day 90 for each benefit period up to 60 days over your lifetime. *Beyond lifetime number of reserve days:* All costs are covered by 20% of the Medicare-approved amount for mental health services you get from doctors and other providers while you are an inpatient at a hospital (Medicare, 2018).
7. *Skilled nursing facility stay:* Costs for Days 1–20: $0 for each benefit period. Costs for Days 21–100: $167.50 coinsurance per day of each benefit period. Costs for *Days 101 and beyond:* All costs (Medicare, 2018).

Part B Coverage Costs

In 2018, the majority of individuals paid the Part B premium of $134 each month. If an individual's modified adjusted gross income as reported on his or her Internal revenue service (IRS) tax return from 2 years before is above a certain amount, the individual will be required to pay a higher premium.

The standard Part B premium amount is $134.00 or higher depending on one's income. Individuals pay a different premium amount if:

- Enrolled in Part B for the first time in 2016.
- Not collecting Social Security benefits.
- Being directly billed for their Part B premiums.
- On Medicare and Medicaid, and Medicaid pays their premiums. The state where the Medicare beneficiary lives will pay the standard premium amount of $121.80.
- One's modified adjusted gross income as reported on the IRS tax return from 2 years previous is above a certain amount.
- An individual is in one of the 5 groups identified in Table 6.3, which depicts the amounts paid for Part B premiums across different income levels.

Table 6.3 Premiums for Medicare Part B, Based Upon Income Bracket

If filing status and yearly income in 2018 was			
File Individual Tax Return	**File Joint Tax Return**	**File Married and Separate Tax Return**	**One Pays (in 2018)**
$85,000 or less	$170,000 or less	$85,000 or less	The plan premium
Above $85,000 up to $107,000	$170,000 up to $214,000	Not applicable	$187.50
Above $107,000 up to $133,500	$214,000 up to $267,000	Not applicable	$267.90
Above $133,500 up to $160,000	Above $267,000 and up to $320,000	Not applicable up	$348.30
Above $160,000	Above $320,000	Above $85,000	$482.60

Source: Social Security Administration. (2018). Retrieved from https://www.ssa.gov

Late Enrollment Penalty

The majority of individuals who do not sign up for Part B when first eligible will have to pay a late enrollment penalty for as long as they maintain Part B coverage. The monthly premium for Part B may go up 10% for each full 12-month period that one was eligible to have had Part B but had not signed up for it.

Part B Costs for Those Qualifying for Original Medicare

Part B Annual Deductible

The Part B deductible for 2018 is $183 per year. After the deductible has been met, the beneficiary will usually pay 20% of the Medicare-approved amount for most physician services, including those services received as an inpatient at a hospital, outpatient therapy, and durable medical equipment.

- *Relevant Part B services include:*
  - The beneficiary pays $0 for Medicare-approved services.
- *Home health services*
  - $0 for home healthcare services, and 20% of the Medicare-approved amount for durable medical equipment.
- *Medical and other services*
  - The Medicare beneficiary will pay 20% of the Medicare-approved amount for most doctor services, along with most doctor services while a hospital inpatient, outpatient therapy, and durable medical equipment.
- *Outpatient mental health services*
  - The beneficiary will pay $0 for a yearly depression screening if the doctor or provider accepts assignment. Accepting assignment means that the doctor or provider is accepting of the amounts that Medicare approves to pay for services.
  - 20% of the Medicare-approved amount is paid for doctor visits or other healthcare providers to diagnose or treat the patient's condition. The Part B deductible applies here.

    - An individual who is receiving services in a hospital outpatient clinic may have to pay an additional copayment or coinsurance amount to the hospital. The amount will vary depending on the service provided but will be between 20% and 40% of the Medicare-approved amount.
    - *Partial hospitalization mental health services*: The Medicare beneficiary will pay a percentage of the Medicare-approved amount for each service received from a doctor or other qualified mental health professionals if the healthcare professional accepts assignment.
    - The beneficiary will pay coinsurance for each day of partial hospitalization services provided in a hospital outpatient setting or community mental health center, and the Part B deductible applies.
- *Outpatient hospital services*
    - The Medicare beneficiary generally pay 20% of the Medicare-approved amount for the doctor or other healthcare provider's services, and the Part B deductible applies.
    - For all other services the beneficiary will generally pay a copayment for each service performed in an outpatient hospital setting; a beneficiary will pay more for services received in a hospital outpatient setting than for the same care in a doctor's office.
    - For some of the screenings and preventive services, coinsurance, copayments, and the Part B deductible does not apply, and the beneficiary pays nothing.

Medicare Part C

Medicare Part C is a program that combines one's hospital coverage (Part A) and medical coverage (Part B) through a health maintenance organization (HMO) or preferred provider organization (PPO). This plan is designed to enable private insurance companies approved by Medicare to provide coverage to subscribers at a cost that may be lower than the original Medicare plan, with some additional benefits. The down side of this plan is that individuals must see physicians within the group assigned to provide coverage. Such a scheme works well for individuals who may be stationary, and remain within their home-based community; however, for people who travel frequently, or spend a portion of their time at a second residence, this plan may not offer the flexibility necessary.

Three specific options are available within the Part C Medicare Advantage Plans, each of which operates slightly differently. For the most part, providers are paid per enrollee, regardless of whether services are used or not. Within each of the three plans—PPO, HMO, or private fee for service plan (PFFS)—there are also some slight variations, and enrollees should consider their needs and which plans would work best. In most cases, prescription drugs are covered in all three of the schemes (PPO, HMO, and PFFS). In the HMO scheme one must see a primary care physician in order to receive a referral elsewhere. Under the PPO and PFFS schemes, personal autonomy is limited in choosing a primary care physician.

Since 2007, Medicare Medical Savings Account (MSAs) Plans are offered. These plans are similar to the Health Savings Account Plans available outside of Medicare and have two distinct parts. The first part, known as the Medicare Advantage Health Plan, does not begin to pay covered costs until a subscriber has met the annual deductible (which varies by plan). The second part is a Medical Savings Account into which Medicare deposits money that a subscriber can use to pay healthcare costs (CMS, 2018).

How Is Medicare Managed Care Different From Other Managed Care Plans?

Medicare Part C, known as Medicare+ Choice, was the result of the Balanced Budget Act in 1997. In this component of the plan, recipients enroll in an HMO plan; however, many plans have been found to discriminate against older adults (Etheredge, 1999; Rural Policy Research Institute [RPRI], 1999a). The act expanded prevention services and created incentives for managed care plans to enter underserved rural areas, bringing a real asset to improving access to care within these areas.

Part C Coverage Costs

The Part C monthly premium varies by plan. The amount one will pay for Part C deductibles, copayments, and/or coinsurance also varies by plan.

One will be charged a late enrollment penalty if one goes without a Medicare Prescription Drug Plan (Part D), or without a Medicare Advantage Plan (Part C) (like an HMO or PPO) or other Medicare health plan that offers Medicare prescription drug coverage. In addition, going without creditable prescription drug coverage for any continuous period of 63 days or more after the initial enrollment period is over may subject one to additional fees through a late enrollment penalty.

In general, one is expected to pay this penalty for as long as he or she has a Medicare drug plan. The cost of the late enrollment penalty depends on how long the individual went without Part D or creditable prescription drug coverage (Medicare, 2018)

Medicare Part D

Medicare Part D offers prescription drug coverage for everyone eligible to enroll and utilize Medicare. This coverage was intended to help lower prescription drug costs and help protect against higher costs in the future. It can give enrollees greater access to drugs that can be used to prevent medical complications of diseases and to promote health and wellness. These plans are run by insurance companies and other private companies approved by Medicare. While Part D is optional, but one may face a penalty if enrolling at a date than the initial enrollment period within which one is eligible. Individuals with limited income and resources can qualify for extra help paying Part D costs. If one's income is below $14,700 (or $19,800 if married and living with a spouse) the individual may qualify for extra help. One's total assets generally must be limited to $11,500 (or $23,000 if married and living with a spouse).

Once an enrollee has spent $4,850 out-of-pocket in 2018, the individual is deemed to be out of the coverage gap. This stage of payment for prescription drugs is called the "donut hole." Once out of the coverage gap (Medicare prescription drug coverage), the individual automatically gets "catastrophic coverage." This protection assures that the enrollee will pay only a small coinsurance/copayment for covered drugs for the remainder of the year (Medicare, 2018).

HOW DOES MEDICARE AFFECT ACCESS TO HEALTHCARE, COST CONTAINMENT, AND QUALITY?

Medicare costs have been rising steadily, causing concern to governmental authorities. According to Brown, Clement, Hill, Retchin, and Bergeron (1993), costs savings accrued through reduced utilization of healthcare services do not balance the high overhead rates charged by HMOs, resulting in no net savings to the Medicare program. Quality is also inconsistent across providers. Finally, fraud has risen steadily since 2000.

WHAT IS MEDICAID AND HOW DOES IT DIFFER FROM MEDICARE?

A program designed to enable individuals who are below the poverty line to pay for healthcare was designed by and is delivered through the program instrument known as Medicaid. This provision is actually a title under the Social Security Act (Title XIX). Medicaid was designed to provide insurance for older adults, people with disabilities, dependent children, and mothers. States participate in the Medicaid program on a voluntary basis, although all states participate. To receive federal funding, states must provide a range of prescribed services. However, each state identifies eligibility criteria, remuneration schedules, and poverty guidelines. Although individual states may establish their own eligibility criteria, note that reimbursement from the federal government will not occur for services provided beyond the currently established guidelines (Government Accountability Office [GAO], 1998; Rosenbach & Lamphere, 1999).

Eligibility

The Medicaid program has some mandatory and optional eligibility criteria. The mandatory criteria target five specific categories of poor- or low-income people

- Pregnant women
- Children
- Older adult Medicare recipients
- Adults under 65 with dependent children
- Children and adults with disabilities

The Social Security Act authorizes multiple waiver and demonstration oversight authorities to allow individual states flexibility in operating Medicaid programs. Each authority has a distinct purpose, and distinct requirements. Within the legislation, some specific sections provide for waivers to enable some flexibility to individual states to develop their own demonstration projects or carve out specific Medicaid opportunities that can meet specific community needs. These specific components of the act include Sections 1115, which addresses research and demonstration projects, and Section 1915, which addresses managed care waivers or home- and community-based services waivers.

Medicaid Waiver Opportunities

Section 1115: Research and Demonstration Projects

Section 1115 gives the Secretary of Health and Human Services broad authority to approve projects that test policy innovations likely to further the objectives of the Medicaid program. These may include innovative primary care health and preventative healthcare delivery options to meet the needs of the elderly who have been subject to low income.

Section 1915(b) Managed Care/Freedom of Choice Waivers

Section 1915(b) provides the secretary authority to grant waivers that allow states to implement managed care delivery systems or otherwise limit individuals' choice of provider under Medicaid. Under this option, older adults may be guaranteed some providers if living below the poverty level, and these providers may care for the healthcare needs of the elderly, especially in medically designated shortage areas.

Section 1915(c) Home- and Community-Based Services Waivers

Section 1915(c) provides the secretary authority to waive Medicaid provisions to allow long-term care services to be delivered in community settings. This program is the Medicaid alternative to providing comprehensive long-term services in institutional settings. This waiver program expands the possibilities for community living and assisted living opportunities for older adults who live in the community, who may otherwise be limited in their housing options or options for community-based care and assistance.

In summary, these options within the Medicaid legislation provide for the opportunities to carve out and develop innovations within the healthcare service delivery networks for low-income older adults. This section also enables individual states to develop model programs that address the cultural and economic contexts of their population base.

THE EFFECTS OF REIMBURSEMENT ON HEALTHCARE QUALITY, ACCESS, AND COSTS

Despite the fact that services are available to meet the medical needs of older adults and the elderly poor, Medicaid and State Children's Health Insurance Programs (CHIP) reimbursement rates are not always consistent with the cost of delivering services. Hence, providers are often dubious about providing services to older adults on Medicaid. Certain neighborhoods in urban areas and certain rural communities may not have access to providers who will accept Medicaid. Prolonged periods of time to wait for reimbursements lead to disinterest in serving as a provider.

CHALLENGES FOR THE FUTURE

Although comprehensive in nature, Medicare faces a number of dilemmas when we look toward the future. Healthcare expenses appear to be most costly during one's last year of life, thus pouring a financial burden onto the current Medicare system. Challenges for the future include the burden of costs of financing a comprehensive healthcare system, the rationing of healthcare services, and accessibility of healthcare services to older adults living in medically designated shortage areas (GAO, 1998; RPRI, 1999b).

An Empty Pot at the End of the Rainbow?

Medicare has been perceived by many to be the "pot of gold" at the end of the rainbow, or a benefit to be treasured in retirement. It was intended to provide medical coverage to older adults, upon retirement age and beyond; however, with the costs of healthcare exploding over the past two decades (since the year 2000), will this pot be empty in years to come, or will it be limited? Healthcare economists predict that the costs of care will far exceed the monies available for reimbursement to physicians and for hospital inpatient treatment. In addition, a number of services are currently not covered which are not necessarily elective services, but necessary and required. Prevention and screening services are not covered, nor is there any expectation that these services will be covered in the near future. In addition, Medicare covers only about 20% of all healthcare expenses. Thus, these issues leave one to wonder whether the pot will continue to "evaporate" over the years to come and become empty. Unfortunately, experts (Barusch, 2002; Derickson, 2005) who have critiqued the system argue that this pot may be close to empty, if not empty, in years to come.

Rationing of Healthcare Services—To Be or Not to Be?

A second challenge for the future is the rationing of healthcare services. At present, rationing does not occur in most states, although it has been argued that Oregon's protocol for healthcare delivery prioritizes care and procedures based upon life tables, in effect, care is rationed as one moves across the life span. This approach is also apparent in some countries that provide socialized medicine, such as Britain. As the cost of healthcare continues to increase, and as our cohort of older adults (people 65+ years of age) continues to grow, will the rationing of healthcare services come to be? Since the philosophical paradigm underlying Medicare at the time of its inception was that "healthcare was a right," will this concept of rationing come to pass, or will another philosophical paradigm prevail that can lead to a rationing of healthcare for older adults through the Medicare program?

SUMMARY

Medicare, a healthcare program perceived to be a universal program rather than one based upon a needs test, currently provides healthcare to people who reach the age of 64. Comprised of four parts, it can provide hospital care, general healthcare, hospice care, home healthcare, and prescription drug coverage. This chapter provides an overview of the Medicare program, its various components, and aspects of healthcare that are covered through its component parts. Although there are currently no needs tests or limitations as to who qualifies for services, the chapter concludes with some dilemmas for the future of healthcare coverage, including "an empty pot at the end of the rainbow" and rationing of healthcare services and procedures.

CASE STUDY DISCUSSION

Consider the following scenarios. What components of Medicare would each utilize? How would services be similar or different between our consumers who have a disability and those who are older adults? How would the pathway to securing Medicare be similar or different for the two groups of consumers?

Ida: Ida, a resident of a Medicaid funded long-term care facility in Denton, Texas, has lived with symptoms of multiple sclerosis since she was 52 years old. Now 80 years of age, Ida is a widow, and her stepchildren look after her needs. Her stepchildren are spread throughout the Dallas area, while her daughter June and four grandchildren reside in Washington state.

Gerry: Gerry was born with cerebral palsy and hydrocephalus. During the first year of his life, a shunt was surgically implanted into his skull; however, the shunt needs to be replaced periodically. Gerry is on Social Security disability and receives funding monthly. Gerry lives in a rural community, attends master level classes in rehabilitation studies at a local university, and mobilizes himself with an electric wheelchair, and is 38 years of age, 1 year younger than Jack Benny!

Lorraine: Lorraine is a 96-year-old Holocaust survivor who currently lives in Fort Myers, Florida. Lorraine moved into an assisted living facility 2 years ago, when she lost her driving privileges and had been reported to be falling within her home. She is renting her family home to her adult grandson. Lorraine, a divorcee, lived in an abusive relationship for most of her 27 years of marriage.

Joan: Joan currently lives in Ohio, and manages independently, despite a car accident that left her with a severe head injury 36 years ago. Joan became a parent shortly after her head injury and often suffers from aphasia. She currently lives in her own home, with her adult son. Disabled for 36 years, Joan makes use of services from Medicare and her state Medicaid program.

DISCUSSION QUESTIONS

1. What philosophical paradigms play a role in the establishment of Medicare and the services provided?
2. Do you think that specific groups may have played a role in exercising their influence power when it comes to the services not allowed under Medicare Part A and B? If so, which groups may have played a role and why?
3. What impact has the Affordable Care Act had on Medicare and its beneficiaries?
4. What components of Medicare are currently under threat?

ADDITIONAL RESOURCES

Websites

Medicare: www.medicare.gov

This governmental website is orchestrated through the healthcare financing administration and provides an overview of Medicare and its programs, and a user's guide is available.

Medicaid: www.cms.hhs.gov

This governmental web site is orchestrated through the healthcare financing administration and provides an overview of the Medicaid program, guidelines for use, and issues for debate. An overview of the Medicaid programs is provided, and a user's guide is available.

Kaiser Family Foundation: www.kff.org

This site for the Kaiser Family Foundation provides a background of current studies and up-to-date information on both the Medicaid and Medicare programs.

Strengthening Medicare: www.whitehouse.gov/infocus/medicare/

This White House site provides an overview of initiatives, speeches, and key summaries of roundtable discussions related to Medicare and Medicare modernization.

Medicare Publications Search: www.medicare.gov/publications/#results

This site provides a range of up-to-date publications and fact sheets that help simplify the process of understanding Medicare and its component parts.

YouTube Resources Related to Medicare

Medicare Made Clear: www.youtube.com/user/medicaremadeclear

This YouTube video provides a condensed view of the various parts of Medicare.

Medicare Choices: www.youtube.com/watch?v=WZVQSFBq2uw

This YouTube video explains the difference between Medicare and Medicare Advantage plans.

Podcast

George Lowery discusses living with a disability and Medicare. **Listen now:** https://bcove.video/2DynyYd

REFERENCES

Alliance for Retired Americans. (2018, January 17). 2018 Social Security and Medicare factsheet. Retrieved from http://retiredamericans.org/2018-social-security-medicare-factsheet/

Ball, R. M. (1996). Medicare's roots: What Medicare's architects had in mind. *Generations*, *20*(2), 13–18.

Barusch, A. (2002). *Foundations of social policy: Social justice, public programs, and the social work profession*. Itasca, IL: Peacock.

Brown, R. S., Clement, D. G., Hill, J. W., Retchin, S. M., & Bergeron, J. W. (1993). Do health maintenance organizations work for Medicare? *Health Care Financing Review*, *15*(1), 7–23.

Centers for Medicare & Medicaid Services. (n.d.). *Key milestones in CMS programs*. Retrieved from https://www.cms.gov/About-CMS/Agency-Information/History/downloads/CMSProgramKeyMilestones.pdf

Centers for Medicare & Medicaid Services. (2018). *Medicare and you, 2018: Official government handbook*. Baltimore, MD: Government Printing Office. Retrieved from https://www.medicare.gov/sites/default/files/2018-09/10050-medicare-and-you.pdf

Derickson, A. (2005). *Health security for all: Dreams of universal health care in America*. Baltimore, MD. Johns Hopkins Press.

DiNitto, D., & Johnson, D. (2016). *Social welfare*. Thousand Oaks, CA: Sage.

Etheredge, L. (1999). Medicare's governance and structure: A proposal: One expert's prescription for fixing what ails the management of Medicare and other federal health programs. *Health Affairs*, *19*(5), 60–71. doi:10.1377/hlthaff.19.5.60

Government Accountability Office. (1998). *Medicaid: Early implication of welfare reform for beneficiaries and states*. Washington, DC: U.S. Government Printing Office.

Rosenbach, M. L., & Lamphere, J. (1999). *Public policy institute: Bridging the gaps between Medicare and Medicaid: The case of QMBs and SLMBs*. Washington, DC: AARP.

Rural Policy Research Institute. (1999a). *A rural perspective on Medicare policy: An initial assessment of the premium support approach*. Columbia, MO: Author.

Rural Policy Research Institute. (1999b). *Taking Medicare into the 21st century: Realities of a post BBA world and implications for rural health care*. Columbia, MO: Author.

Social Security Administration. (2018). Website. Retrieved from https://www.ssa.gov

7

The Older Americans Act

LEARNING OBJECTIVES

At the end of this chapter, readers will:

1. *Understand the history of the Older Americans Act (OAA).*
2. *Understand specific components of the OAA.*
3. *Understand how the OAA provides resources to older adults and people with disabilities.*

Theresa and Erica have decided that they want to investigate what programs and services can be offered at the state, regional, and local levels to meet the needs of some of the consumers that they have encountered in their "speak out" sessions during their cross-country tour of aging services and consumers. They were particularly drawn to two consumers and the individual needs of these consumers. A thumbnail sketch of these consumers follows.

Gerry: Gerry was born with cerebral palsy and hydrocephalus. During the first year of his life, a shunt was surgically implanted into his skull. However, the shunt needs to be replaced periodically, and was recently replaced leaving Gerry somewhat incapacitated and unable to cook for himself, do laundry, and clean his house. Initially, he needed someone to help him with bathing and dressing. Gerry is on Social Security Disability and receives funding monthly, which should qualify him for in-home support services.

Lorraine: Lorraine is a 96-year-old woman who has survived the Holocaust and currently lives in Fort Myers, Florida. Lorraine moved into an assisted living facility 2 years ago, when she lost her driving privileges and had been reported to be falling within her home. Lorraine needs assistance with shopping for groceries and household chores such as laundry and cleaning her apartment. She has also been having some flashbacks recently from her days in the Holocaust. Her unemployed son has also been receiving frequent donations from Lorraine, which appear to be more than a casual occurrence.

Hence, our "investigative team" decided to explore the Older Americans Act (OAA) and what options mandated services within this piece of federal legislation has to offer. Before we arrive at their conclusions, let us understand some of the history and components of the OAA.

© Springer Publishing Company DOI:10.1891/9780826128393.0007

BACKGROUND AND OVERVIEW

Prior to the 1920s, limited attention was placed on aging services or older adults' needs and concerns. The passage of the Civil Service Retirement Act provided for a retirement system for a number of government employees and served as a pioneering effort to consider social welfare needs for aging adults. However, this act did not provide for any programs or services to meet the needs of older adults living in the community. No development was apparent in this area until 1950, when President Harry Truman initiated the first National Conference on Aging, sponsored by the Federal Security Agency. This conference resulted in the first federal funds being appropriated for social service programs for older people (1952); however, these funds were appropriated under the Social Security Act. In 1956, a special staff on aging was established and housed within the Office of the Secretary of Health, Education, and Welfare, with its main function to coordinate responsibilities for the aging. In addition, a Federal Council on Aging was created by President Eisenhower. Legislation introduced in Congress in 1958 called for a White House Conference on Aging, which was held in 1961. This led to legislation introduced in Congress to establish an independent and permanent Commission on Aging. A direct result of this commission was the development of the Older Americans Act (OAA) of 1965.

THE OLDER AMERICANS ACT OF 1965

The OAA (PL 89–73) signed into law on July 14, 1965, has been the cornerstone of community services for older adults in the United States and served as the first blueprint for community-based services to meet the needs of older adults. It is based upon 10 objectives that identify how older adults should be valued and treated, including:

- Conditions for an adequate income in concert with a standard of living in the United States.
- The most up-to-date physical and mental healthcare guided by scientific findings.
- Affordable and suitable housing.
- Complete rehabilitative or restorative services for people in institutional care.
- Opportunities for nondiscriminatory employment, regardless of age.
- A retirement that offers dignity and honor in return for one's contribution to the nation's economy.
- Participation in meaningful activity within the widest available range of civic, cultural, education/training, and recreational opportunities.
- Efficient community services that enable access to supported living arrangements and social assistance, thus making it easier to coordinate and maintain a continuum of care for vulnerable older individuals.
- Immediate benefit from proven research knowledge, which in turn sustains and improves health and happiness.
- The freedom for autonomy and independence and sufficient and effective community care services that promote independence.

In the original act, these principles are defined through six specific titles.

Title I: Definitions

In the original OAA, Title I outlined the objectives and defined the administrative oversight for the OAA. In addition to laying the groundwork to assure that the programs and services preserve the dignity and worth of the individual, Title I provides definitions for the administrative structure to carry out the OAA. This organization includes the Secretary, Commissioner, and the role that individual states will take on in the administration of the act.

Title II: Administration on Aging

Title II establishes the infrastructure for the administration of aging services and outlines the main activities of this administrative structure. The Administration on Aging (AoA) is housed within the Department of Health, Education, and Welfare (as of 2007 known as the Department of Health and Human Services) and is headed by a commissioner, appointed by the president. The functions of the AoA include:

- To provide a clearinghouse of information related to aging.
- To assist the secretary on all matters that pertain to aging and aging issues.
- To administer grants provided by the OAA.
- To develop, plan, execute, and disseminate research and demonstration programs within the field of aging.
- To provide consultation and technical assistance to individual states on issues related to aging.
- To prepare, publish, and disseminate information that relates to older adults.
- To collect data on issues pertinent to aging, which was not currently collected by other federal authorities.
- To encourage the use of services to promote healthy aging.

Title III: Grants for Community Planning, Services, and Training

Title III outlines the authorization process of appropriations for the purpose of community planning, services, and training. Outlined within this title are allotments, reallotments, and monies available for grants, time limitations for grants, and an outline of ways state plans filter into the grants process. This title also outlines ways state agencies can administer a plan, the development of programs and activities, personnel, and ways to prioritize projects and maintain records. An appeals process for state-based entities is also outlined.

Title IV: Research and Development Projects

Under Section 401 of the original OAA, the secretary can authorize grants for the purpose of conducting research and development projects in up to four specific areas: (a) to study patterns and living conditions of older adults to assure and maximize their well-being; (b) to develop new approaches, techniques, and models of service delivery that will promote the well-being and maximize the potential for healthy lifestyles for older adults; (c) to evaluate approaches to promote and maximize service delivery models for community-based services; and (d) to promote best practice methods in social welfare.

Title V: Training Projects

Under Section 502 of the original OAA, Title V outlines the provision of funds for training projects to benefit individual states, which are identified within the specific state's plan of priorities. Funds are appropriated from the Secretary of the AoA, sanction must also be provided for by the individual state to receive funds.

Title VI: General

Title VI outlines the advisory committees that govern the administration of the OAA. Membership on the advisory committee, the terms of office, compensation and travel expenses, and guidelines for the publication of informational materials are also outlined.

Although the OAA is still in operation and serves as the mandate to guide service delivery for community-dwelling older adults, a number of legislative amendments have been enacted since 1965. The next section provides a thumbnail sketch of some of these amendments, including the most recent amendments of 2006 to the OAA.

AMENDMENTS TO THE OLDER AMERICANS ACT: 1967–2000

Since the inception of the OAA, a number of amendments have been passed that have both extended the initial appropriations and expanded the amounts budgeted for the act. However, with many of the amendments, the act has been expanded to address new issues or additional concerns for older adults living within communities. In 1967, for example, with the first set of amendments, the OAA was extended for 2 years, with an expansion of the original act to study the personnel needs within the aging field. Two years later, amendments, to the act included the provision of funds for foster grandparent and retired senior volunteer programs and model demonstration projects. The development of nutrition programs resulted following the amendments of 1972, when Title VII was created to authorize funds for such programs for the elderly. The establishment of Area Agencies on Aging (AAA) was the result of the 1973 comprehensive services amendments. Title V authorized grants to community agencies for multipurpose senior centers and created community service employment grants for people 55 years of age and older and considered in a low-income bracket.

Title III of the OAA was expanded in 1974 to include transportation, and in 1975, grants were authorized for Indian tribal organizations. In addition, priority services were defined in the areas of transportation, home care, legal services, and home renovation/repair.

Changes to Title VII made in 1977 focused on nutrition programs. These changes led to nutrition sites, making use of surplus commodities through the Department of Agriculture. Further changes were seen in 1978, when OAA Amendments consolidated the Title III area agency on aging administration and social services (Code of Federal Regulations, n.d.), the Title VII nutrition services, and the Title V multipurpose senior centers into a new Title III and added a new Title VI for grants to Indian tribal organizations. The former Title V became the Community Service Employment grant program for low-income persons, age 55 and older (created under the 1978 amendments as Title IX). In addition, in 1978, amendments mandated each state to develop a long-term care (LTC) ombudsman program to address issues of concern from residents and their families in nursing homes.

Amendments to the OAA that took place in the 1980s emphasized the support for community-based care and the principle of maintaining independence within the community. In 1981, the ombudsman program was expanded to provide coverage to board and care homes through OAA amendments. The subsequent reauthorizations that took place in 1984 reaffirmed the roles of the state and the local AAA to coordinate community-based services, and to assure funding to enable state and local entities to maintain accountability and funding of nationally prioritized services such as legal assistance, in-home care, and accessibility. The reauthorization of the OAA added six additional distinct appropriations for services: in-home services for the frail elderly; LTC ombudsman; assistance for special needs; health education and promotion; prevention of elder abuse, neglect, and

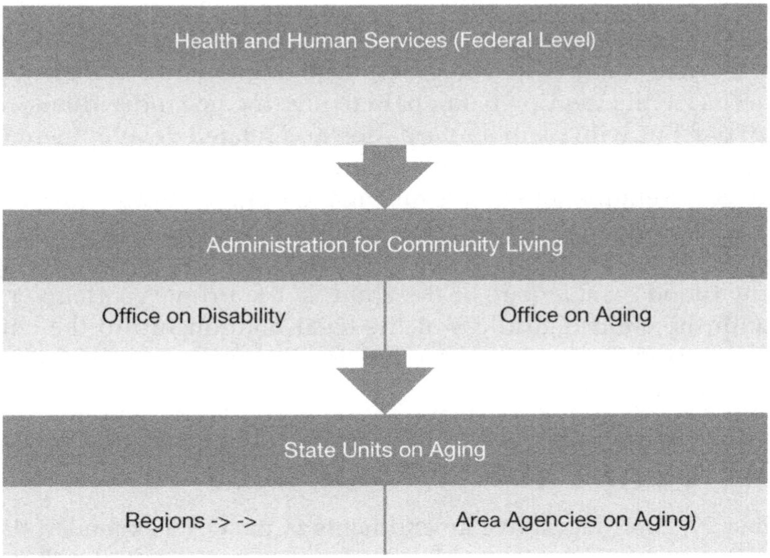

Figure 7.1 An overview of the Administration for Community Living and Aging Network.

exploitation; and outreach activities for persons who may be eligible for benefits under supplemental security income (SSI), Medicaid, and food stamps. Additional emphasis was given to serving those in the greatest economic and social need, including low-income minorities. In addition, the OAA reauthorization charged states to guarantee ombudsman access to facilities and patient records, provided important legal protections, authorized state ombudsmen to designate local ombudsman programs, and required that ombudsman programs have adequate legal counsel. See Figure 7.1.

OAA Amendments of 2000 (PL 106–501), which reauthorized the OAA for 5 years, was signed into law on November 13, 2000. It included the establishment of the National Family Caregiver Support Program (Lexis-Nexis Congressional Universe, 2000).

The National Family Caregiver Support Program

Caregivers provide a tremendous service to individuals requiring support, and they are often not regarded as an integral component of a service delivery system when examining care strategies. The National Family Caregiver Support Program (originally devised as a component of the OAA but later passed as a separate law that is discussed in Chapter 9) acknowledges this vital role and provides assistance to family caregivers. Within the National Family Caregiver Support Act, a family caregiver is defined as an adult family member, or other individual, who is an informal provider of in-home and community care to an older individual. This definition provides some scope and flexibility in order to meet the needs of those responsible for caring for their loved ones. It also acknowledges the fact that other relatives, friends, neighbors, and domestic partners will also share the responsibility of caring for loved ones.

The National Family Caregiver Support Program provides services within five areas of support service, including (a) information about services available; (b) assistance in gaining access to these services; (c) counseling, organization of support groups, and caregiver training; (d) respite care; and (e) supplemental services on a limited basis to augment the care provided by caregivers. The act also places a high priority for services to (a) older caregivers who demonstrate the greatest social and economic needs (with attention being paid to low-income individuals), and (b) older caregivers of persons with mental retardation and related developmental disabilities. The act also allows each state to use no more than 10% of its total funds to provide support services to eligible caregivers raising their grandchildren (under the age of 18 years). It should be noted that an eligible grandparent caregiver would be defined as someone who is at least 60 years of age or older; is a grandparent, step-grandparent, or relative by blood or marriage of the child; is the primary caregiver of the child; and lives with the child regardless of the legal relationship to the child (National Caregiver Support Program, 2006). A more detailed discussion of this piece of legislation is found in Chapter 11.

LEGISLATIVE AMENDMENTS OF 2006

On September 29, 2006, legislative amendments to the OAA expanded the existing act and moved toward assuring that older Americans could maintain their dignity and independence, while segments of the act sought to put prevention efforts into place for services (N4A, 2006). Amendments known as Public Law 109–365 bring some specific new areas for consideration to include:

- Enhanced coordination of LTC services to be developed in home- and community-based settings.
- Support for community planning efforts at the state level in order to begin to address some of the LTC needs that the baby boom generation will face.
- An increased focus on prevention and treatment of psychiatric disorders.
- An expansion of the category of caregivers served under the National Family Caregiver Support Program.
- An increased focus on civic engagement and volunteerism.
- An expansion of programs designed to address elder abuse, neglect, and exploitation.

The amendments of 2006 expanded on the president's New Freedom Commission Initiative and affirmed the commitment to some specific values. These values included health promotion and disease prevention, independence, empowerment, and community-based care.

The OAA Amendments of 2006 are the primary source for the delivery of social and nutrition services for older individuals. First enacted in 1965, the act's programs include supportive services; congregate and home-delivered nutrition services; community service employment; the LTC ombudsman program; and services to prevent the abuse, neglect, and exploitation of older individuals. The act also provides grants to Native Americans and research, training, and demonstration activities (Walker, Burns & Wren, 2006).

Title I

Title I of the OAA sets broad social policy objectives to improve the lives of all older Americans. Although the definitions have been updated in order to be consistent with other statutes and proposals, the objectives have been retained and remain unchanged

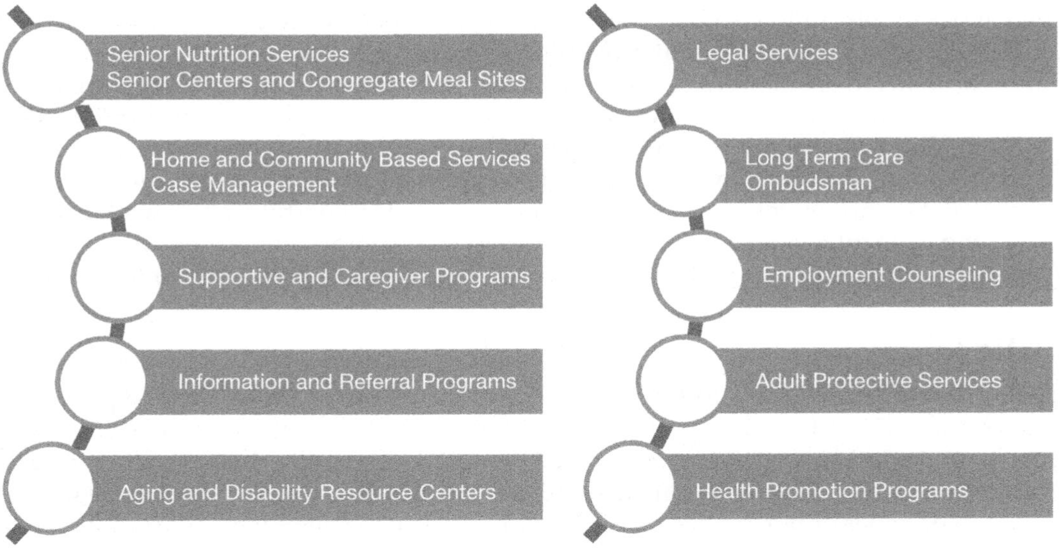

Figure 7.2 Aging Services Network at a regional level.
Source: Administration for Community Living, https://acl.gov.

from previous legislation. It recognizes the need for an adequate income in retirement, the importance of physical and mental health, employment in community services for older individuals, and LTC services. Definitions related to assistive technology have been made consistent with the Assistive Technology Act of 1998. The definitions for elder abuse, neglect, and exploitation have also been made consistent with the definitions used by the Justice Coalition in the Elder Justice Act. See Figure 7.2.

Title II

Title II establishes the AoA, within the Department of Health and Human Services, to be the primary federal advocate for older individuals and to administer the provision of the OAA. It also establishes the National Eldercare Locator Service to provide nationwide information with regard to resources for older individuals, the National Long-Term Care Ombudsman Resource Center, the National Center on Elder Abuse, the National Aging Information Center, and the Pension Counseling and Information Program. The 2006 amendments authorize the designation of a person to have responsibility for elder abuse prevention to develop a long-term plan and national response to elder abuse prevention, detection, treatment, and intervention. It also authorizes the assistant secretary to designate an individual to be responsible for administration of mental health services and authorizes Aging and Disability Resource Centers (ADRCs). Further, the 2006 amendments strengthen the leadership of the Department of Health and Human Services through an interagency coordinating committee to guide policy and program development across the federal government with respect to aging and demographic changes.

Within Title II, definitions for numerous key issues impacting older adults have been expanded within the new legislative amendments. These include exploitation, self-neglect, and at risk for institutional placement, which were not included in the past. The definition of disease prevention and health promotion was changed to include an evidence-based approach, includes examples of chronic disease, and adds to the examples of health promotion activities: "falls prevention, physical activity, and improved nutrition." ADRCs (see Chapter 8 for a more comprehensive description) have also been added to the list of definitions. The functions of AoA are also expanded to include elder abuse prevention, benefits enrollment, choices for independence, federal partnerships, mental health, civic engagement, evidence-based nutrition services, and private pay options. Healthy lifestyles are also promoted through evidence-based disease prevention interventions.

Title III

Title III authorizes grants to fund 655 AAA and more than 29,000 service providers nationwide. Title III services are targeted to those with the greatest economic and social need, particularly low-income minority persons and older individuals residing in rural communities. The 2006 amendments authorize organizations with experience in providing volunteer opportunities for older individuals to be eligible to enter cooperative arrangements; require state agencies to promote the development and implementation of state systems that enable older individuals to receive LTC and community-based settings in accordance with needs and preferences; encourage both states and AAA to plan for population changes; improve access to supportive services that help foster independence; require nutrition projects to prepare meals that comply with the most recent dietary guidelines; and reauthorize the National Family Caregiver Support Program.

The reauthorization of the National Family Caregiver Support Program broadens the population to be served and now includes caregivers of individuals with Alzheimer's disease; grandparents or older relation caregivers who are 55 years of age or older (the former minimum age was 60 years) caring for a child related by blood, marriage, or adoption; and individuals responsible for an adult child with a disability.

Title IV

Title IV supports a wide range of ongoing research and demonstration activities that enhance innovation, identify best practices, and provide technical assistance for older individuals. The 2006 amendments permit competitive grants for planning activities that benefit the aging population and assessment of technology-based models to aid in remote health monitoring systems, communication devices, and assistive technologies. These activities include naturally occurring retirement communities (NORCs); innovations to improve transportation, mental health services, and screening; and civic engagement. Further, the amendments include Hispanic-serving institutions among those eligible to compete for grants to provide education and training in the field of aging; reauthorize grants to improve transportation services for older individuals; ensure increased awareness of mental health disorders among older individuals; and authorize development of innovative models of service delivery to ensure older individuals may age in place, as they are able and as they choose.

Title V

Title V authorizes the community service employment program for older Americans—known as the Senior Community Service Employment Program (SCSEP)—to promote part-time opportunities in community service for unemployed, low-income persons who are 55 years old or older and who have poor employment prospects. It is administered by the Department of Labor. This program represents approximately one-quarter of OAA funds—$432 million out of $1.78 billion in fiscal year (FY) 2006. This program is operated by states, and national grantees were awarded competitive grants, supporting 61,050 jobs and serving approximately 91,500 individuals in FY 2005. The 2006 amendments establish 4-year grant cycles for the competitive program and prohibit poor-performing grantees from competing during the next grant cycle. It expands participation for eligible individuals who are underemployed and establishes a 48-month time limit for participation in the program, with a waiver for particularly hard-to-serve individuals. It establishes an overall grantee average participation cap of up to 27 months and authorizes a waiver of up to 36 months.

Titles VI and VII

Title VI provides funds for supportive and nutrition services for older Native Americans. The 2006 amendments increased the Native American caregiver support program through 2011. Also, Title VII authorizes programs for the LTC ombudsman; elder abuse, neglect, and exploitation prevention; legal service developers; and vulnerable Native American elder rights. The 2006 amendments enhanced the elder abuse prevention activities by awarding grants to states and Indian tribes, which enabled them to strengthen LTC and provide assistance for elder justice and elder abuse prevention programs. It created grants for prevention, detection, assessment, treatment of, intervention in, investigation of, and response to elder abuse; safe havens demonstrations for older individuals; volunteer programs; multidisciplinary activities; elder fatality and serious injury review teams; programs for underserved populations; incentives for LTC facilities to train and retain employees; and other collaborative and innovative approaches.

Finally, the National Resource Center for Women and Retirement was a highly successful program run by the Women's Institute for a Secure Retirement (WISER)—a nonprofit organization dedicated to ensuring the security of women's retirement income through outreach, partnerships, and policy development. We know that many older Americans lack financial knowledge, and that financial education is needed. This program provides a helpful service and has continued to be funded in subsequent reauthorizations of OAA so as to expand its various programs for older Americans, including financial literacy.

The 2010 Reauthorization

In 2010, the Older American's Act was reauthorized for an additional 3 years. It took an additional 3 years for the next reauthorization to take place.

LEGISLATIVE AMENDMENTS OF 2016 (PL 114–144)

President Barack Obama signed the OAA Reauthorization Act of 2016 into law on April 19, 2016. A number of innovations and expansions of the OAA resulted in the amendments of 2016. They include innovations to the ADRCs, Senior Centers, Adult Protective Services, and funding formulas. The following section addresses these changes.

Aging and Disability Resource Centers

The OAA Amendments and reauthorization of 2016 also impacted the ADRCs in a few ways. Firstly, OAA reauthorization focused on improving the coordination with AAA with a goal of promoting independent living and home and community-based services. The Assistant Secretary of the Administration of Community Living is responsible for implementing ADRCs to provide accessible assistance regarding LTC options, navigating Medicare and Medicaid programs, and informing consumers about available home- and community-based services. This assistance to consumers assures that the older adult consumer population can retain broad autonomy and discretion when making choices about their care intervention.

The change from AoA, to the Administration for Community Living (ACL) brought into the fold individuals with disabilities. Thus, the language promoting the target population served by ADRC's also needed to be changed to better reflect the population of people with disabilities. Further amendments for the OAA reauthorization of 2016 included a change in definition of target consumers and moved from specifically having ADRCs serve primarily people who were older adults to "for older individuals and individuals with disabilities . . . and the caregivers of older individuals and individuals with disabilities."

Finally, additional language was added to ensure that ADRCs cooperate with AAA, centers for independent living, and other community-based organizations to support individuals "who are at risk for residing in, or who reside in, institutional settings, so that the individuals have the choice to remain in or to return to the community."

With the reauthorization, greater emphasis has been placed on providing assistance that includes information about federal and state home- and community-based services, and there were some minor changes on how person-centered counseling is defined. Language was also added that showed support for the value of home- and community-based services as part of the range of long-term support services.

Area Plans

Area plans are conducted every 3 years by AAAs and are used to help define and prioritize programs and services for delivery within the AAAs' catchment areas. The reauthorization of 2016 outlined more succinctly how AAAs should conduct area plans. It explicitly states that that AAAs should include in their plans activities and procedures to increase public awareness and remove barriers to prevention and investigation of, and response to, elder abuse, neglect, and exploitation in coordination with states, Title VII funding and activities, and other appropriate partners.

Disease Prevention and Health Promotion Services

Programs for disease prevention and health promotion should be "evidence based" if used within AAA or programs/services receiving funds from the local/regional AAAs. The addition of "oral health" to the OAA Title I definition of disease prevention and health promotion highlights that oral health is a crucial component of the health and wellness of older adults.

Behavioral health is also incorporated into the mental health provision of the OAA. In addition, substance abuse and suicide prevention are identified as components of the mental health spectrum.

Elder Abuse

The 2016 OAA reauthorization includes two new examples of activities that would be allowable uses of a state's Section 721 funding: the collection and submission of data related to abuse, neglect, and exploitation; and support and study of innovative practices to address abuse, neglect, and exploitation. Unfortunately, this additional language does not mandate the services or mean that they are required to be provided, so despite the expansion of ombudsman services, they may not be implemented as presented in the reauthorization.

Funding Formula

The formula grant distributions for Title III, Parts B, C1, C2, and D depend on the amount of funding appropriated for each, compared to the funding appropriated in the previous FY. During FY 2017–2019, all "hold harmless states/territories" received 99% of the prior year's funding amount. The "hold harmless" clause guarantees that each state/territory loses no more than 1% of its Title III funding (National Conference of State Legislatures [NCSL], 2016). Starting in FY 2020 and going forward (until there is a new reauthorization), the hold harmless amount will be the FY 2019 amount. Depending on the amount of the increase, some of these states/territories may no longer be included in the hold harmless category and instead may receive additional allocations based on the new population data. All other "population states/territories" will receive allocations based on new population data, after the minimum/hold harmless state/territory amounts are calculated. If the new FY's appropriation decreases by 1% or more compared to the previous FY, each state/territory will receive the prior year's funding, minus the same percentage as the overall decrease. These authorization levels are intended to provide guidance regarding the appropriate amount of funds to carry out the authorized activities of a program. The amount appropriated by Congress in each FY will determine the funding levels for ACL-funded programs.

Holocaust Survivors

Per the provision in Section 10 of the OAA, ACL will engage experts and organizations serving Holocaust survivors to solicit comments and input regarding this new provision. The goal of including this provision for funding in the reauthorization is to preserve the voices and experiences of this specific group of older adults (ACL, 2017; NORC, 2016).

Home- and Community-Based Services

Title IIIB, home- and community-based services, includes the terms "chronic condition self-care management, or falls prevention services." This language affirms that Title IIIB supportive services may include programs and services that relate to chronic condition self-care management and falls prevention. These activities were never excluded from Title IIIB services, but the new terminology and language now makes their inclusion clear.

Long-Term Care Ombudsman Program

The 2016 OAA reauthorization also made multiple changes and clarifications to the LTC Ombudsman Program authorized under Title VII of the Act. The changes in the 2016 reauthorization require the LTC Ombudsman Program to serve and protect all residents of LTC facilities without age limitations. Changes in the new reauthorization also helps protect confidentiality of the resident. Each ombudsman participating in the state ombudsman program is also required to undergo training provided by the National Ombudsman Resource Center. In addition, a provision within the 2016 reauthorization pushes the ACL to collect and analyze the reports received through its National Ombudsman

Reporting System (NORS) related to abuse, neglect, and exploitation in LTC facilities. These reports include numbers of complaints in these topic areas as well as narratives of case examples and systems-level advocacy work. ACL has made revisions to NORS' data collection tables that will be used starting on October 1, 2019 (NORC, 2018). These revised data instruments would collect additional relevant information (including information on perpetrators in abuse, neglect, or exploitation complaints) and significantly improve ACLs' ability to analyze complaint-related data (through collection of disaggregated data).

National Family Caregiver Support Program

Changes to the National Family Caregiver Support Program include updates in language to incorporate people with disabilities. The provision now includes individuals with disabilities, replaces "grandparents" as caregivers with "older relative caregivers," and also includes people 55 and older who are parents of people with disabilities. These definitions are intended to provide more opportunity for inclusivity.

Other changes include a language revision to clarify that a state may use not more than 10% of the total (both federal and nonfederal) dollars available to the state to provide support services to older-relative caregivers (Section 373 (g)(2)(C)).

Nutrition Services

The 2016 reauthorization included some changes to language related to home delivered meals, which now includes some supplemental foods that should be included *with* the meals, and not *in addition to* the meals. These may include nutritional supplements that are designed to enhance the nutritional status, but not supplement the foods. Another innovation is the use of a dietitian. Formerly, they were to provide advice on senior meal programs; however, this was revised in the current amendments to read to "utilize the expertise of a dietician or other individual with equivalent education and training . . . " This change means that states must use ("utilize") the expertise of such an individual, rather than just ask for ("solicit") that expertise.

Legal Assistance

Statutory language governing the Legal Assistance Development Program was retained, and the program is still in effect under Title VII Section 731 and Section 307(a)(13). The Section 702(c) authorization of appropriations specifically for the Legal Assistance Development Program was struck, and a new authorization for appropriations was added, combining Chapters 3 (Elder Abuse Prevention) and 4 (Legal Assistance Development) of the legislation.

Any nonprofit organization experienced in providing support and technical assistance on a nationwide basis to states, AAA, legal assistance providers, ombudsmen, elder abuse prevention programs, and other organizations interested in the legal rights of older individuals may receive an award under the revised language in Section 420(c).

Title IV Demonstration Projects

The OAA reauthorization also repealed three Title IV demonstration projects: computer training, multidisciplinary centers and multidisciplinary systems, and ombudsman and advocacy demonstration projects. Primarily, these changes related to out-of-date language. Since technology has grown in use by older adults, it was perceived that this training was no longer relevant for older adults. Although this rationale may be true in urban centers, there are still many older adults living in rural areas who do not have access to computers. Many of the other demonstration project initiatives have now moved into permanent components of the act.

PHILOSOPHICAL PARADIGMS IMPACTING LEGISLATIVE AMENDMENTS

In view of these legislative amendments to the OAA, one can ponder the philosophical paradigms that have been influential in these amendments. The OAA changed slowly and incrementally since the passage of the original act; thus, one can suggest that the philosophical paradigm known as *incrementalism* is at play. *Social welfare as a right* is also a philosophical paradigm at play within the development of the actual legislation and within the amendments over time, since the OAA was developed with the idea in mind that older adults deserve programs and services, given that they contributed to society and, with these programs and services, can remain healthy and living in their own homes. In addition, one may argue that street-level bureaucrats may have an influence on how the act is administered, since area and state plans have a tremendous influence in how services are prioritized and delivered from state to state and region to region.

SUMMARY

The OAA has been a significant piece of legislation that has impacted the face of services for older adults and enabled older adults at risk of institutionalization to remain within their homes and communities. Since the passage of the original act, the range of services has grown, and its reach has extended to a number of services within the community and noninstitutionalized environments.

USEFUL WEBSITES

Websites

The AoA's official website: www.aoa.gov

This is the official AoA website and provides an overview of specific links related to the administration of the OAA.

Family Caregiver Alliance, National Center for Caregiving: www.caregiver.org

This website provides an overview of the National Caregiver Support Program and materials and resources associated with this program. The program is one supported through amendments to the OAA.

ACL: Support to Caregivers: www.acl.gov/programs/support-caregivers

This website provides caregiver support information through the ACL. Resources include the National Family Caregiver Support Program, which funds services available to family and informal caregivers of older adults; and the Lifespan Respite Care Program, which aims to improve the quality and delivery of respite services that caregivers provide for older adults and people with disabilities.

National Association of AAA: www.n4a.org/

This is the official website of the national body organizing individual AAA. The organization attempts to provide some unity to local entities and helps bring policy to practice and from a national to local level.

YouTube Videos

OAA of 1965: www.bing.com/videos/search?q=utube+videos+on+the+older+americans+act&&view=detail&mid=0CF54E6D6A89FAFE59A50CF54E6D6A89FAFE59A5&rvsmid=44F1194B16747ED68ACE44F1194B16747ED68ACE&FORM=VDRVRV

This video presents an overview of the Older Adults Act of 1965 and provides the viewer with a rationale for the act and background to the issues which the act addresses for older adults.

OAA Reauthorization passes: www.bing.com/videos/search?q=utube+videos+on+the+older+americans+act&view=detail&mid=35952F84EABAE937CC7435952F84EABAE937CC74&FORM=VIRE

This video reviews the passage of the 2016 Amendments to the OAA and provides some of the backdrop to the stall tactics related to the OAA.

The OAA testimony by Bernie Sanders:www.bing.com/videos/search?q=utube+videos+on+the+older+americans+act&view=detail&mid=44F1194B16747ED68ACE44F1194B16747ED68ACE&FORM=VIRE

This video provides a presentation by then-Representative Bernie Sanders of Vermont, who introduced the Older Adult Act reauthorization to the House for reauthorization.

Podcast

John Smith discusses services from the Area Agencies on Aging. **Listen now:** https://bcove.video/2OTBv5d

DISCUSSION QUESTIONS

1. What programs and services would Gerry and Lorraine (cases presented at the beginning of the chapter) benefit from resulting from the OAA?
2. How are the programs and services similar and different for people if they are disabled versus older (60 years of age and older) resulting from the OAA?
3. Programs such as Meals on Wheels have been identified as not presenting positive outcomes for the users and criticized for not being cost effective. If you were Erica or Theresa, how would you begin to identify strategies to promote the effectiveness of this program?
4. What needs currently exist in your community that are not being met by either the OAA or the funding formula that disperses funds for the execution of programs and services related to mandates under the OAA?

REFERENCES

Administration for Community Living. (2017). *ACL guidance to the Aging Services Network: Outreach and service provision to Holocaust survivors*. Retrieved from http://www.acl.gov/sites/default/files/about-acl/2017-04/FINAL%20FOR%20POSTING%20-%20ACL%20Guidance%20-%20Holocaust%20Survivor%20Services%20-%201-12-17.pdf

Code of Federal Regulations. (n.d.). *Older Americans Act: Title III Regulations* (Title 45, 4, 45CFR1321). Washington, DC: Government Printing Office.

LEXIS-NEXIS Congressional Universe. (2000). *Older Americans Act*. Retrieved from http://web.lexis-nexis.com/congcomp/document

National Association of Area Agencies on Aging. (2006, July 10). *Side by side comparison of House and Senate Older Americans Act reauthorization bills*. Retrieved from http://www.i4ainfo.org/OAAsidebyside060710.pdf

National Conference of State Legislatures. (2016). *Summary of S. 192: The Older Americans Act Reauthorization Act of 2016*. Retrieved from http://www.ncsl.org/documents/standcomm/schealthhum/OAA_Reauth_ES.pdf

National Long-Term Care Ombudsman Resource Center. (2016). *Sec. 10. Guidance on serving Holocaust survivors*. Retrieved from http://ltcombudsman.org/uploads/files/issues/Section10-OAA-Reauthorization-Act-2016.pdf

National Long-Term Care Ombudsman Resource Center. (2018). *Revised NORS data collection effective October 1, 2019*. Retrieved from http://ltcombudsman.org/omb_support/nors/revised-nors-data-collection

Older Americans Act of 2006, Public Law No. 109–365, Congressional Record, Vol. 152, USC 3001, 2006.

Walker, E., Burns, F., & Wren, J. (2006). *Amendments to the Older Americans Act, PL 109–365. A presentation to the United States Administration on Aging*.

Yeo, T. (2016). Key changes of the Older Americans Act Reauthorization Act of 2016. *Bifocal*, *37*(6), 120–121.

8

The Americans With Disabilities Act

LEARNING OBJECTIVES

At the end of this chapter, readers will:

1. *Understand the history of the Americans with Disabilities Act (ADA).*
2. *Understand specific components of the ADA.*
3. *Understand how the ADA provides resources to older adults and people with disabilities.*

Erica and Theresa are trying to understand how the Americans with Disabilities Act (ADA) has had an impact for people within both urban and rural communities. They explore the dynamics and provisions of the Public Law, and at the same time, understand how the Act provides opportunities for people with disabilities. The two cases they examined were "Susan" and "Joan."

Susan: Susan is a 57-year-old woman who has sustained a work-related injury that has affected her knees and mobility. In addition to her own mobility impairment, she lives with her older parents, Irma and Gus. Gus was diagnosed with early stages of Alzheimer's disease about 10 years ago, and it has progressed to the point where he is mobility impaired and needs constant supervision. Irma is a brittle diabetic and cannot handle the care needs of her husband, so she relies mostly on Susan for help. They lived on a farm, but now the family has moved to a metropolitan area. Susan has five adult siblings, but she is the only one who lives with their parents. Susan is able to work at a full-time job as a result of the ADA.

Joan: Joan currently lives in Ohio, and manages independently, despite a car accident that left her with a severe head injury 36 years ago. Joan became a parent shortly after her head injury, and she often suffers from aphasia. She currently lives in her own home with her adult son.

Joan has been disabled for 36 years, but she has been able to function at home with minimal supports and work as an emergency care foster worker, thanks to the ADA. She also received assistance with shopping and utilizing public services and enjoys frequent travel to see her son in St. Louis or present at local, regional, and national conferences for the Head Injury Association. These opportunities would not be possible without utilizing benefits afforded through the ADA.

 DOI:10.1891/9780826128393.0008

THE INTERSECTION BETWEEN DISABILITY AND AGING

Increasingly, people with activity limitations (one or more limitations to their activities of daily living), or limitations to mobility due to chronic disabilities, will opt to remain in the community. Consequently, community-based options have been influenced by the philosophical paradigms driving the independent living movements over the past half-century. Increasingly, Centers for Independent Living are also providing resources to adults over the age of 60 for the sole purpose of making their lives more comfortable within a community-based setting.

HISTORY OF THE DISABILITY MOVEMENT

Prior to World War II, people with disabilities or chronic healthcare needs were dehumanized and often left to the care of the Poor House or Settlement Movement, despite the prevailing notion that these individuals should be cared for by the state, an idea resulting from the Elizabethan Poor Laws. Despite these acts of charity, returning soldiers from World War I were not content with the status quo arrangement to be admitted and remain in a nursing home. Hence in the late 1940s activists began to argue for training the veteran to be a productive citizen and to be a part of their entire community (Jurkowski, 1987). Despite the provisions of the Rehabilitation Act of 1978, some people were not able to return to productive work: thus they returned to a nursing care facility. Lex Frieden, a paraplegic himself, questioned the validity of this approach and made the argument that every person deserved the right to remain in the community with community-based supports (Jurkowski, 1987). This then led to the development of the Independent Living Movement, which gained momentum and popularity following the civil rights legislation in the 1960s (Albrecht, 1992; Essex-Sorlie, 1994), and a prelude to the Americans with Disabilities Act (ADA).

The Rehabilitation Act of 1973 was a precursor to the ADA. It was considered at the time, a piece of civil rights legislation which provided some recognition for the need to address architectural barriers and environmental conditions which would limit the ability for people to travel freely within the built environment and community. The Rehabilitation Act of 1973 (Dinitto, 2016) also addressed the need for training/retraining for civilians in need of academic training or upgrades in order to become competitive within the workplace. However, despite individual with disabilities being qualified for jobs, discrimination still existed in terms of the employment sector, and the Rehabilitation Act of 1973 did not go far enough in terms of addressing employer discrimination.

The Individuals with Disabilities Education Act (IDEA) of 1975 provided for educational opportunities to reach children with disabilities within public settings. However, the upper limits of education ended once students reached 21 years of age (Dinitto, 2016). Once again, the limits of this piece of legislation did not address the needs of people once they aged out of the educational system, leaving countless people with disabilities marginalized and segregated from community opportunities.

THE JOURNEY TOWARD THE AMERICANS WITH DISABILITIES ACT

In the later 1980s, prior to the signing of the ADA, more than 43 million Americans had one or more physical disabilities and it was anticipated that as people age, this number would only increase. Coupled with this staggering number was the reality that historically, society has had a tendency to isolate and/or segregate people with disabilities.

Regardless of movements such as the Independent Living movement (DeJong, 1979) discrimination and segregation toward people with disabilities continued to be a pervasive social issue. In addition, discrimination against people with disabilities had a pervasive impact financially both in terms of dependency and under-productivity for people with disabilities. These issues grew as people with disabilities were considered across the life span, and people who were older adults and those with a disability were more likely to be discriminated against.

THE AMERICANS WITH DISABILITIES ACT OF 1990

The ADA of 1990 was established to fulfill a fourfold purpose

1. To provide a clear and comprehensive national mandate for the elimination of discrimination against individuals with disabilities.
2. To provide clear, strong, consistent, enforceable standards addressing discrimination against individuals with disabilities.
3. To ensure that the federal government plays a central role in enforcing the standards established in this act on behalf of individuals with disabilities.
4. To invoke the sweep of congressional authority, including the power to enforce the Fourteenth Amendment and to regulate commerce, in order to address the major areas of discrimination faced day-to-day by people with disabilities (U.S. Department of Justice, 1999).

Disability, within ADA, refers to a physical or mental impairment that substantially limits one or more major life activities for a person. ADA's basic definition of "disability" is an impairment that substantially limits one or more major life activities; a record of such an impairment; or being regarded as having such an impairment. However, it changes the way that the statutory terms should be interpreted. The ADA excludes people with substance use or chronic drug histories from being addressed or covered within this Act (U.S. Department of Labor, 2007).

The ADA of 1990 (Public Law 101–336), signed into law by President George H. W. Bush, consists of five specific titles. Title I lays out provisions within the area of employment; Title II relates to public services; Title III focuses upon public accommodations and services operated by private entities; Title IV relates to accommodations; and Title V relates to miscellaneous provisions. This segment will lay out some of the provisions within each of the titles.

Title I: Employment

Title I attempts to ensure that individuals are not discriminated against within the employment sector as a result of their disability. Reasonable accommodations must be made for individuals with a disability who are qualified to perform the essential functions of a specific job. Reasonable accommodations are also specified within Title I, which includes making existing job resources accessible to the individual and restructuring the job so as to accommodate the handicapping condition for the individual. Accommodation also includes acquiring or modifying equipment or devices, adjusting training materials to provide for the person with a disability, or providing qualified readers and interpreters when necessary. Employers can be exempt, however, if they can prove undue hardship financially on their business if accommodations are pursued.

An employer is required to make an accommodation to the known disability of a qualified applicant or employee if it would not impose an "undue hardship" on the operation of the employer's business. Undue hardship is defined as an action requiring significant difficulty or expense when considered in light of factors such as an employer's size, financial resources, and the nature and structure of its operation. An employer is not required to lower quality or production standards to make an accommodation, nor is an employer obligated to provide personal use items such as glasses or hearing aids.

Title II: Public Services

Title II of ADA provides for accommodations within the transportation arena. According to Title II of ADA, all new public transit buses and rail cars ordered after August 26, 1990 must be accessible to individuals with disabilities. In addition, local transportation authorities must provide comparable paratransit or other special transportation services to individuals with disabilities who cannot use fixed route bus services, unless they can prove that an undue burden would result from providing these services. Rail transportation systems existing at the time of the signing of the ADA were required to have at least one accessible car per train by July 26, 1995. While there is not much that can be expected of existing train and bus stations, new bus and train stations were to be accessible. Within this segment of Title II, key stations in rapid, light, and commuter rail systems had to be made accessible by July 26, 1993, with extensions up to 20 years for commuter rail (30 years for rapid and light rail). All existing Amtrak stations had to be accessible by July 26, 2010. State and local governments may not discriminate against qualified individuals with disabilities. All government facilities, services, and communications must be accessible consistent with the requirements of Section 504 of the Rehabilitation Act of 1973. As of 2018, some of these deadlines have been met, with at least some of the carriers and some of the accessibility required for the disabled. As rail cars, buses, and other public transportation modalities are upgraded, their replacements are now and have been accessible.

Title III: Public Accommodations and Services Offered Through Private Entities

Within Title III of the ADA, private entities such as restaurants, hotels, and retail stores may not discriminate against individuals with disabilities; this requirement has been in effect since January 26, 1992. Reasonable modifications must be made to policies, practices, or procedures to avoid discriminating unless a fundamental alteration to the nature of the goods or services would result. In addition, auxiliary aids and services must be provided to ensure effective communication with individuals with disabilities that substantially limit the ability to communicate, such as vision, hearing, or speech impairments, unless an undue burden or a fundamental alteration would result. Physical barriers in existing facilities must be removed if removal is readily achievable. If not, alternative methods of providing the services must be offered if they are readily achievable. All new construction and alterations of facilities had to be accessible as of 1998.

Title IV: Telecommunications

Companies offering telephone service to the general public must offer telephone relay services to allow communications access for people with speech and hearing impairments who cannot use telephones. Closed captioning is also required by "any television public service announcement that is produced or funded in whole or in part by any agency or instrumentality of Federal Government" for public service announcements.

Title V: Miscellaneous Provisions

Title V of the ADA covers items such as building construction, prohibition against retaliation and coercion, federal wilderness areas, treatment of transvestites, the illegal use of drugs, amendments to the Rehabilitation Act of 1973, coverage of Congress and the agencies of the legislative branch, and alternative means of dispute resolution and severability.

IMPLICATIONS OF THE AMERICANS WITH DISABILITIES ACT ON THE AGING AND OLDER ADULT POPULATIONS

The ADA, although originally intended for a community-based population of individuals with disabilities, also has numerous implications for older adults who acquire mobility and sensory disabilities. A number of implications can be identified within each of the titles. In the next segment of this chapter, we review implications of the ADA for an older adult population.

Title I: Employment

Individuals qualify for services under the Older Adults Act when they reach 60 years of age. Ironically, the same definition of older adult is not followed in the administration of retirement benefits from Social Security, whose effective date is becoming later and will eventually be at least 67 years of age. It is possible that one may develop some mobility or sensory problems during the course of this lapse in time, in which case job modifications will be required. Older adults may also develop chronic health issues, such as stroke or sensory impairment, that would require employers to provide job modifications in order to accommodate them. Under Title I, individuals with some physical and sensory impairments could not be discriminated against when seeking employment on the basis of some condition that may be detected during a company physical. This can also be an advantage for older adults, since many health conditions begin to emerge in one's 40s, 50s, and 60s. Hence, the ADA and its provisions under Title I can be a real asset to protect older workers.

Title II: Public Services

The implications of Title II for older adults have the most impact in the area of transportation and preserving one's dignity and autonomy. Lack of ability to travel in one's own vehicle, or the loss of one's driver's license can be a tremendous blow to one's autonomy and impact one's ability to travel independently through one's community. Transportation systems within both urban and rural communities that can accommodate people with disabilities can be a tremendous asset to maintaining one in their home and within their community. In addition, transportation systems such as rail and air can assure that older adults continue to travel and maintain recreational outlets previously enjoyed by people in their younger years. With the increase in family mobility these days, more and more older adults travel and want to remain active with their loved ones. Accommodations to public transportation services make this possible and increase the likelihood that people with some mobility impairments are able to travel freely using rail or public transportation systems.

Title III: Public Accommodations and Services Offered Through Private Entities

Title III also promotes the inclusion of older adults into community-based activities. Public accommodations such as parking spaces, curb cuts, and longer period of time to travel across streets with traffic lights, although simple changes, make it possible for older adults to continue to participate within the community. Accommodations available to older adults to assist with some "instrumental activities of daily living" (Katz, 1983) can include assistance within stores when shopping, banking, doing laundry at public facilities, or traveling to churches or local recreational events. Architectural barriers are also minimized as a result of Title III and can have a profound effect on one's ability to navigate a community.

Title IV: Telecommunications

Title IV enables older adults the opportunity to enjoy major communication with a wealth of resources, which may not necessarily be possible without this piece of legislation. Aging individuals with sensory impairments will be able to enjoy television as a result of the closed caption subtitles. People who have hearing deficits will be able to carry on conversations with loved ones or conduct business transactions as a result of Text Telephone (TTY) relay equipment.

In the decades to come, the ADA will become much more significant within the lives of people who are aging with a disability. As more people who are aging and who have disabilities remain living in the community, increasing numbers of people will utilize services from the disability resource community. One specific provision for access has occurred through the Aging and Disability Resource Centers (ADRCs) legislated by Congress in 2002.

THE AMERICANS WITH DISABILITIES ACT AMENDMENTS OF 2008

The ADA Amendments Act of 2008 broadened the scope of who is considered disabled under the law passed in 1990. When considering whether a person is disabled, the law required that people ignore the beneficial effects of any mitigating measures (except ordinary eyeglasses and contact lenses) the person uses. Within the consideration of whether one is substantially limited in a major life activity that would make the individual disabled under the law, the 2008 amendments required the consideration of bodily functions as well as other major life activities, and having one major life activity substantially limited is sufficient to be recognized as disabled. For those whose condition is episodic or in remission, the law requires consideration of the person's limitations as they are when the condition is in an active state.

Some of the specific amendments within the 2008 legislation include expansion of accessibility requirements for recreational facilities such as swimming pools, golf courses, exercise clubs, and boating facilities. They also set standards for the use of wheelchairs and other mobility devices in public spaces and changed the standards for things such as selling tickets to events and reserving accessible hotel rooms to accommodate for patrons with disabilities. The new rules also clearly defined "service animal" as "any dog that is individually trained to do work or perform tasks for the benefit of an individual with a disability, including a physical, sensory, psychiatric, intellectual, or other mental disability." This portion of the law also states that the services the service animal provides must be "directly related to the handler's disability" and dogs that provide only emotional support or crime deterrence cannot be defined as service animals.

Specific changes within the titles include the following.

Title 1

The impact on the legislation amendments of 2008 on Title I has largely helped clarify what types of functionality and behavioral components should be addressed in order to understand when and how a person is or is not functioning within the workplace. It also helps clarify what types of issues require address within the workplace when modifications are required for specific accommodations.

Title II

Although the provisions to public service entities such as publicly funded railways, airlines, government services, and so on did not change, but the definition of disability did change to provide more clarity as to what a disability is. Consequently, it becomes easier to identify when a person with a specifically defined disability is or is not being served appropriately and when that person is being discriminated against.

Title III

Under Title III, private services, while there is no specific expansion of the types of services which require address. The clarification within the definition of disability makes it less confusing to identify when one is being discriminated against. Title III prohibits discrimination among individuals living with a disability in places of public accommodation. Public accommodations include privately owned, leased or operated facilities such as hotels, restaurants, retail merchants, doctor's offices, golf courses, private schools, day care centers, health clubs, sports stadiums, and movie theaters. The title also sets the minimum standards for accessibility for alterations and new construction of commercial facilities and privately owned public accommodations and the public accommodations are required to remove barriers in existing buildings where easy to do so without difficulty or expense.

Title IV

Title IV of the ADA is controlled by the Federal Communication Commission and requires closed captioning of federally funded public service announcements. In addition, telephone and Internet companies are required to provide a nationwide system of interstate and intrastate telecommunications relay service that allows for communication over the telephone by individuals with hearing and speech disabilities as result of the updates to the original ADA of 1990.

Title V

Under Title V, definitions of disability and requirements for construction are more clearly laid out and articulated. Provision for retaliation and dispute are also addressed with the legislation. Some specific regulations (Sections 508 and 511) prevent sexual orientations and gender identity disorders from being defined as disabilities. Title V also more clearly articulates provisions for discrimination.

Erica and Theresa considered the case scenarios of Susan and Joan. Using these as case studies, they decided that these scenarios benefited from at least the first four titles of the Americans with Disabilities Act (ADA). For example, Susan required workplace modifications in order for her to retain her position with her employer. Under the ADA, she benefited from a workplace where accommodations to her knee injuries were made to her job so that she could continue to work without being on her feet for most of the workday. Her parents benefited because they were able to utilize government offices that had elevators and offices within short walking distances. Joan was also able to take her parents to local establishments to enjoy dinner and theater (private accommodations under Title III). Lastly, her hard-of-hearing father was able to use closed captioning (Title IV) when watching movies while she and her mother quilted in the quiet of their fabric paradise.

A review of this case provided both Erica and Theresa with some ideas of how the ADA would enhance the lifestyles and community integration of people with mobility and ability challenges. Ericka and Theresa both felt that they were beginning to understand more fully how the ADA provided enhanced opportunities for community living.

AGING AND DISABILITY RESOURCE CENTERS

In response to the growing numbers of older adults with disabilities found in communities, the Centers for Medicaid and Medicare, in conjunction with the Administration on Aging, have developed a cooperative grant program to support and assist states in efforts to create a single coordinated system of care and long-term support. This system provides funding for ADRCs. The goal of these centers is to provide a single, coordinated system of information and access for people seeking long-term support. This approach reduces confusion and maximizes opportunities for older adults and their families to make informed choices. As of fall 2006, 43 states had received ADRC initiative grants. Planning grants were awarded in 2003, 2004, and 2005, with another round awarded in 2006. By 2017, all states had access to ADRCs and over 1,300 now exist across the country. Table 8.1 lists states that have been awarded the original ADRC grants, which is important because these states were pioneer in their efforts to provide ADRC resources. This concept had become so popular, that the most current reauthorization of the Older Americans Act (see Chapter 7) included funds to encourage the aging community to build resources and collaborate with the disability movement and Centers for Independent Living on initiatives toward building ADRCs. Appendix E provides a contact list for all current ADRCs in the United States.

Some of the activities undertaken through the ADRCs include information, referral, and educational services. Some of the anticipated outcomes of these projects include the following

- Maximize the abilities of older people, persons with physical disabilities, and persons with developmental disabilities to make informed choices and to meet their long-term care needs.
- Provide direct assistance to family caregivers in planning for the future needs of family members who have physical disabilities and/or developmental disabilities.
- Enable consumers to choose services tailored to their needs through tools connecting them to streamlined assessment.
- Enable consumers to experience less confusion and enhance their choices since they will receive information in a timelier way.

Table 8.1 Original States That Have Received ADRC Grants

State	Year Grant Received
Louisiana	2003
Maine	2003
Maryland	2003
Massachusetts	2003
Minnesota	2003
Montana	2003
New Hampshire	2003
New Jersey	2003
Pennsylvania	2003
Rhode Island	2003
South Carolina	2003
West Virginia	2003
Alaska	2004
Arkansas	2004
California	2004
Florida	2004
Georgia	2004
Illinois	2004
Indiana	2004
Iowa	2004
New Mexico	2004
North Carolina	2004
Northern Marina Islands	2004
Wisconsin	2004
Alabama	2005
Arizona	2005
Colorado	2005
District of Columbia	2005

(*continued*)

Table 8.1 Original States That Have Received ADRC Grants (*continued*)

State	Year Grant Received
Guam	2005
Hawaii	2005
Idaho	2005
Kansas	2005
Kentucky	2005
Michigan	2005
Mississippi	2005
Nevada	2005
Ohio	2005
Tennessee	2005
Texas	2005
Vermont	2005
Virginia	2005
Washington	2005
West Virginia	2005

ADRCs, Aging and Disability Resource Centers.

- Enable the long-term care system of services to be managed through a single, coordinated method of intake, assessment, and eligibility with quality monitoring through centralized data collection and evaluation.
- Develop databases that will enable professionals to have access to a single, coordinated system of intake, assessment, and eligibility.
- Improve capacity for state and local governments to connect consumers to needed services and supports from publicly and privately funded services.
- Increase the number of physicians and other professionals who refer their patients and clients to the resource centers.
- Develop nonstigmatizing public places of service that can be used to promote independence and accessibility by a range of diverse people.
- Promote the accessibility of information and assistance by both public- and private-pay individuals.
- Develop a sustainable single coordinated system of information and access for all persons seeking long-term support.
- Increase the numbers of elderly/disabled individual living in their own homes in their own communities.

- Increase early planning for long-term care.
- Increase referrals of persons over 60 to community mental health centers (CMHC).
- Streamline access to long-term support services.
- Improve outreach to underserved populations.
- Empower individuals in need, or planning for long-term supports, to make informed choices.
- Reduce and potentially eliminate barriers to community living and support consumer-driven home- and community-based service options.
- Develop technology systems, forms, software, and other necessary tools to provide streamlined access to all long-term care services.
- Increase collaboration among providers of services to the aging and people with disabilities.
- Improve marketing and public awareness campaigns related to aging and disability.
- Increase requests for information, referral to services, and enrollments in home- and community-based service.
- Improve knowledge for health and long-term support professionals and others providing services to the elderly and people with disabilities.
- Maximize consumer choice and provide services in a consumer-friendly manner, respecting and ensuring dignity of all served.
- Create a more balanced system of long-term care to include more home- and community-based services.

Key stakeholder groups involved within the aging and disability networks include the following

- Representatives of aging and disability advocacy groups
- Departments on aging
- Departments of human services
- Departments of public aid
- Departments of public health
- Departments of rehabilitation services
- Area agencies on aging
- Benefit-planning assistance outreach programs
- State health assistance programs
- Employment centers
- Alzheimer's associations
- Community service providers
- Long-term care ombudsmen
- Developmental disabilities councils
- Independent living centers
- State assistance technology projects
- Housing development authorities
- AARP
- Local university and community college programs

The ADRC Technical Assistance Exchange (TAE) supports ADRC program grantees. Some of the resources that the TAE will provide for the ADRC include technical assistance for one-on-one support, weekly newsletters, semiannual ADRC national meetings, and monthly Webcasts (Table 8.2).

Table 8.2 An Overview of Components and Elements of an ADRC

I&R/A
- Formal marketing plan for all ages, income levels, disability types - Marketing to and serving private paying populations - Systematic information and referral processes provided across all operating organizations - Follow-up on information and referral services - Online comprehensive resource database, public and searchable
Options counseling and assistance
- \Formal standards and protocols guiding delivery to all income levels and disabilities - Short-term support in crisis/urgent situations (preventing institutionalization) - Follow-up on options counseling services - Futures planning for LTSS needs
Streamlined eligibility determination for public programs
- Coordinated/integrated process for financial and functional eligibility - Standardized intake and screening across all operating organizations - Uniform criteria to assess risk of institutionalization - Functional eligibility determined on-site or through seamless referral process - Personalized assistance in financial application completion - Financial eligibility determined on-site or through electronic exchange - Applicants tracked through determination process; follow-up with ineligible individuals
Person-centered transition support
- Formal agreements with critical pathway providers and protocols for providing transitions support, referral processes, and staff training - Local contact agency designation (MDS 3.0 Section Q)
Consumer populations, partnerships, and stakeholder involvement
- Staff with capacity and training to serve all ages and disability types - Consumer involvement in program design, operation, and quality improvement - Formal partnership agreements, protocols, or contracts with • Critical Aging and Disability Organizations • Medicaid • SHIP, APS, and 2-1-1 • VA Medical Center(s)
Quality assurance and continuous improvement

(*continued*)

Table 8.2 An Overview of Components and Elements of an ADRC (*continued*)

- Formal sustainability plan with diverse funding sources
- Adequate staffing and management
- Continuous quality improvement plan and procedures in effect
- IT/MIS supports all program functions and routine state level performance tracking
- Routine local level performance tracking

ADRC, Aging and Disability Resource Centers; APS, Adult Protective Services; I&R/A, Information, referral, and awareness; SHIP, State Health Insurance Assistance Program; VA, Veteran's Administration.

Source: Aging and Disability Resource Center: Technical Assistance exchange. Retieved from https://www.nasuad.org.

SUMMARY

The ADA, while groundbreaking, was not initially intended for people with disabilities rather than for older adults. As time progressed, however, the benefits of the ADA were much more far-reaching than originally intended, especially for aging adults with disabilities. The individual titles of the ADA have had some dramatically positive and specific impact for older adults wishing to remain in their homes or in their communities as long as possible. Although the ADA is still in its young adulthood, the benefits of the ADA have only grown as new and further linkages, such as the ADRCs, have developed in all regions of the United States.

USEFUL WEBSITES

Disability Resources—Office of Disability Employment Policy, U.S. Department of Labor: www.disability.gov

This online connection provides a link to the U.S. government's disability-related information and resources. It serves as a one-stop Web site for information to a range of groups including people with disabilities, their families, employers, service providers, and others. This site was developed following President George W. Bush's New Freedom Initiative, in an effort to support its goals.

ADA Guidelines: www.access-board.gov

This website provides a comprehensive listing of accessibility guidelines as defined in the ADA accessibility standards.

ADA Technical Assistance Program: www.ada.gov/taprog.htm

This website provides a comprehensive resource for information on the ADA and information about accessible technology. The site enables one to use a drop-down menu to find a specific state and secure information specific to that state.

U.S. Department of Justice, ADA Home Page: www.ada.gov

This website, a federal resource, provides a comprehensive guide to standards, regulations, and status in the implementation of the ADA. It includes information on ADA design standards; ADA information line; technical assistance programs; enforcement of the ADA; ADA business connection; new and proposed regulations, ADA mediation programs, and links to other federal agencies with ADA responsibilities, including the Equal Employment Opportunity Commission (EEOC), Department of Transportation (DOT), telephone relay service (FCC), education, healthcare, and labor.

ADRCs: www.n4a.org/adrcs
This website provides a link to information about ADRCs and the TAE. It provides contact information for consumers, information about the ADRC grant program, information about the TAE program, and links to helpful background information that supports the ADRC.

ADDITIONAL RESOURCES

YouTube Videos

The ADA of 1990: www.youtube.com/watch?v=eq0pBEJoCvY
This video goes through a short summary of the components of the ADA of 1990. It provides a visual representation of many of the specific innovations that transform society through this legislation for people with disabilities.

The Signing of the ADA, July 26, 1990: www.youtube.com/watch?v=dFKicqqVME8
This YouTube video goes through a series of vignettes that showcase the process and victory of the signing of the ADA. It includes a number of key stakeholders and key actors in the process leading up to the signing of the ADA of 1990.

What the ADA Means for People Living in Communities: www.youtube.com/watch?v=FFoKBF6MRHY
This video showcases specific aspects of our community and provides an overview of the impacts of the ADA for people living within communities.

Life Before the ADA: www.youtube.com/watch?v=pa1UH__mqv0
This video, narrated by Senator Tom Harkin, summarizes how life existed for people with disabilities prior to the passage of the ADA. It provides the viewer with specific aspects of American life and how they were impacted for people with disabilities by not having a specific set of laws to protect them from discrimination.

Podcasts

Kathy Hughes discusses living with a head injury and the Americans with Disabilities Act. **Listen now:** https://bcove.video/2OUItqk

Dr. Anthony Agbeh discusses dealing with travel accommodations through the Americans with Disabilities Act. **Listen now:** https://bcove.video/2DzKc2w

DISCUSSION QUESTIONS

1. The text reviews some of the impacts and advantages of the *Americans with Disabilities Act* (ADA) for Susan and Joan. Can you think of other areas for which the legislation provides both protection and benefits to these two women in their everyday lives?
2. Although the ADA was initially designed for people with disabilities, the legislation benefits people across the lifespan and has benefits for people advancing in age. Can you identify some benefits in addition to the ones discussed in this chapter?

(*continued*)

DISCUSSION QUESTIONS *(continued)*

3. Take a few hours and explore your campus and business community to identify innovations in the community to make accessibility easier for people with disabilities. What specifically are these innovations? How do these innovations help people be more fully integrated into community life?
4. What gaps still exist in your community with respect to providing accessibility? What recommendations can you make to have these gaps addressed?

REFERENCES

Albrecht, G. L. (1992). *The disability business: Rehabilitation in America*. Thousand Oaks, CA: Sage.

DeJong, G. (1979). Independent living: From social movement to analytic paradigm. *Archives of Physical Medicine and Rehabilitation, 60*, 435–446.

Dinitto, E. (2016). *Social welfare and social policy*. San Francisco, CA: Cengage.

Essex-Sorlie, D. (1994). The Americans with Disabilities Act: History, summary, and key components. *Academic Medicine, 68*(7), 519–524. doi:10.1097/00001888-199407000-00001

Jurkowski, E. T. (1987). *Leadership and community participation for people with and without disabilities*. Ann Arbor, MI: Dissertation Abstracts International.

Katz, S. (1983). Assessing self-maintenance: Activities of daily living, mobility, and instrumental activities of daily living. *Journal of American Geriatric Sociology, 31*, 721–727. doi:10.1111/j.1532-5415.1983.tb03391.x

Aging and Disability Resource Center: Technical Assistance exchange. (n.d.) Retieved from https://www.nasuad.org

U.S. Department of Justice. (1999). *ADA regulations and technical assistance*. Retrieved from http://www.usdoj.gov/crt/ada/publicat.html

U.S. Department of Labor. (2007). *The Americans with Disabilities Act of 1990*. Retrieved from http://www.dol.gov/esa/regs/statutes/ofccp/ada.htm

9

Mental Health: The Community Mental Health Act

LEARNING OBJECTIVES

At the end of this chapter, readers will:

1. *Understand the history of the Community Mental Health Centers Act and other mental health (MH)-related legislation.*
2. *Understand specific components of the Community Mental Health Act and other MH-related legislation.*
3. *Understand how legislation related to MH provides resources to older adults and people with disabilities.*

Nora: *Nora is both a caregiver to her 87-year-old father and disabled due to an orthopedic injury while riding a bicycle. Her recent knee replacement surgery has left her with less mobility in her right knee than prior to her surgery. Being caregiver to her father leaves her with limited emotional resources at the end of a day. Nora's father is legally blind, suffers from Crone's disease, and has had a series of mini strokes. They live together in the three-bedroom family home and receive in-home services to support Nora in her caregiving role. Nora's mother passed away 10 years ago, and she also helps in the caregiving role for her two grandsons. Nora's father was emotionally distant to her while growing up as an only child. Nora's father also attends a day program 3 days per week.*

Gerry: *Gerry was born with Cerebral Palsy and Hydrocephalus. During the first year of his life, a shunt was surgically implanted into his skull, however the shunt needs to be replaced periodically. Gerry is on Social Security Disability and receives funding monthly. Gerry lives in a rural community, attends Master level classes in Rehabilitation Studies at a local university, and mobilizes himself with an electric wheelchair. He boasts that he is 38 years of age—1 year younger than Jack Benny!*

Lorraine: *Lorraine is a 96-year-old woman who has survived the Holocaust and currently lives in Fort Myers, Florida. Lorraine moved into an Assisted Living facility 2 years ago, when she lost her driving privileges and had been reported to be falling within her home. She is renting her family home to her adult grandson. Lorraine, a divorcee lived in an abusive relationship for most of her 27 years of marriage.*

© Springer Publishing Company DOI:10.1891/9780826128393.0009

How would the MH needs of both Nora and her father be dealt with in this case scenario considering MH needs? Let us look at the concept of MH in this chapter and identify at the end of the chapter how to handle these case situations.

WHAT IS MENTAL HEALTH?

The concept of mental health (MH), especially MH for older adults, has evolved over time. The same holds true of legislation to play a role in the preservation of MH conditions for older adults. This chapter explores some of the changes in legislation over time and some of the currently mandated/legislated programs available for older adults in the United States.

Definition of Mental Health

MH can be defined as the successful performance of mental function, resulting in productive activities, fulfilling relationships with other people, and the ability to adapt to change and to cope with adversity, from early childhood to late life (United States Department of Health and Human Services [USDHHS], 1999). The *Surgeon General's Report on Mental Health* was a seminal report released in 1999, which provided a blueprint for the development of services, research, and policy in the MH arena, including older adults. There are four overarching themes in the report

1. A public health perspective.
2. The realization that mental disorders are disabling.
3. The realization that MH and illness are on a continuum.
4. The realization that the mind and body are inseparable.

Although the concepts of utilizing a public health perspective, considering mental disorders as potentially chronic, and moving from a labeling perspective to a continuum of care seem obvious and practical, these are actually new concepts and paradigms, which have not a been historically valued or represented in legislative efforts.

Paradigms of Mental Health

As we move through history, various paradigms have affected legislative efforts within the MH legislative arena (Geller, 2000). Institutionalization was once the preferred mode of intervention, and thus legislative efforts focused on institutional care rather than community care. Elements of this paradigm probably affected the development of institutions that housed people with mental illness and older adults with chronic depression or mental illness.

The medical model prevails within most of the legislative efforts since disease-specific diagnostic categories generally serve as eligibility criteria. In the medical model, disease or illness is treated medically and is not otherwise reversible. In many of the early legislative efforts for MH initiatives, the concept of disease prevailed and played a critical role in the eligibility for disability benefits through Social Security Insurance (SSI).

The advent of psychotropic medications led to the deinstitutionalization movement and paradigm. In this paradigm, hospital care is limited, and the notion of having people move back into their home environments is the key. The advent of psychotropic medications unleashed the potential for chronically mentally ill patients to participate in the community. An example of where this paradigm plays a role is with Medicare options for mental healthcare. Within Medicare Part A, inpatient day treatment is limited, with partial hospitalization being the preferred mode of care and treatment. Many of the community day hospital programs and community MH programs administered through the Community Mental Health Act are based on the deinstitutionalization paradigm since the goal is to treat people outside the institution and within community settings.

The rehabilitation paradigm makes the argument that people have the potential to be capable of returning to meaningful activities outside of a treatment setting and within the community, given the appropriate therapeutic options. This concept places value and dignity upon individuals and their unique value to their community and social support network.

The civil rights movement paradigm sets the tone for treatment options to be a right, not a privilege for individuals. This paradigm flows directly from the civil rights movement, whereby individuals regardless of color, ability, or gender should be granted the same rights and privileges as people considered in the dominant majority of the population. This movement, which piggybacked onto the Vietnam War protests, used the "window of opportunity" to push forward issues for people representing diverse groups.

The self-help and peer support paradigm relies upon peer helpers and supports to move through or assist in the rehabilitation process, rather than relying solely on professional intervention. Some state-based programs that operate with gero-psychiatry also operate peer support groups modeled after either the Alcoholic Anonymous concept or the GROW group (https://grow.ie/the-12-steps-to-recovery) concept.

Demedicalization is a paradigm that attempts to move issues outside of the medical arena and examine the person in the environment, pointing to environmental causes for specific issues of concern.

Consumerism is a paradigm that suggests the consumer is a key player and/or partner in the rehabilitation or intervention process. Consumers are at the forefront of the planning and evaluation process within service development and delivery. President Bush's Freedom Commission Initiative is based upon the paradigm of consumerism.

The independent living paradigm makes the argument that all people, regardless of their functioning level, have the ability to participate in the community with the right community-based supports (DeJong, 1979). Assertive community treatment programs work with this paradigm in mind.

HISTORY OF LEGISLATIVE EFFORTS AFFECTING OLDER ADULTS AND OTHERS WITH MENTAL DISORDERS

The earliest indications of legislative efforts within a progressive venue for people with MH issues and older adults suffering from mental illness can be seen with the initial federal legislation that provided land grants for mental institutions, initially on the East Coast, and eventually across the United States. This initiative was spearheaded by a social change reformer, Dorothea Dix. Dix lobbied for the appropriation of land grants from the federal government to state governments in order to provide for land that could be used to build state-based institutions. In 1840, there were only eight asylums for the insane in the United States. Dorothea Dix's crusading led to establishment or enlargement of 32 mental hospitals and transfer of the mentally ill from poorhouses and jails. These institutions would thus serve to protect people with MH issues and provide them a place to convalesce. The paradigms of institutionalization and medical model can be seen as prevalent themes within the context of care here; however, at the point in history when these programs were developed, it seemed reasonable to develop structural opportunities within which people could be somewhat protected from the stigma that prevailed in communities (Gollaher, 1995).

The Community Mental Health Act of 1946 laid the groundwork for policies to address institutionalization and hospitalization for people suffering from mental illness or psychiatric conditions. Through this act, the general status of MH was addressed in order to improve the MH of U.S. citizens through research into the causes, diagnosis, and treatment of psychiatric disorders. The Act also authorized the Surgeon General to support research, training, and assistance to state MH programs (Pub. L. No. 79–487, 60 Stat. L. 421). The National Institute of Mental Health (NIMH) was established under the authority of this law on April 15, 1949. This was followed shortly thereafter with the Hospital Survey and Construction Act (Hill–Burton Act), which authorized grants to the states for construction of hospitals and public health centers, for planning construction of additional facilities, and for surveying existing hospitals and other facilities (Pub. L. No. 79–725, 60 Stat. L. 1040).

In 1962, President John Kennedy appointed a group of experts and community representatives to spearhead the President's Commission on Mental Illness. This 19-member task force set forth to examine the face of services for people afflicted with mental illness and to make recommendations for legislation, service delivery, and intervention efforts. One outgrowth of the President's Commission on Mental Illness report was a recommendation for community-based treatment and outpatient centers, currently known as community MH centers (Ozarin & Sharfstein, 1978).

Kennedy expressed great optimism in his special message to Congress on February 5, 1963, in which he proposed a national MH program to inaugurate "a wholly new emphasis and approach to care for the mentally ill." The Mental Retardation Facilities and Community Mental Health Centers Construction Act of 1963 (Pub. L. No. 88–164) was signed just a few weeks before President Kennedy's assassination. This legislation led the legislative mandate for community MH treatment centers and to their construction. These centers were intended for the target group of people who had been deinstitutionalized and moved from institutional care to community-based care. Funding from the federal government to state-based governments came in the form of Medicaid funds, to support efforts related to treatment for people with severe, persistent mental illness. The context for the Community Mental Health Centers Act is important to consider, as it has played a role ever since. For example, this piece of legislation was originally intended to address the needs of individuals who were institutionalized and chronically mentally ill and served as a strategy to provide humane community-based treatment for this target group. In addition, it was perceived that the cost of community-based care was a fraction of institutional care.

A closer analysis of the legislation reveals that no mention or appropriation is given to individuals who were aging. In fact, since mental illness is not a normal part of the aging process, chronic care for people suffering from mental illness or some MH condition, and who are older adults, is not a component of the Community Mental Health Centers Construction Act. Thus, this omission imposes some interesting concerns about service delivery for older adults with MH issues (Ray & Finley, 1994). Currently, there is a limited legislative mandate to address these issues. However, the Older Americans Act Amendments of 2006 and onward provide a legislative mandate to provide screening and detection services for MH issues among older adults.

The 1973 National Rehabilitation Act (HR 8070) provides for funds to support programs and services to assist people with disabilities to return to the community and promotes maximum independence. The issue at hand, however, is that this legislation is framed to consider individuals whose goal is to become self-sufficient economically, through paid work. Since the goal for many people who are in their golden years is retirement, rather than full employment, many individuals who are older adults are excluded from services and provisions allotted through the 1973 National Rehabilitation Act.

President Ronald Reagan signed the Omnibus Budget Reconciliation Act (OBRA) of 1981. This act repealed the Mental Health Systems Act and consolidated devolved funding for treatment and rehabilitation service programs into a single block grant that enabled each state to administer its allocated funds. With the repeal of the community MH legislation and the establishment of block grants, the federal role in services to the mentally ill became one of providing technical assistance to increase the capacity of state and local providers of MH services. The target group most impacted as a result of OBRA, relative to MH services, was older adults. Service delivery was retrenched and cut back to assure that the initial priority and target group (people at risk of institutionalization and/or chronically mentally ill) were served first and foremost. This further eroded aspirations for a system of care that would be responsive to people with some MH conditions, especially acute conditions, and who are older adults.

The Paul Wellstone and Pete Domenici Mental Health Parity and Addiction Equity Act of 2008 (Pub. L. No. 110–343) advanced treatments to people received care for MH concerns and provide parity to care for MH or substance use disorders to the same level as medical and surgical benefits. The Act required health insurers as well as group health plans to guarantee that financial requirements on benefits, including co-pays, deductibles, and out-of-pocket maximums, and limitations on treatment benefits such as caps on visits with a provider or days in a hospital visit, for MH or substance use disorders are not more restrictive than the insurer's requirements and restrictions for medical and surgical benefits.

The Patient Protection and Affordable Care Act of 2010 (Pub. L. No. 111–148) also had some provisions to address MH needs (Frank, Beronio, & Glied, 2014). It established a unit within the office of the director of the National Institutes of Health (NIH) to examine patient-centered outcomes research. It also established a unit to examine pain outcomes and conduct research within the area (a precursor to understanding the opioid epidemic that was designated as a national crisis by President Donald Trump in 2017).

The 2000 National Family Caregivers' Support Program

The National Family Caregiver Support Program became law in November 2000 as part of the reauthorization of the Older Americans Act. The program gives federal grants to states to provide information and referral, training, counseling, respite care, and other supportive services to (a) people caring at home for chronically ill, frail, elderly relatives or relatives with mental deficiencies, or other developmental disabilities and (b) grandparents and other relatives caring for children at home. The states must provide the services through their existing Area Agencies on Aging (AAA), established by the Older Americans Act of 1965. Local AAAs or their contractors will provide the services, which include caregiver counseling and some respite services, as well as information and referral services. Specifically, the AAAs must provide

1. Information about available services;
2. Help in accessing the services;
3. Training, counseling, and support groups to help caregivers make decisions and solve problems concerning their caregiving roles;

4. Temporary relief from caregiver responsibilities through respite care; and
5. Limited supplemental services not available through other programs (to be defined by each state).

Under the program, states must give priority to services for older people with the greatest social and economic need (with particular attention to low-income older people) and to older people who are taking care of relatives with mental retardation or other related developmental disabilities.

The New Freedom Commission on Mental Health

The New Freedom Commission on Mental Health was established by President George W. Bush in April 2002 to examine in a comprehensive manner the status of the U.S. MH service delivery system and to develop a series of recommendations based on the commission's findings. The president directed the commission to identify policies that could be implemented by federal, state, and local governments to maximize the utility of existing resources, improve coordination of treatments and services, and promote successful community integration for adults with serious mental illness and children with a serious emotional disturbance.

Perhaps one of the more significant pieces of legislation has been the Ronald Reagan Alzheimer's Breakthrough Act of 2004 (S2533, HR 4595). Clearly this piece of legislation took advantage of the window of opportunity in its passage. Some of the features of this legislation to benefit older adults include the doubling of funding for NIH Alzheimer's research by increasing authorization levels to $1.4 billion beginning in 2005. In addition, funding to assure a hosted national summit and the codification of three existing Alzheimer's research programs into law are all features of this legislation.

INFLUENCES TO CONSIDER IN THE DEVELOPMENT OF MENTAL HEALTH LEGISLATION

A number of influences on the treatment process are significant in the development of legislation that affects older adults. Some of these influences are patterns of service utilization, who uses services and where these services thus are located, health beliefs, the role of culture, family influences, the role of location (rural vs. urban), and family/consumer movements.

Patterns of Service Utilization

Although the legislative base may suggest that services be provided regardless of location and socioeconomic environment, the reality is that patterns of service utilization may differ, based upon the availability of trained MH professionals. Rural communities are more likely to face a lack of trained professionals to begin with, because the census count often does not make it attractive to build a practice for specialty psychiatrists within rural communities.

Health Beliefs and the Role of Culture

Furthermore, service delivery within rural communities may also be affected by the reality that older adults associate the receipt of mental healthcare with institutional care and feel somewhat concerned that their health beliefs will guide their need for more severe intervention than may actually be required.

The role of culture and MH services plays a role in both the development of legislation and programs/services. Increasingly, the health disparities gap is widening due to cross-cultural issues and differences in health status. MH legislation needs to consider cultural differences. Health beliefs, perceptions of services and outcomes, and perceived seriousness of potential mental illness and its conditions all require consideration as legislation is drafted as efforts to ensure that the role of culture is considered in the intervention process.

A CURRENT MENTAL HEALTH PROFILE OF OLDER ADULTS AND PEOPLE WITH DISABILITIES IN THE UNITED STATES

It is predicted that disability due to mental illness in individuals over 65 will become a major public health problem in the near future because of demographic changes (USDHHS, 1999; World Health Organization, 2017). This problem is magnified in rural communities because of the various barriers that play a role in accessing care for rural residents (New Freedom Commission on Mental Health, 2004). Consequently, the solution to the burgeoning issue may not rest with professionals, but with the voice of the consumers themselves, older adults.

A CLOSER VIEW OF THE MEANING OF MENTAL HEALTH

According to former U.S. Surgeon General David Satcher, MH is "the successful performance of mental functions and the ability to be productive in one's life, to have positive relationships, to have the ability to deal with adversity, and to be flexible in a changing environment" (USDHHS, 1999). Hence, if this definition is considered, the notion of MH and aging will take into consideration how people adapt to the changes in their life and the tasks of late life. MH intervention should focus on recognition that people are somewhere on the continuum and need assistance to move forward. Successful interventions will require the partnership of the older adult, physician, and/or social service provider.

Despite the thought that all older adults have the same needs, several researchers and social scientists have made the distinction between the young old, middle old, and old old. The needs and issues may not be similar for the three different categories of older adults. Bernice Neugarten (1984), a well-known developmental psychologist argued that the young old are vigorous and competent, while the old old suffer from physical, mental, or social losses and require a range of supportive and restorative health services. Neugarten also argued that ageist attitudes prevail in the MH system and cause a challenge in providing adequate services. Given these premises, what are the perspectives toward MH services, older adults, and physicians/providers of services?

MH, Older Adults, and Physicians

Sarkisian, Hays, Berry, and Mangione (2001) studied expectations regarding aging among older adults and physicians who cared for older adults. They found that physicians perceived that their domains of concern were physical function, cognitive function, social function, pain, and sexual function. In contrast, they found that older adults differed in their expectations and areas of concern. The older adults were concerned about issues related to MH such as anxiety, emotional well-being, happiness, sleep, and their own mortality.

Kaplan, Adamek, and Martin (2001) studied the knowledge and attitude of physicians related to assessing MH issues for older adults. Their findings suggest that the physician's own confidence in assessing depression was the strongest predictor in whether assessment, diagnosis, and treatment would occur. Hence, the older adult who may be feeling depressed may or may not receive treatment, despite their requests, and treatment would be largely determined by the physician's own comfort level.

The attitudes, knowledge, and behavior of family physicians regarding depression in older adults was studied by Gallo, Ryan, and Ford (1999). They found that physicians recognized the value of treatment for older adults; however, they also found that physicians' intervention of choice was medication-based. Physicians did not see the value of psychotherapy or "talk therapy." These authors also found a need for stronger collaboration among the physician and practitioner and older adult in treatment.

The goals of caregivers and clinicians were examined by Bogardus et al. (2001) to determine whether there was a difference in the goal related to MH treatment by each group. They found that there were clear differences in goals between caregivers and physicians. Caregivers were interested in behavioral and emotional health, while physicians were interested in day-to-day physical functioning of the caregiver or patient.

Mackenzie, Gekoski, and Knox (1999) examined whether family physicians treated mental disorders in older patients differently than in their younger patients. The findings suggested that there were differences that may contribute to lower use of MH services by older adults. Findings also suggest that physicians reported being less prepared to deal with older adults.

Patterns of care for depressed older adults in a large Health Maintenance Organization (HMO) were studied by Unutzer et al. (1996). They found older adults were less likely than younger adults to receive more than two primary care visits for depression. Their findings also suggest that older adults were less likely to receive specialty mental healthcare following antidepressant medications.

Other findings that suggest barriers to treatment for older adults have been identified by several researchers. Older adults are more likely to seek treatment from physicians than MH agencies because of the labels and stigma. Older adults are under-represented in treatment for MH issues (Bane, 1997; Henderson et al., 2014; Stewart, Jameson & Curtin, 2015). Rural communities face additional barriers to treatment, which include stigma, lack of trained professionals, and barriers of availability and accessibility (Bane, 1997; Kessler, Agines & Bowen, 2015).

MH, Older Adults, and Social Services

The differences in service use between urban and rural services for memory-related problems in older adults were studied by Chumbler, Cody, Booth, and Beck (2001). This group of researchers found that rural residents were more likely to seek treatment from their primary care physician, and these same rural residents were less likely to seek help from MH specialists. Interestingly, travel difficulties and lack of providers seem to account for the differences.

Bane (1997) examined issues of case management in rural settings for older adults. In his work, he found that older adults are underrepresented as recipients of MH services. In addition, he found that barriers such as stigma and lack of access could be broken down by case managers. Finally, Bane concluded that a key role for case managers included outreach and education in order to break down these barriers.

Mickus, Colenda, and Hogan (2000) examined the general awareness of MH services of the older adult population. They found that people over 65 would initially seek treatment from the primary care provider. In addition, their findings corroborated with the work of Chumbler et al. (2001) and Bane (1997). They found that older adults in rural communities were not likely to seek care from MH providers or seek counseling or educational care.

THE EPIDEMIOLOGY OF MH ISSUES OF OLDER ADULTS

How prevalent are MH conditions for older adults? Is there cause for concern? Actually, over 40% of older adults may suffer from some form of psychiatric condition, as reported in the U.S. *Surgeon General's Report on Mental Health* (USDHHS, 1999). These may take the form of any anxiety disorder (11%), simple phobias (7.3%), severe cognitive impairments (6.6%), any mood disorder (4.4 %), a major depressive episode (3.8%), or agoraphobia (4.1%; USDHHS, 1999).

The incidence and prevalence of psychiatric disorders is similar between urban and rural centers (Kessler et al., 1994); however, people residing in rural communities have much more limited access to services (Illinois Rural Health Association [IRHA], 2006; Lambert, 1995; USDHHS, 2000). Furthermore, rural residents are less likely to have financial or insurance benefits to access MH services (Mueller, Kashinath, & Ullrich, 1997). In addition, programs to specifically train and promote the placement of rural MH professionals are not available, and those that do exist are often not located in rural areas (Bird, Dempsey, & Hartley, 2001). In 2017, there has been little change in these figures (NIMH, 2017).

Depression in Older Adults

Despite the popular perception that MH is not a major issue within both urban and rural communities, it is not clear that healthcare professionals have an accurate reading on the full extent of depression and other symptoms of psychopathology among adults in our aging population. According to the Centers for Disease Control (CDC)'s Trends in Health and Aging (2006), only 2.8% of the population of people 65 years of age and older visited a MH professional in the year preceding 2004. When this figure was age adjusted, it was reported that 3% sought help from a MH professional in the 65 to 74 age group, as compared to 2.9% in the 75 and older age group. Females were more likely to seek treatment than males. These data are amplified by the data found in the 2014 Health and Retirement Study, which utilized the Center for Epidemiologic Study Depression Scale (C-ESD) to screen for depression within an elderly population. These data found that 14.9% of women and 10.1% of men were screened with clinically relevant depressive symptoms. When age adjusted, it was found that the 65- to 69-year-old age group showed 13.4% of women and 11.3% of men to be displaying symptoms; within 70- to 74-year-olds, 13.4% of women as compared to 7.0% of men; within the 75- to 79-year-olds 15.9% of women as compared to 8.7% of men; within the 80- to 84-year-olds, 18.7% of women as compared to 12.7% of men and within the 85-year-old and over age group 16% of women as compared to 13.9% of men. Figure 9.1 illustrates and compares these prevalence rates.

Ironically, a problem with diagnosis is that diagnosis usually is conducted through the *Diagnostic and Statistical Manual of Mental Disorders* (*DSM-5*; American Psychiatric Association, 2013) symptoms of major depression, and an individual would have to have at least four of the eight behavioral criteria for a sustained period of time (at least 2 months) in order to be diagnosed with a major depression. Since older adults often do not meet the full criteria for major depression, a new diagnostic entity of minor depression has been proposed to in order to characterize some of these patients. "Minor depression," a component form of depression, has not yet recognized as an official

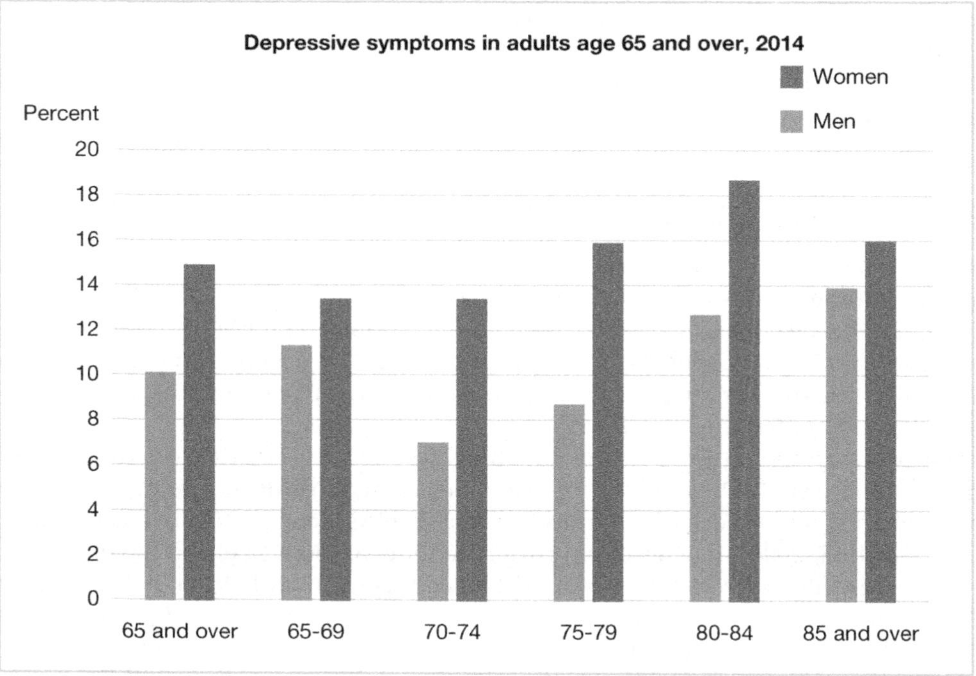

Figure 9.1 Percentage of people age 65 and over with clinically relevant depressive symptoms, by age group and sex, 2014.

Notes: This reflects the percentage of people age 65 years and older with depression with clinically relevant symptoms, 2002.

The definition of "clinically relevant depressive symptoms" is four or more symptoms out of a list of eight depressive symptoms from an abbreviated version of the CES-D, adapted by the Health and Retirement study.

The CES-D scale is a measure of depressive symptoms and is not to be used as a diagnosis of clinical depression. A detailed explanation concerning the "four or more symptoms" cutoff can be found in the following documentation:

hrsonline.isr.umich.edu/sitedocs/userg/dr_005.pdf. Percentages are based on weighted data using the preliminary respondent weight from HRS 2014.

Reference population: These data refer to the civilian noninstitutionalized population.

CES-D, Center for Epidemiological Studies Depression scale

Source: Federal Interagency Forum on Aging-Related Statistics. (2016). *Older Americans 2016: Key indicators of well-being.* Washington, DC: U.S. Government Printing Office; Health and Retirement Study, https://hrs.isr.umich.edu/about.

disorder, and the architects of the *DSM-5* propose further research on it prior to its official recommendation.

According to some studies (Alexopoulos, 1997; Field, 2017; Gallo & Lebowitz, 1999) this form of minor depression is much more common than major depression and anywhere from 8% to 20% of the older adult population living in the community can be found with some form of minor depression. The *Surgeon General's Report on Mental Health* (USDHHS, 1999) suggests that given depression is more difficult to assess and detect in older adults, more research is needed to define the clinical features that might help identify older adults at increased risk for sustained depressive symptoms and suicide.

Late-Onset Depression

According to the *Surgeon General's Report on Mental Health* (USDHHS, 1999, p. 347), "Major or minor depression diagnosed with first onset later than age 60 has been termed *late-onset depression.*" Patients with late-onset depression display greater apathy (Krishnan, Hays, Tupler, George, & Blazer, 1995) and less lifetime personality dysfunction (Abrams, Rosendahl, Card, & Alexopoulos, 1994). Cognitive deficits may be more prominent, with more impaired executive and memory functioning (Salloway et al., 1996) and greater medial temporal lobe abnormalities on MRI, similar to those seen in dementia (Greenwald et al., 1997). It has also been predicted that one is more likely to suffer from a reoccurrence of depression once there has been depression after the age of 60 (Reynolds, 1998).

Some known risk factors that have been identified for late-onset depression include widowhood (Harlow, Goldberg, & Comstock, 1991; Hummel et al., 2017; Mendes de Leon, Kasl, & Jacobs, 1994; NIMH, 2018; Zisook & Shuchter, 1991; University of Cambridge, School of Clinical Medicine, 2012), physical illness (Cadoret & Widmer, 1988; Harlow et al., 1991), high school or less education (Gallo, Royall, & Anthony, 1993; Wallace & O'Hara, 1992), problems with one's activities of daily living (Bruce & Hoff, 1994), and the use of alcohol (Brelow, Faden, & Smothers, 2003; Choi, Dinitto, & Marti, 2015; Memmet, 2003; National Institute on Alcohol Abuse and Alcoholism. n.d.; Saunders et al., 1991).

Alzheimer's Disease

Prevalence and Incidence

Alzheimer's disease is a recognized disorder associated with aging and has become more of a concern in the press following the passing in 2004 of former President Ronald Reagan, who was diagnosed with the disease. Approximately 8% to 15% of people over age 65 have Alzheimer's disease (Ritchie & Kildea, 1995). It is also anticipated that the prevalence of dementia (most of which is accounted for by Alzheimer's disease) nearly doubles with every 5 years of age after age 60 (Jorm, Korten, & Henderson, 1987). Apparently, more women than men are diagnosed with Alzheimer's disease (that is, the *prevalence* of the disease appears to be higher among women), but this may be an artifact of the reality that women have a longer life span than men (Lebowitz, Pearson, & Cohen, 1998). Incidence studies also reveal age-related increases in Alzheimer's disease (Aevarsson & Skoog, 1996; Breteler, Claus, van Duijn, Launer, & Hofman, 1992; Hebert et al., 1995; Johansson & Zarit, 1995; Paykel et al., 1994). In the 2011 National Health and Aging Trends (NHATS) study, 5% of men and 3% of women age 65 to 74 are affected with dementia. Additionally, the percentage of affected adults is 11% of men and 13% of women age 75 to 84, and 24% of men and 30% of women age 85 and older (Federal Interagency Forum on Aging-Related Statistics [FIFARS], 2016).

The "graying of America" is likely to result in an increase in the number of individuals with Alzheimer's disease, yet shifts in the composition of the affected population also are anticipated. Increased education is correlated with a lower frequency of Alzheimer's disease (Hill et al., 1993; Katzman, 1993; Stern et al., 1994), and future cohorts are expected to have attained greater levels of education. For example, the portion of those currently 75 years of age and older—those most vulnerable to Alzheimer's disease—with at least a high school education is 58.7%. Of those currently age 60 to 64 who entered the period of maximum vulnerability by the year 2010, 75.5% have at least a high school education. A higher educational level among the at-risk cohort may delay the onset of Alzheimer's disease and thereby decrease the overall frequency of Alzheimer's disease (by decreasing the number of individuals who live long enough to enter their period of maximum vulnerability). However, this trend may be counterbalanced or overtaken by greater longevity and longer survival of affected individuals. Specifically, improvements in general health and healthcare may lengthen the survival of dementia patients, increase the number of severely affected patients, and raise overall levels of comorbidity. Similarly, through dissemination of information to patients and clinicians, better detection, especially of early stage patients, is expected. Some authors suggest that the increased use of protective agents, such as vitamin E, also may increase the number of patients from progressing beyond the middle phases of the illness (Cummings & Jeste, 1999).

Anxiety Disorders

Anxiety symptoms and syndromes are important but understudied conditions in older adults. It has been estimated that in the community, about 11.4% of adults aged 55 years and older meet criteria for an anxiety disorder in 1 year (Reynolds, Pietrzak, El-Gabalawy, Mackenzie, & Sareen, 2015). Phobic anxiety disorders are among the most common mental disturbances in late life according to the National Epidemiological Survey and Alcohol and Related Conditions (NESARC), Wave 2. Prevalence studies of panic disorder (1.4%) and obsessive-compulsive disorder (6.5%) in older samples reveal low rates (Reynolds et al., 2015). There was also a 2.8% prevalence of generalized anxiety disorder. Other studies showed a range of 1.1% to 17.3% higher than that reported for panic disorder or obsessive-compulsive disorder (NIMH, 2017; Skoog, 1993). Worry or "nervous tension," rather than specific anxiety syndromes, may be more important in older people. Since many of the symptoms of anxiety mirror symptoms of heart-related disease, anxiety is often underdiagnosed or misdiagnosed within an older adult cohort group.

Schizophrenia in Late Life

Although schizophrenia is commonly thought of as an illness of young adulthood, it can both extend into and first appear in later life. Diagnostic criteria for schizophrenia are the same across the life span, and *DSM-5* places no restrictions on age of onset for a diagnosis to be made. Symptoms include delusions, hallucinations, disorganized speech, disorganized or catatonic behavior, as well as affective flattening. Symptoms must cause significant social or occupational dysfunction, must not be accompanied by prominent mood symptoms, and must not be uniquely associated with substance use.

One-year prevalence of schizophrenia among those 65 years or older is reportedly only around 1% to 2%, about one-half the 1-year prevalence of the 1.3% that is estimated for the population aged 18 to 54 (USDHHS, 1999).

MH and Older Adults

Depressive symptoms are an important indicator of general well-being and MH among older adults. People who report many depressive symptoms often experience higher rates of physical illness, greater functional disability, and higher healthcare utilization (Mehta, Yaffe, & Covinsky, 2002; Wells et al., 1989). MH issues and substance abuse disorders often co-occur for both adults and children (Regier et al., 1990). Although older adults may be at increased risk or vulnerability to experiencing MH-related problems, they often do not seek or are not successful at linking with the necessary MH services (USDHHS, 1999). A variety of factors can account for this outcome including stigma of mental illness; ageism; complexity and fragmentation of services; lack of coordination between medical, MH, and aging systems of care; lack of professional staff trained in geriatric MH; and inadequacy of health insurance coverage (USDHHS, 1999). Consequently, there is a poorly coordinated system of care and lack of integration between systems (especially aging, MH, and primary healthcare).

While most older people prefer to live in the community, mental disorders have been implicated as one of the major risk factors to institutionalization (Katz & Parmelee, 1997; USDHHS, 1999). Despite this risk, community-based services to meet the needs of older adults in community-care settings have largely been provided through the general medical sector since the MH organizations have focused primarily on persons with severe persistent MH disorders. However, the focus of primary care is often medical and acute care; thus, MH issues are often overlooked (George, 1992; USDHHS, 1999). Home health agencies provide limited short-term care (Meeks & Murrell, 1997; Meeks et al., 1997; Robinson, 1990).

MH in Rural Communities Versus Urban Communities

The realities that specialty MH services for older adults have been underutilized is identified in the literature (National Institute on Aging [NIA], 2000; Proctor, Morrow-Howell, Rubin, & Ringenberg, 1999; Proctor et al., 2003; Taube, Morlock, Burns, & Santos, 1990). In addition, general health has served in fact as the MH system of care for older adults (Regier, Goldberg, & Taube, 1978). Social services have in fact been under-utilized by older adults who are in need of MH services (Proctor et al., 1999); however, older adults with physical care needs and comorbid medical conditions were more likely to be in need of MH services (Proctor et al., 2003). Patients living in rural areas were less likely to use certain MH services than their urban counterparts, but the need was documented to be similar in nature across both locations.

SOCIAL WORK, MENTAL HEALTH, AGING, AND SERVICE UTILIZATION

Despite the dearth of research and efficacy studies on the benefits of various treatment modalities for MH issues and older adults, *Mental Health: The Report of the Surgeon General* (USDHHS, 1999) argues for a range of services that can be an adjunct to the formal treatment setting. This report supports the concept of health education and health promotion strategies to create an awareness of the aging process and MH functioning within the aging process. A range of interventions that have largely not been evaluated can be used to help improve the MH of older adults living in the community. These may include peer support, wellness programs, life reviews, bereavement groups, health promotion, and health education programs (Cohen, 1995; Haight, Michel, & Hendrix, 1998; Rowe & Kahn, 1997; Scott-Lennox & George, 1996; Waters, 1995). Social workers can play a major role in this educative process if they understand MH and older adults, as well as the role that health disparities can play in the continuum of MH functioning. The intersection between disability, chronic physical conditions, and depression is not well understood or underscored often by social workers working in community-care settings. These issues may be compounded with the location of one's residence and socioeconomic status. This study begins to address these issues conceptually and lay the foundation for pilot data that can be utilized to better prepare social workers working in community-care and home health settings.

From our previous studies, we can see that we need programming to meet the MH needs of older adults. The next section addresses programs available to meet these needs.

PROGRAMS AVAILABLE TO MEET THE MENTAL HEALTHCARE NEEDS OF OLDER ADULTS AND PEOPLE WITH DISABILITIES

Medicare

Medicare has a small provision for mental healthcare in its original plan. Under the original plan, Medicare Part A, some expenses related to mental healthcare given in a hospital are covered, which include one's room, meals, nursing care, and other-related services and/or supplies. Medicare Part A has a lifetime cap on the number of days for which it will pay for care in an inpatient psychiatric facility. Although there is no lifetime limit for inpatient care provided through a general hospital, Medicare will cover only up to 190 days of inpatient psychiatric hospital services care during one's lifetime.

Medicare Part B helps pay for MH services generally given outside a hospital, including visits with a doctor, clinical psychologist, clinical social worker, clinical nurse specialist, nurse practitioner, and/or physician's assistant and for lab tests. These services, however, are paid for by Medicare only when provided by a health professional who has been approved to accept Medicare reimbursement.

Medicare Part B also helps pay for outpatient MH services or services provided for through an outpatient or MH clinic, physician's office, therapist's office, or outpatient hospital department. In addition, services such as individual and group therapies approved by one's local or state government, family counseling in relation to the older adult's treatment plan, lab work and psychological assessments, occupational therapy related to one's treatment plan, individual patient training, and education and diagnostic tests are all covered.

A number of services are not covered within the Medicare plan. Some of these services that are not covered include any meals and transportation to or from MH treatment, support groups that are offered in nonmedical settings for peer support, and any testing/job training that has not been a part of the prescribed MH plan.

Partial hospitalization programs are also funded through Medicare Part B. This type of therapeutic program provides intensive psychiatric care through active treatment but differs from counseling or outpatient care in its intensity, duration, and depth of treatment available from one's physician or therapist. Partial hospitalization treatment offers day treatment and does not require any inpatient overnight stays. Generally, these partial hospitalization programs are provided through either hospital outpatient departments or local community MH centers. Medicare can pay for partial hospitalization programs on the condition one's physician can make the case that without such a program, the consumer would require an inpatient stay for treatment. In addition, the physician and partial hospitalization program need to be provided by a recognized Medicare provider in order to receive reimbursement.

Medicare is a program available to individuals who have worked up to 40 quarters and contributed through payroll tax into a plan. In the event that one does not have this plan to qualify for, or lives below a specific income level, MH services are still available under the Medicaid program.

Medicaid

Generally, one can qualify for resources through Medicaid or public aid MH services if one's resources or monthly income are less than $1,464 for a couple or $1,097 for an individual, and total bank accounts, stocks, bonds, or other resources are worth less than $6,000 for a couple or $4,000 for an individual. *Note*: These are 2017 income amounts and may change on January 1 of each succeeding year. Alaska and Hawaii also have slightly higher income limits. Generally speaking, therapists working with older adults and receiving state public aid or Medicaid funding may be required to provide therapeutic treatment based upon an evidence-based best practice model. These are intervention strategies that have been approved by the Substance Abuse and Mental Health Services Administration (SAMHSA) and NIMH as being interventions guided by successful clinical trials and an evidenced-based approach to treatment. Not all state public aid/Medicaid sources require these intervention approaches, and some states, such as Illinois, currently allow therapists to utilize their professional judgment as to which intervention strategies work best for a specific diagnosis and patient.

Area Agencies on Aging

Under the Older Americans Act of 2000, some funding was available to area agencies for short-term supportive counseling for MH needs. However, these funds did not cover the areas of screening and assessment for older adults adequately and were designated for pilot initiatives rather than long-term programs. The Older Americans Act Amendments of 2006 (Pub. L. No. 109–365) expand the delivery of MH services. MH services or MH screening replace the terms health screening or health services in the act, including Section 306. The amendments of 2006 also include new Mental Health Multidisciplinary Centers under Title IV. The House bill amends section 419 by adding new language requiring centers to collect information on best practices in long-term care service delivery, housing, and transportation. It also requires MH multidisciplinary centers to provide training and technical assistance to support community-based MH services to older people. The Senate bill, S. 3570, amended Section 419 by authorizing new grants to states on a competitive basis for the development and delivery of systems for MH screening and treatment services for older individuals. Such grants support programs that (a) increase public awareness related to benefits of prevention and treatment of MH conditions faced by people 60 years of age and older and (b) target stigma associated with mental disorders and other barriers that impact the diagnosis and treatment of MH disorders. If state agencies receive such funds they will be required to allocate the funds through AAA to carry out the programs. The Reauthorization of 2016 expanded these services to a greater extent.

SERVICE DELIVERY SETTINGS FOR MENTAL HEALTHCARE FOR OLDER ADULTS

Traditionally, services for mental healthcare for older adults have been constrained and limited to settings designed for chronically mentally ill adults, and specialized services for treating the older adult has been limited. The *Surgeon General's Report on Mental Health* (USDHHS, 1999) provided an overview of settings within which MH treatment occurs. They suggest that MH services for older adults within communities occurs within homes, group homes, retirement communities, primary care and general medical care sectors, outpatient therapy, board and care homes, assisted living facilities, and community MH centers. Institutional settings for MH treatment of older adults occurs within nursing homes, general hospitals with psychiatric units, general hospitals without psychiatric units, state mental hospitals, and Veterans Affairs hospitals.

Unfortunately, these settings have tailored interventions to meet the needs of an adult population rather than offering any specializations for an older adult population. In addition, when state funds are limited or budgets are in need of retrenchment, the first target group to be dismissed are older adults who do not fit into the category of chronically mentally ill. This situation calls into question the need to look at alternative treatment modalities and policies that embrace the older adults and build in their unique needs and therapeutic approaches.

Increasingly, primary care settings are also beginning to address MH needs of older adults through screening, assessment, and educational approaches. Several model programs have incorporated social work staff to provide screening and assessment services to patients during their wait for the primary care physician (Field, 2017; Eady, Courtenay & Strydom, 2015; Fulton, 2016; Gum, Dautovich, Green, Hirsch & Schoenfeld, 2015; Katon et al., 1996; Schulberg et al., 1995). While these approaches are still in their infancy, and primary care still requires being addressed before physicians will deal adequately with the older adults' MH needs, these intervention schemes hold great promise. Such approaches minimize the potential for stigma and prejudice on the part of both the provider and the patient. Overall, models that consider the integration of MH treatment into primary care were designed to meet the needs of people with depression, but other disorders may also be targeted within primary care settings. A set of recommendations for appropriate referrals to specialty mental healthcare is available through the American Association for Geriatric Psychiatry (AAGP, 1997).

ISSUES FACING OLDER ADULTS, PEOPLE WITH DISABILITIES, AND MENTAL HEALTHCARE NEEDS

A number of issues currently face older adults with mental healthcare needs residing in the community. These include the financing of mental healthcare for older adults, community-based care, prevention services, screening and detection, and medication management. This section reviews some of these specific issues and showcases areas for further development.

Financing Mental Healthcare for Older Adults

Until the Older Americans Act Amendments of 2006, financing mental healthcare for older adults was an issue that led to a battleground between divisions of aging and MH and substance abuse arenas. Each group perceived that mental healthcare for older adults was not its mandate, and funding for services and resources was limited if existent. Departments on aging perceived MH issues and services to be the role of departments/divisions for mental health (DMH). Conversely, divisions of MH perceived their role to be one of intervention for people with chronic mental illness rather than acute, short-term issues. DMHs also perceived that issues related to service delivery for older adults was the mandate of the aging directorates, regardless of specialty area need. Consequently, financing (or lack of financing) is and remains an issue for older adult service delivery settings.

Financing also plays a critical role when delivering services, either assessment or intervention. Ultimately, one must work with an older adult with a different set of approaches than one would take when working with children, teenagers, or younger adults. Older adults may require a longer time period within which to complete assessments because of the need for a slower-paced interview, and a longer period of time to develop rapport or engage the individual in the therapeutic relationship. This situation becomes difficult for caseworkers, who may be reimbursed per session as opposed to per case. Effective models of financing assessments may revert to using a block-funded approach to service delivery rather than a case-by-case approach.

Community-Based Care

Community-based care for MH concerns has largely been delivered through local community MH centers. The centers were originally developed to meet the needs of the deinstitutionalized long-term psychiatric patients, who moved into local communities following the passage of the Community Mental Health Centers Act of 1966 (Pub. L. No. 88–164). These settings have aged along with their constituents, and now many of the young adults with chronic MH problems have also aged and are in the older adult (60+) target group. Unfortunately, the funding schemes and the modus operandi are very much focused on providing community-based services to stabilize individuals with chronic MH needs, rather than older adults with acute and short-term care needs. Conversely, the settings are often stigmatizing and unfavorable to older adults with short-term MH needs. Treatment groups available through partial hospitalization programs often target the younger patient, and older adults often feel out of place. These issues become compounded when considering a smaller rural community setting, where privacy is limited, and one would not be able to maintain anonymity when confronted with visiting a community MH center.

Models for Gero-Psychiatry

A number of models are beginning to develop around the United States for gero-psychiatry. These model demonstration projects hold promise for innovative ways to provide screening, detection, education, and intervention services for older adults. Such approaches will be imperative for the effective treatment of older adults. These models will also aim to provide for a nonstigmatizing approach to dealing with older adults and will also improve the specialty areas for intervention services for older adults. These model approaches will also require some legislative base and intervention to provide a legislative mandate for individual states to create these services.

Prevention Services

Currently, federal legislation does not have any provisions for prevention-oriented services. The legislative base behind Medicare and the Older Americans Act (2000 amendments) do not provide for preventative services. Individual states and funded initiatives through NIMH, NIA, and SAMHSA have provided funds to develop evidence-based prevention interventions; however, these approaches are often not funded federally; once they are deemed effective, individual states may introduce them into their systems for their constituents. It is hoped that the 2006 amendments to the Older Americans Act will facilitate some prevention-oriented approaches particularly to target the onset of depression or target substance use issues for older adults. SAMHSA's Action Plan for Older Adults, Fiscal Years 2006 and 2007 begins to address these needs.

Screening and Detection

The ideal venue for an older adult to be assessed for MH needs (e.g., depression, cognitive impairment, or substance use/misuse) would be during an initial assessment for home health services or within primary care settings. Currently, not all community-care settings screen for these MH issues during their initial assessments or follow-ups. In addition, not all home health caseworkers are trained to understand the behavioral symptoms associated with the *DSM-5* diagnostic groups. Without training of caseworkers or primary care health providers, many signs of mental disorders may go undetected or untreated. The screening and assessment tools also used for this population group are limited and require further development. Last, many of the tools for screening and assessment were normed and developed using a nursing home and institutionalized population, but given the needs of a community-dwelling, noninstitutionalized population, we have been seeing an increased focus on community-based assessment tools and interventions.

Medications

Medications for the treatment of psychiatric disorders are often tested within clinical trials on a younger adult population; hence, there is limited information about how these metabolize within an older adult's system. It is quite common for people over the age of 60 to require several attempts with different medications prior to finding the one that will best work within one's body and among the other drugs one may be taking. One may be required to pursue a variety of medications prior to finding one that will work effectively. Challenges are that we have a limited understanding of clinical trials that can be used with an older adult population. Second, with Medicare Part D enrollment periods only once per year, one may have greater out-of-pocket expenses than anticipated because of different medication prescriptions required to stabilize an acute MH condition. Medications are also leading to opioid addictions, which have become a crisis across the life span.

People With Chronic Mental Health Needs Who Are Aging

There is an important distinction to be made between the needs of individuals with chronic mental illness who are older adults and older adults with acute MH needs. People with chronic MH needs who are aging have multiple health and MH issues that result in the use of institutionalized services as compared to older adults with brief periods of instability.

Oppressed Groups and Visible Minorities

The seminal work articulated in *Mental Health: Culture, Race, and Ethnicity: A Supplement to Mental Health: A Report of the Surgeon General* (USDHHS, 2001) points out that culture, race, and ethnicity are not addressed adequately at all within MH service delivery settings in the United States. If one adds an additional variable of age into the equation, it becomes relatively clear very quickly that older adults who are visible minorities or from traditionally oppressed groups may be less likely to have access to culturally sensitive and relevant services. Clinical trials need to include individuals who are older adults and representative of minority groups when the development of new medications is under consideration. Approaches to evidence-based treatment require the inclusion of people who are minorities and older adults. Effective treatment interventions could also be expanded through a more concrete understanding of the role culture plays in one's health behaviors and help-seeking behavior. People from minority groups also need to be able to assure language access, and investigation is required to better understand the role that culture and ethnicity play in relation to shame, stigma, and discrimination. The area of understanding cultural minorities and mental healthcare is an area that can present opportunity for development (Kawaii-Bogue, Williams & MacNea, 2017; Lim et al., 2015; Streed, Arroyo & Goldstein, 2018).

MODEL PROGRAMS AND BEST PRACTICE APPROACHES TO MENTAL HEALTH SERVICE DELIVERY

Although a range of behavioral health approaches exist to meet the MH and substance misuse needs of older adults, the concept of evidence-based interventions is becoming widely prescribed by behavioral health service providers. Levkoff, Chen, Fisher, and McIntyre (2006) have developed a guide to the implementation of such programs. The section that follows presents some specific programs, recognized by the SAMHSA for potential intervention strategies and best practice models for MH service delivery.

The Center for Older Adult Recovery at Hanley Center

In 1998, the Hanley Center in West Palm Beach, FL opened its pioneering Center for Older Adult Recovery after developing an age-responsive model of treatment of alcohol and chemical addictions (Emlet, Hawks, & Callahan, 2001). Hanley's outcomes suggest that the older adult target group can be the most successful with recovery rates when compared to any other age group. The program offers prevention for late-onset addiction as well. Situated in lush tropical enclaves, Hanley Center offers its older adult consumers a Serenity Fountain and Garden and a homey, comfortable residence. Hanley's holistic treatment model addresses patients' physical and mental status as well as the values of this generation.

After an initial thorough evaluation, individualized treatment takes on a slower pace because of the normal aging process, as well as chronic medical conditions, cognitive impairment, and possible dual diagnosis. Hanley's interdisciplinary team of highly skilled professionals provides holistic treatment in the areas of medicine, psychiatry, psychology, and counseling, wellness, spirituality, and expressive arts. Continuing care plans are put into place prior to patients' discharge and are specific to each individual's special needs (USDHHS, 2006b).

The Gatekeeper Program

The Gatekeeper model seeks at-risk older adults who typically do not come to the attention of the formal MH, substance abuse, and aging service delivery systems. This volunteer program was developed in 1978 by the late Raymond Raschko, MSW, at Elder Services Mental Health, Spokane, Washington. The program recruits and trains community businesses and organizations to identify high-risk older adults who may be exhibiting signs and symptoms that indicate they need assistance. Gatekeepers may include meter readers, bank tellers, postal carriers, first responders, utility workers, and many others. Following a referral, a geriatric MH specialist makes a home visit to conduct a comprehensive assessment and evaluation. Appropriate linkages are made to MH, substance abuse, aging, medical, and other social services. Research has shown the Gatekeeper model to be an effective outreach model for identifying socially isolated older adults who show signs of psychiatric symptoms (USDHHS, 2005).

MENTAL HEALTHCARE CHALLENGES FOR THE FUTURE

MH challenges for the future are many, and although this chapter touches upon several, this section is definitely not exhaustive. The biggest challenge will probably be the very nature of financing to meet the community-based noninstitutionalized population. Prevention, screening, detection, and intervention strategies to meet the needs of baby boomers as they advance further into old age will be another challenge. Models of service delivery that are innovative, preventative in nature, and nonstigmatizing will also be an important goal to strive toward. Establishing systems of care that are not fragmented and provide seamless service delivery will also be an important goal for MH, healthcare, and public health service delivery systems.

There are a number of issues for consideration when looking toward the need for resources and policy development to promote the MH of older adults and people with disabilities. One of the first and significantly important is the need to continue to build an evidence base and best practice interventions through legislated initiatives. The issue of stigma still surfaces and prevents individuals and/or their aging loved ones from seeking MH treatment. Hence, the need for legislation and funding to support and improve public awareness of effective treatment interventions is also paramount.

In an effort to ensure the supply of MH services and providers, legislative initiatives that examine workforce issues will be a necessary future consideration. This will include support and benefits to medically designated shortage areas to help build both the professional workforce and also a workforce that is aware and trained in the delivery of state-of-the-art treatments.

Finally, legislative efforts within the MH arena should assure that we tailor treatments to age, race, gender, and culture. Financial resources that can support clinical trials when developing norms for interventions specific to older adults and their caregivers should also be considered.

SUMMARY

Despite attempts to develop legislation to meet the needs of people with mental illness throughout history, these legislative efforts have had limited benefit to older adults and some people with disabilities, unless the person has been afflicted with a long-standing chronic mental illness. This chapter presents a brief overview of some legislative efforts within the MH arena and examined their limitations and application with respect to older adults and people living with mental illness.

This chapter also takes us through a journey to examine the current status of MH and older adults, with a particular emphasis on cognitive impairments, depression, anxiety, and schizophrenia. Programs and services are reviewed, and issues still outstanding within the MH arena are discussed. This chapter concludes with laying out some challenges for the future in the area of MH and older adults.

ADDITIONAL RESOURCEES

Websites

Mental Health America: www.nmha.org

This website provides consumer-oriented information on a range of MH topics by audience, issue, disorders, treatments, and medications. It also provides links to a range of policy issues and MH topics.

Suicide and Depression Fact Sheets: www.nimh.gov/publicat/elderlydepsuicide.cfm

This website provides an excellent set of fact sheets on older adults, depression, and suicide. It is written on a level that enables the reader to glean some behavioral signs and symptoms about suicide and identify whether they or a loved one is at risk. The fact sheets are a product of the NIMH.

NIMH: www.nimh.nih.gov

This website provides up-to-date health information on a range of disorders including anxiety disorders, posttraumatic stress disorder, depression, and eating disorders, with some vantage points for older adults.

SAMHSA: www.samhsa.gov

This website provides a matrix of services for older adults. It includes information and linkages to the Older Americans Substance Abuse and Mental Health Technical Assistance Center, and campaigns for public awareness. Current campaigns at the time of the writing of this book include a "Caring for Every Child's Mental Health," "HHS 5-Point Strategy to Combat the Opioid Crisis," "Mental Health First Aid for Adults," and an "underage drinking prevention" campaign. The site also provides links to professional resources that can be useful in gleaning current knowledge in the area and developing resources for professional development and public education.

SAMHSA Fact Sheets on drugs of interest: www.oas.samhsa.gov/drugs.cfm

This website provides fact sheets on various drugs, with up-to-date medical background information.

Senior Health Online Depression information: nihseniorhealth.gov/depression/toc.html

This website provides an overview of numerous health topics of interest, including depression in older adults. Since approximately two million Americans age 65 or older suffer from major depression, and another five million suffer from less severe forms, a collaborative effort between the NIA and the National Library of Medicine (NLM) worked conjointly to develop this senior-friendly medical Web site.

Older Adult Technical Assistance Network: www.samhsa.gov/OlderAdultsTAC/

Through work with national experts and researchers, federal agencies and national aging organizations, the Older Americans Substance Abuse and Mental Health Technical Assistance Center is collecting, reviewing, and assessing the best available knowledge, research, and programmatic efforts around substance abuse and MH science for older adults.

John F. Kennedy Special Message to the Nation on Mental Illness and Mental Retardation: www.presidency.ucsb.edu/ws/index.php?pid = 9546

This website provides an interesting background and the presidential speech from John F. Kennedy, and his vision for the legislative efforts impacting mental illness and mental retardation.

YouTube Videos

Mental Health America: www.youtube.com/user/mentalhealthamerica

This YouTube video provides a short overview of MH screening and needs. It is a wonderful introductory video for users to understand the nature and impact of MH concerns.

Mental Health Crisis in America: www.youtube.com/watch?v=jBqyuQGvcTgwww.youtube.com/watch?v=jBqyuQGvcTgwww.youtube.com/watch?v=jBqyuQGvcTgwww.youtube.com/watch?v=jBqyuQGvcTg

This video addresses the current crisis in the United States related to MH concerns. It also addresses issues that have been ignored by legislators and policy development.

The Community Mental Health Act of 1963: www.youtube.com/watch?v=OtHD-IG-VKoowww.youtube.com/watch?v=OtHD-IGVKoowww.youtube.com/watch?v=OtHD-IG-VKoowww.youtube.com/watch?v=OtHD-IGVKoo

This video describes the Community Mental Health Act of 1963 and provides a brief discussion of the strengths of the legislation and deficits.

Deinstitutionalization: What is it and its impacts: www.youtube.com/watch?v=kVPz96PwDXE

This YouTube video provides an overview of the process of deinstitutionalization and its impacts for people living within the United States.

Podcast

Helen Hogue discusses mental health policy and services. **Listen now:** https://bcove.video/2ziCKG5

DISCUSSION QUESTIONS

1. Looking back at the three cases presented at the outset of this chapter, what pieces of legislation will have an impact on Nora, Gerry, and Lorraine? Can you revise the case to show specific mental health (MH) diagnoses and how each person would receive or not receive appropriate treatment?
2. What programs and services are available for each of the individual cases detailed at the beginning of this chapter?
3. What legislation is currently needed to address the MH needs of people growing older, people living with chronic persistent mental healthcare needs and those with acute mental healthcare needs? Should this legislation be targeted at a state level or at the federal level?
4. Consider the *Healthy People 2020* objectives for MH, which are available in Appendices B and C. Which three objectives do you think are realistic to address in your community, region, or state? How would you go about addressing these objectives?

REFERENCES

Abrams, R. C., Rosendahl, E., Card, C., & Alexopoulos, G. S. (1994). Personality disorder correlates of late and early onset depression. *Journal of the American Geriatrics Society*, *42*, 727–731. doi:10.1111/j.1532-5415.1994.tb06532.x

Aevarsson, O., & Skoog, I. (1996). A population-based study on the incidence of dementia disorders between 85 and 88 years of age. *Journal of the American Geriatrics Society*, *44*, 1455–1460. doi:10.1111/j.1532-5415.1996.tb04070.x

Alexopoulos, G. S. (1997, November 6). *Epidemiology, nosology and treatment of geriatric depression*. Paper presented at Exploring Opportunities to Advance Mental Health Care for an Aging Population, meeting sponsored by the John A. Hartford Foundation, Rockville, MD.

American Association for Geriatric Psychiatry. (1997). *Recommendations from primary care physicians: When to refer depressed elderly patients to a geriatric psychiatrist* Bethesda, MD: Author.

American Psychiatric Association. (2013). *Diagnostic and statistical manual of psychiatric disorders* (5th ed.). Washington, DC: Author.

Bane, S. D. (1997). Rural mental health and aging: Implication for case management. *Journal of Case Management*, *6*(4), 158–161.

Bird, D. C., Dempsey, P., & Hartley, D. (2001). *Addressing mental health workforce needs in underserved rural areas: Accomplishments and challenges*. Portland, ME: Maine Rural Health Research Center, Muskie Institute, University of Southern Maine.

Bogardus, S. T., Bradley, E. H., Williams, C. S., Maciejewski, P. K., Doorn, C. V., & Inouye, S. K. (2001). Goals for the care of frail older adults: Do caregivers and clinicians agree? *The American Journal of Medicine, 110*(2), 97–102. doi:10.1016/S0002-9343(00)00668-9

Brelow, R. A., Faden, V. B., & Smothers, B. (2003). Alcohol consumption by elderly Americans. *Journal of Studies on Alcohol, 64*(6), 884–892. doi:10.15288/jsa.2003.64.884

Breteler, M. M., Claus, J. J., van Duijn, C. M., Launer, L. J., & Hofman, A. (1992). Epidemiology of Alzheimer's disease. *Epidemiology Review, 14*, 59–82. doi:10.1093/oxfordjournals.epirev.a036092

Bruce, M. L., & Hoff, R. A. (1994). Social and physical health risk factors for first-onset major depressive disorder in a community sample. *Social Psychiatry and Psychiatric Epidemiology, 29*(4), 165–171.

Cadoret, R. J., & Widmer, R. B. (1988). The development of depressive symptoms in elderly following onset of severe physical illness. *Journal of Family Practice, 27*(1), 71–76.

Centers for Disease Control and Prevention. (2006). *Trends in health and aging*. Washington, DC: Government Printing Office.

Choi, N.G., DiNitto, D.M., & Marti, C.N. (2015). Alcohol and other substance use, mental health treatment use, and perceived unmet treatment need: Comparison between baby boomers and older adults. *American Journal on Addictions, 24*(4), 299–307. doi:10.1111/ajad.12225

Chumbler, N. R., Cody, M., Booth, B. M., & Beck, C. K. (2001). Rural-urban difference in service use for memory-related problems in older adults. *Journal-Behavior Health-Services and Research, 28*(2), 212–221. doi:10.1007/bf02287463

Cohen, G. D. (1995). Mental health promotion in later life: The case for social portfolio. *American Journal of Geriatric Psychiatry, 3*(4), 277–279. doi:10.1097/00019442-199503040-00001

Cummings, J., & Jeste, D. (1999). Alzheimer's disease and its management in the year 2010. *Psychiatric Services, 50*(9), 1173–1177. doi:10.1176/ps.50.9.1173

DeJong, G. (1979). Independent living: From social movement to analytic paradigm. *Archives of Physical Medicine and Rehabilitation, 60*, 435–446.

Eady, N., Courtney, K., & Strydom, A. (2015). Pharmacological management of behavioral and psychiatric symptoms in older adults with Intellectual disability. *Drugs and Aging, 32*(2), 95-102. doi:10.1007/s40266-014-0236-7

Emlet, C., Hawks, H., & Callahan, J. (2001). Alcohol use and abuse in a population of community dwelling, frail older adults. *Journal of Gerontological Social Work, 35*(4), 21–33. doi:10.1300/j083v35n04_03

Evans, D. A., Funkenstein, H. H., Albert, M. S., Scherr, P. A., Cook, N. R., Chown, M. J., … Taylor, J. O. (1989). Prevalence of Alzheimer's disease in a community population of older persons. Higher than previously reported. *Journal of the American Medical Association, 262*(18), 2551–2556. doi:10.1001/jama.262.18.2551

Federal Interagency Forum on Aging-Related Statistics. (2016). *Older Americans 2016: Key indicators of well-being*. Washington, DC: U.S. Government Printing Office.

Field, T.A. (2017). Clinical mental health counseling: A 40 year retrospective. *Journal of Mental Health Counseling, 39*(1), 1–11. doi:10.17744/mehc.39.1.01

Frank, R. G., Beronio, K., & Glied, S. A. (2014). Behavioral health parity and the Affordable Care Act. *Journal of Social Work in Disability & Rehabilitation, 13*(1–2), 31–43. doi:10.1080/1536710X.2013.870512

Fullen, M. C. (2016). Medicare advocacy for the counselor advocate. *Adultspan Journal, 15*(1), 3–12. doi:10.1002/adsp.12015

Gallo, J. J., & Lebowitz, B. D. (1999). The epidemiology of common late-life mental disorders in the community: Themes for the new century. *Psychiatric Services, 50*(9), 1158–1166. doi:10.1176/ps.50.9.1158

Gallo, J. J., Royall, D. R., & Anthony, J. C. (1993). Risk factors for the onset of depression in middle age and later life. *Social Psychiatry and Psychiatric Epidemiology, 28*(3), 101–108. doi:10.1007/bf00801739

Gallo, J. J., Ryan, S. D., & Ford, D. (1999). Attitudes, knowledge, and behavior of family physicians regarding depression in late life. *Archives of Family Medicine, 8*(3), 249–255. doi:10.1001/archfami.8.3.249

Geller, J. L. (2000). The last half-century of psychiatric services as reflected in psychiatric services. *Psychiatric Services, 51*(1), 41–67. doi:10.1176/ps.51.1.41

George, L. K. (1992). Community and home care for mentally ill older adults. In J. E. Birren, R. B. Sloane, G. D. Cohen, N. R. Hooyman, B. D. Lebowitz, & M. I. Wykle (Eds.), *Handbook of mental health and aging* (2nd ed., pp. 793–813). San Diego, CA: Academic Press.

Goldsmith, J. S., & Kurpius, S. R. (2015). Older Adults and integrated health settings. Opportunities and challenges for mental health counselors. *Journal of Mental Health Counseling, 37*(2), 124–137. doi:10.17744/mehc.37.2.q57403638j4671n0

Gollaher, D. (1995). *Voice for the mad: The life of Dorothea Dix.* New York, NY: Free Press.

Greenwald, B. S., Kramer-Ginsberg, E., Bogerts, B., Ashtari, M., Aupperle, P., Wu, H., … Patel, M. (1997). Qualitative magnetic resonance imaging findings in geriatric depression. Possible link between later-onset depression and Alzheimer's disease? *Psychological Medicine, 27*(2), 421–431. doi:10.1017/s0033291796004576

Gum, A.M., Dautovich, N.D., Green, J., Hirsh, A., & Schoenfeld, L. (2015). Improving home-based providers' communication to primary care providers to enhance care coordination, *Aging & Mental Health, 19*(10), 921–931. doi:10.1080/13607863.2014.977772

Haight, B. K., Michel, Y., & Hendrix, S. (1998). Life review: Preventing despair in newly relocated nursing home residents' short- and long-term effects. *International Journal of Aging and Human Development, 47*(2), 119–142. doi:10.2190/A011-BRXD-HAFV-5NJ6

Harlow, S. D., Goldberg, E. L., & Comstock, G. W. (1991). A longitudinal study of risk factors for depressive symptomatology in elderly widowed and married women. *American Journal of Epidemiology, 134*, 526–538. doi:10.1093/oxfordjournals.aje.a116125

Health and Retirement Study. (2014).

Hebert, L. E., Scherr, P. A., Beckett, L. A., Albert, M. S., Pilgrim, D. M., Chown, M. J., … Evans, D. A. (1995). Age-specific incidence of Alzheimer's disease in a community population. *JAMA, 273*(17), 1354–1359.

Henderson, J., Crotty, M. M., Fuller, J., & Martinez, L. (2014). Meeting unmet needs? The role of a rural mental health service for older people. *Advances in Mental Health, 12*(3), 182–191. doi:10.5172/jamh.2014.12.3.182

Hill, L. R., Klauber, M. R., Salmon, D. P., Yu, E. S., Liu, W. T., Zhang, M., & Katzman, R. (1993). Functional status, education, and the diagnosis of dementia in the Shanghai survey. *Neurology, 43*, 138–145. doi:10.1212/WNL.43.1_Part_1.138

Hummel, J., Weisbrod, C., Boesch, L., Himpler, K., Hauer, K., Hautzinger, M., . . . Kopf, D. (2017). AIDE–acute illness and depression in elderly patients. cognitive behavioral group psychotherapy in geriatric patients with comorbid depression: A randomized, controlled trial, *JAMDA, The Journal of Post-Acute and Long-Term Care Medicine, 18*(4), 341-349. doi:10.1016/j.jamda.2016.10.009

Illinois Rural Health Association. (2006). *Mental health in rural Illinois: Recovery is the goal: An analysis of mental health care in rural Illinois.* Springfield, IL: Author.

Johansson, B., & Zarit, S. H. (1995). Prevalence and incidence of dementia in the oldest old: A longitudinal study of a population-based sample of 84–90 year olds in Sweden. *International Journal of Geriatric Psychiatry, 10*(5), 359–366. doi:10.1002/gps.930100504

Jorm, A. F., Korten, A. E., & Henderson, A. S. (1987). The prevalence of dementia: A quantitative integration of the literature. *Acta Psychiatrica Scandinavica, 76*(5), 465–479. doi:10.1111/j.1600-0447.1987.tb02906.x

Kaplan, M. S., Adamek, M. E., & Martin, J. L. (2001). Confidence of primary care physicians in assessing the suicidality of geriatric patients. *International Journal of Geriatric Psychiatry, 16*(7), 728–734. doi:10.1002/gps.420

Katon, W., Robinson, P., Von Korff, M., Lin, E., Bush, T., Ludman, E., … Walker, E. (1996). A multifaceted intervention to improve treatment of depression in primary care. *Archives of General Psychiatry*, 53(10), 924–932. doi:10.1001/archpsyc.1996.01830100072009

Katz, I. R., & Parmelee, P. A. (1997). Overview. In R. L. Rubinstein & M. Lawton (Eds.), *Depression in long term and residential care* (pp. 1–28. New York, NY: Springer Publishing.

Katzman, R. (1993). Education and the prevalence of dementia and Alzheimer's disease. *Neurology, 43*(1), 13–20. doi:10.1212/WNL.43.1_Part_1.13

Kawaii-Bogue, B., Williams, N. J. & & MacNear, K. (2017). Mental health care access and treatment in African American communities: An integrative care framework. *Best Practices in Mental Health, 13*(2), 11–29.

Kessler, E., Agines, S., & Bowen, C. E. (2015). Attitudes towards seeking mental health services among older adults: personal and contextual correlates. *Aging & Mental Health. 19*(2), 182–191. doi:10.1080/13607863.2014.929399

Kessler, R. C., McGonagle, K. A., Zhao, S., Nelson, C. B., Hughs, M., Ehleman, S., … Kendler, K. S. (1994). Lifetime and 12-month prevalence rates of DSM-III-R psychiatric disorders in the United States. *Archives of General Psychiatry, 51*, 8–19. doi:10.1001/archpsyc.1994.03950010008002

Khaiaila, R., & Cohen, M. (2016). Emotional suppression, caregiving burden, mastery, coping strategies and mental health in spousal caregivers. *Aging & Mental Health, 20*(9), 908–917. doi:10.1080/13607863.2015.1055551

Kofoed, L. L. (1984). Abuse and misuse of over-the-counter drugs by the elderly. In R. M. Atkinson (Ed.), *Alcohol and drug abuse in old age* (pp. 49–59. Washington, DC: American Psychiatric Press.

Krishnan, K. R., Hays, J. C., Tupler, L. A., George, L. K., & Blazer, D. G. (1995). Clinical and phenomenological comparisons of late-onset and early-onset depression. *American Journal of Psychiatry, 152*, 785–788. doi:10.1176/ajp.152.5.785

LaGreca, A. J., Akers, R. L., & Dwyer, J. W. (1988). Life events and alcohol behavior among older adults. *The Gerontologist*, *28*(4), 552–558. doi:10.1093/geront/28.4.552

Lambert, D. (1995). Access of rural AFDC Medicaid beneficiaries to mental health services. *Health Care Financing Review*, *17*, 133–145.

Lanoye, A., Stewart, K. E., Rybarczyk, B. D., Auerbach, S, M., Sadock, E., Aggarwal, A., & Austin, K. (2017). The impact of integrated psychological services in a safety net primary care clinic on medical utilization. *Journal of Clinical Psychology, 73*(6), 681–692.

Lebowitz, B. D., Pearson, J. L., & Cohen, G. D. (1998). *Clinical geriatric psychopharmacology*. Baltimore, MD: Williams & Wilkins.

Levkoff, S. E., Chen, H., Fisher, J. E., & McIntyre, J. S. (2006). *Evidence-based behavioral health practices for older adults: A guide to implementation*. New York, NY: Springer Publishing.

Lim, M. L., Lim, D., Gwee, X., Nyuntm, Z., Kumar, R., & Ng, T. P. (2015). Resilience, stressful life events, and depressive symptomatology among older Chinese adults. *Aging and Mental Health, 19*(11), 1005–1014. doi:10.1080/13607863.2014.995591

Mackenzie, C. S., Gekoski, W. L., & Knox, V. J. (1999). Do family physicians treat older patients with mental disorders differently from younger patients? *Canadian Family Physician*, *45*, 124–129.

McDonald, B. Kulkarni, M., Andkhoie, M., Kendell, J., Gall, S., Chelladurai, S., & Farag, M. (2017). Determinants of self-reported mental health and utilization of mental health services in Canada. *International Journal of Mental Health, 46*(4), 299–311. doi:10.1080/00207411.2017.1345045

Meeks, S., Carstensen, L. L., Stafford, P. B., Brenner, L. L., Weathers, F., Welch, R., & Thomas F. (1997). Mental health needs of the chronically mentally ill elderly. *Psychology and Aging*, *5*(2), 163–171. doi:10.1037//0882-7974.5.2.163

Meeks, S., & Murrell, S. A. (1997). Mental illness in late life: Socioeconomic conditions, psychiatric symptoms, and adjustment of long-term sufferers. *Psychology and Aging*, *12*, 296–308. doi:10.1037//0882-7974.12.2.296

Mehta, K. M., Yaffe, K., & Covinsky, K. E. (2002). Cognitive impairment, depressive symptoms, and functional decline in older people. *Journal of the American Geriatrics Society*, *50*(6), 1045–1050. doi:10.1046/j.1532-5415.2002.50259.x

Memmet, J. L. (2003). Alcohol consumption by elderly Americans. *Journal of Studies on Alcohol*, *64*(6), 884–892. doi:10.15288/jsa.2003.64.884

Mendes de Leon, C. F., Kasl, S. V., & Jacobs, S. (1994). A prospective study of widowhood and changes in symptoms of depression in a community sample of the elderly. *Psychological Medicine*, *24*, 613–624. doi:10.1017/s0033291700027768

Mickus, M., Colenda, C., & Hogan, A. (2000). Knowledge of mental health benefits and preferences for type of mental health providers among the general public. *Psychiatric Services*, *51*(2), 199–202. doi:10.1176/appi.ps.51.2.199

Mueller, K., Kashinath, P., & Ullrich, F. (1997). Lengthening spells of "uninsurance" and their consequences. *Journal of Rural Health*, *13*(1), 29–37. doi:10.1111/j.1748-0361.1997.tb00831.x

National Institute on Aging. (2000). *Senior health facts*. Retrieved from www.seniorhealth.gov

National Institute on Alcohol Abuse and Alcoholism. (n.d.) Older Adults. Retrieved from https://www.niaaa.nih.gov/alcohol-health/special-populations-co-occurring-disorders/older-adults

National Institute on Mental Health. (2017, November). Prevalence of any anxiety disorder among adults. Retrieved from https://www.nimh.nih.gov/health/statistics/any-anxiety-disorder.shtml#part_155094

National Institute on Mental Health. (2018, January). Prevalence of panic disorder among adults. Retrieved from https://www.nimh.nih.gov/health/statistics/panic-disorder.shtml#part_155945

Neugarten, B. L. (1984). Psychological aspects of aging and illness. *Psychosomatics*, *25*(2), 123–125. doi:10.1016/s0033-3182(84)73081-7

New Freedom Commission on Mental Health. (2004). *Subcommittee on rural issues: Background paper* (DHHS Publication No. SMA-04-3890). Rockville, MD.

Ozarin, L. D., & Sharfstein, S. S. (1978). The aftermaths of deinstitutionalization: Problems and solutions. *Psychiatric Quarterly, 50*(2), 128–132. doi:10.1007/bf01064812

Paykel, E. S., Brayne, C., Huppert, F. A., Gill, C., Barkley, C., Gehlhaar, E., … O'Connor, D. (1994). Incidence of dementia in a population older than 75 years in the United Kingdom. *Archives of General Psychiatry, 51*(4), 325–332. doi:10.1001/archpsyc.1994.03950040069009

Proctor, E. K., Morrow-Howell, N., Doré, P., Wentz, J., Rubin, E., Thompson, S., & Li H. (2003). Comorbid medical conditions among depressed elderly patients discharged home after acute psychiatric care. *The American Journal of Geriatric Psychiatry, 11*(3), 329–338. doi:10.1097/00019442-200305000-00010

Proctor, E. K., Morrow-Howell, N., Rubin, E., & Ringenberg, M. (1999). Service use by elderly patients after psychiatric hospitalization. *Psychiatric Services, 50*(4), 553–555. doi:org/10.1176/ps.50.4.553

Ray, C. G, & Finley, J. K. (1994). Did CMHCs fail or succeed? Analysis of the expectations and outcomes of the community mental health movement. *Administration and Policy in Mental Health, 21*(4), 283–293. doi:10.1007/bf00709476

Regier, D. A., Farmer, M. E., Rae, D. S., Locke, B. Z., Keith, S. J., Judd, L. L., & Goodwin, M. D. (1990). Comorbidity of mental disorders with alcohol and other drug abuse. *JAMA, 264*(19), 2511–2518. doi:10.1001/jama.1990.03450190043026

Regier, D. A., Goldberg, I. D., & Taube, C. A. (1978). The de facto U.S. mental health service system: A public health perspective. *Archives of General Psychiatry, 35*(6), 685–693. doi:10.1001/archpsyc.1978.01770300027002

Reynolds, C. F., III. (1998, March 8–11). *The challenge of treatment in 70+ year olds with recurrent major depression: Excellent short-term but brittle long-term response.* Annual meeting of the American Association for Geriatric Psychiatry, San Diego, CA.

Reynolds, K., Pietrzak, R. H., El-Gabalawy, R., Mackenzie, C. S., & Sareen, J. (2015). Prevalence of psychiatric disorders in U.S. older adults: Findings from a nationally representative survey. *World Psychiatry, 14*(1), 74–81. doi:10.1002/wps.20193

Ritchie, K., & Kildea, D. (1995). Is senile dementia "age-related" or "ageing-related"? Evidence from meta-analysis of dementia prevalence in the oldest old. *Lancet, 346*(8980), 931–934. doi:10.1016/S0140-6736(95)91556-7

Robinson, G. K. (1990). The psychiatric component of long-term care models. In B. S. Fogel, G. L. Gottlieb, & A. Furino (Eds.), *Mental health policy for older Americans: Protecting minds at risk* (pp. 157–178. Washington, DC: American Psychiatric Press.

Rowe, J. W., & Kahn, R. L. (1997). Successful aging. *Gerontologist, 37*, 433–440. doi:10.1093/geront/37.4.433

Salloway, S., Malloy, P., Kohn, R., Gillard, E., Duffy, J., Rogg, J., … Westlake, R. (1996). MRI and neuropsychological differences in early- and late-life-onset geriatric depression. *Neurology, 46*, 1567–1574. doi:10.1212/wnl.46.6.1567

Sarkisian, C. A., Hays, R. D., Berry, S. H., & Mangione, C. M. (2001). Expectations regarding aging among older adults and physicians who care for older adults. *Medical Care, 39*(9), 1025–1036. doi:10.1097/00005650-200109000-00012

Saunders, P. A., Copeland, J. R., Dewey, M. E., Davidson, I. A., McWilliam, C., Sharma, V., & Sullivan, C. (1991). Heavy drinking as a risk factor for depression and dementia in elderly men. Findings from the Liverpool longitudinal community study. *British Journal of Psychiatry, 159*, 213–216. doi:10.1192/bjp.159.2.213

Schulberg, H. C., Madonia, M. J., Block, M. R., Coulehan, J. L., Scott, C. P., Rodriguez, E., & Black, A. (1995). Major depression in primary care practice: Clinical characteristics and treatment implications. *Psychosomatics, 36*(2), 129–137. doi:10.1016/S0033-3182(95)71682-6

Scott-Lennox, J. A., & George, L. (1996). Epidemiology of psychiatric disorders and mental health services use among older Americans. In B. L. Levin & J. Petrila (Eds.), *Mental health services: A public health perspective* (pp. 253–289. New York, NY: Oxford University Press.

Skoog, I. (1993). The prevalence of psychotic, depressive, and anxiety syndromes in demented and non-demented 85-year olds. *International Journal of Geriatric Psychiatry, 8*(3), 247–253. doi:10.1002/gps.930080308

Stern, Y., Gurland, B., Tatemichi, T. K., Tang, M. X., Wilder, D., & Mayeux, R. (1994). Influence of education and occupation on the incidence of Alzheimer's disease. *Journal of the American Medical Association, 271*, 1004–1010. doi:10.1001/jama.271.13.1004

Stewart, H., Jameson, J. P., & Curtin, L. (2015). The relationship between stigma and self-reported willingness to use mental health services among rural and urban older adults. *Psychological Services, 12*(2), 141–148. doi: 10.1037/a0038651

Taube, C. A., Morlock, L., Burns, B. J., & Santos, A. B. (1990). New directions in research on assertive community treatment. *Hospital & Community Psychiatry, 41*(6), 642–647. doi:10.1176/ps.41.6.642

United States Department of Health and Human Services. (1999). *Mental health and older adults. Chapter five appearing in report of the surgeon general on mental health needs*. Bethesda, MD: U.S. Government Printing Office.

United States Department of Health and Human Services. (2000). *NIA's strategic plan to address health disparities in aging: Fiscal years 2000–2005*. Bethesda, MD: U.S. Government Printing Office.

United States Department of Health and Human Services. (2001). *Mental health: Culture, race and ethnicity, A supplement to mental health: A report to the Surgeon General*. Rockville, MD: U.S. Department of Health and Human Services, Public Health Service, Office of the Surgeon General.

United States Department of Health and Human Services. (2005). Featured program: The gatekeeper model. *e-Communication, 1*(2). Rockville, MD: Substance Abuse and Mental Health.

United States Department of Health and Human Services. (2006a). Featured program: The mental health and aging systems integration initiative. *e-Communication*, 2(1). Rockville, MD: Substance Abuse and Mental Health.

United States Department of Health and Human Services. (2006b). Featured program: The recovery center. *e-Communication*, 2(1). RRockville, MD: Substance Abuse and Mental Health.

University of Cambridge, School of Clinical Medicine. (2012, April 25). Depression linked to longer hospital stays for illness. Retrieved from http://www.phpc.cam.ac.uk/blog/depression-linked-to-longer-hospital-stays-for-illness

Unutzer, J., Katon, W. J., Simon, G., Walker, E. A., Grembowski, D., & Patrick, D. (1996). Depression, quality of life, and use of health services in primary care patients over 65: A 4-year prospective study. *Psychosomatics, 37*, 35.

Wallace, J., & O'Hara, M. W. (1992). Increases in depressive symptomatology in the rural elderly: Results from a cross-sectional and longitudinal study. *Journal of Abnormal Psychology, 101*, 398–404. doi:10.1037//0021-843x.101.3.398

Waters, E. (1995). Let's not wait till it's broke: Interventions to maintain and enhance mental health in late life. In M. Gatz (Ed.), *Emerging issues in the mental health and aging* (pp. 183–209. Washington, DC: American Psychological Association.

Wells, K. B., Stewart, A., Hays, R. D., Burnam, M. A., Rogers, W., Daniels, M., ... Ware, J. (1989). The functioning and well-being of depressed patients: Results from the Medical Outcomes Study. *JAMA, 262*(7), 914–919. doi:10.1001/jama.1989.03430070062031

World Health Organization. (2017). *Mental health of older adults*. Retrieved from http://www.who.int/news-room/fact-sheets/detail/mental-health-of-older-adults

Zisook, S., & Shuchter, S. R. (1991). Depression through the first year after the death of a spouse. *American Journal of Psychiatry, 148*(10), 1346–1352. doi:10.1176/ajp.148.10.1346

10

The Patient Protection and Affordable Care Act

LEARNING OBJECTIVES

At the end of this chapter, readers will:

1. *Understand the history of the Affordable Care Act (ACA) and community prevention.*
2. *Understand specific components of the ACA in relationship to community prevention.*
3. *Understand how community prevention within the ACA prepares the workforce to address the service needs of older adults and people with disabilities.*

Erica and Theresa wanted to explore the extent to which the Patient Protection and Affordable Care Act (ACA) played a role in the lives of people growing older and people with disabilities. They were surprised to learn that the ACA spanned so many areas to include provision of healthcare, protection of elders through the Elder Justice Act, workforce development, prevention of chronic disease, and transparency related to health outcomes. Since improved access to healthcare services in rural and frontier areas was a component of the ACA, the two researchers also wondered how this feature of the act could impact the array of services to be delivered. The pair decided to talk to some older adults to gain an idea of how the ACA impacted them and to help with their own needs assessment related to how to build statewide services, health exchanges, and workforce training.

Lorraine: *Lorraine is a 96-year-old woman who has survived the Holocaust and currently lives in Fort Myers, Florida. Lorraine moved into an Assisted Living facility 2 years ago, when she lost her driving privileges and had been reported to be falling within her home. She is renting her family home to her adult grandson. Lorraine, a divorcee lived in an abusive relationship for most of her 27 years of marriage.*

Joan: *Joan currently lives in Ohio, and manages independently, despite a car accident that left her with a severe head injury 36 years ago. Joan became a parent shortly after her head injury, and often suffers from aphasia. She currently lives in her own home, with her adult son. Disabled for 36 years, she is approaching her 65th birthday and will be eligible to collect Medicare. Despite her disability, she has been able to work in her family's business.*

 DOI:10.1891/9780826128393.00010

THE AFFORDABLE CARE ACT BECOMES LAW

The Patient Protection and Affordable Care Act (ACA), a landmark piece of legislation, originally conceptualized to provide healthcare to at least 35 million people without health insurance, was signed by President Barack Obama on March 23, 2010. To many, it is known by its unofficial name, "Obamacare." Ironically, some people do not realize that they are different names for the same legislation and will variably have different opinions on one as opposed to the other.

The 10 titles of the legislation were staged to be implemented between 2010 and 2014. The passage of the ACA was somewhat controversial because of the way the process was handled. Some of the important highlights in the process of the bill becoming law include the following events within a timeline:

- July 2009: Speaker of the House Nancy Pelosi and a group of Democrats from the House of Representatives reveal their plan for overhauling the healthcare system. It was drafted as H.R. 3962, the Affordable Health Care for America Act.
- August 25, 2009: Massachusetts senator Ted Kennedy, a leading supporter of healthcare reform, dies and puts the Senate Democrats' 60-seat supermajority required to pass a piece of legislation at risk.
- September 24, 2009: Democrat Paul Kirk is appointed interim senator from Massachusetts, temporarily restoring the Democrats' filibuster-proof 60th vote.
- November 7, 2009: In the House of Representatives, 219 Democrats and one Republican vote for the Affordable Health Care for America Act, and 39 Democrats and 176 Republicans vote against it.
- December 24, 2009: In the Senate, 60 Democrats vote for the Senate's version of the bill, called America's Healthy Future Act, whose lead author is Senator Max Baucus of Montana. Thirty-nine Republicans vote against the bill, and one Republican senator, Jim Bunning of Kentucky, does not vote.
- January 2010: Scott Brown, a Republican, wins the special election in Massachusetts to finish out the remaining term of Senator Ted Kennedy, a Democrat. Brown campaigned heavily against the healthcare law and won an upset victory in a state that heavily favors the Democratic Party.
- March 11, 2010: Now lacking the 60th vote needed to pass the bill, Senate Democrats decide to use budget reconciliation in order to get to one bill approved by the House and the Senate. The use of budget reconciliation requires only 51 Senators to vote in favor of the bill in order for it to go to the president's desk for signature.
- March 21, 2010: The Senate's version of the healthcare plan is approved by the House in a 219 to 212 vote. All Republicans and 34 Democrats vote against the plan. This moved the bill to President Obama's desk.
- March 23, 2010: President Obama signs the Patient Protection and Affordable Care Act into public law (Pub. L. No. 111–148).

COMPONENTS OF THE ACA

The Patient Protection and ACA, Public Law 111–148, comprises 10 titles, and the entire piece of legislation spans over 1,000 pages. In the following sections, a short review of each of the 10 titles, helps the reader to understand the context of the Patient Protection and ACA. First, let us look at the actual titles that make up this landmark legislation.

- Title I: Quality, Affordable Health Care for All Americans
- Title II: Role of Public Program
- Title III: Improving the Quality and Efficiency of Health Care
- Title IV: Prevention of Chronic Disease and Improving Public Health
- Title V: Health Care Workforce
- Title VI: Transparency and Program Integrity
- Title VII: Improving Access to Innovative Medical Therapies
- Title VIII: Class Act
- Title IX: Revenue Provision
- Title X: Strengthening Quality, Affordable Health Care for All Americans

The following sections explain some of the legislative highlights, policies, and programs that have been articulated within each of the specific titles of the ACA.

Title I: Quality, Affordable Healthcare for All Americans

The sections addressed within Title I include the following highlights

- Individual and group market reforms.
- Actions to preserve and expand coverage.
- Quality health insurance coverage for all Americans.
- Available coverage choices for all Americans.
- Consumer choices and insurance competition through health benefit exchanges.
- State flexibility related to exchanges.
- Small business tax credit.

A portion of Title I seeks to provide amendments to the existing Public Health Services Act. Within this act is a component that seeks to provide for individual and group market reforms that ultimately will improve coverage for consumers. Among the provisions are no lifetime or annual limits for coverage and coverage for preventive health services (rather than merely acute and curative services). In the past, people may have been denied coverages based upon their salary, a restriction that has now been eliminated from this component. Other areas aimed at improving coverage include an appeals process; health insurance consumer information that is designed to target consumer needs and literacy levels; and a provision to ensure that consumers get value for their money and coverage.

Title I also seems to prohibit the denial of healthcare coverage based upon preexisting conditions and other forms of discrimination based upon health status. People who retire early also can benefit from a form of reinsurance, and immediate information will enable consumers to identify affordable coverage options and opportunities. The improvement in access for consumers includes guaranteed availability of coverage, comprehensive health insurance coverage, and the opportunity to renew coverage regardless of healthcare status.

Title I of the ACA is very committed to ensuring quality affordable healthcare for all Americans. This includes the opportunity for Americans to be guaranteed renewability of coverage, ensuring that people are not discriminated against based on their health status, and ensuring that people have comprehensive health insurance coverage. The legislation also prohibits excessive waiting periods to receive care from healthcare providers.

State exchanges have been used to create pooled options for health insurance. Under this title, states are afforded the flexibility to operate within specific requirements. They are also given the flexibility to be able to develop health programs and coverage for people who are not eligible for Medicaid. A waiver for the provision of innovation is also provided in the legislation. This means that states can take the opportunity to provide for some innovative programming within their own states, based upon their demographics and the resources available for healthcare coverage. This aspect benefits people with disabilities, especially children (Children's Health Insurance Program [CHIP]) and people with low incomes or who qualify for Medicaid coverage, because the paperwork is streamlined within exchanges for these individuals.

Small businesses are also given tax credits in order to provide coverage for their employees, and Title I addresses the benefits and provisions for small business owners. However, because these aspects of Title I do not directly benefit older adults or people with disabilities, they will not be elaborated upon here.

Under the miscellaneous clause within Title I, the legislation enables people, regardless of age and ability, to access the therapies that they prefer. Interestingly, this provision is not commonly addressed within the materials that are publicly available. There is also a provision in the legislation to prohibit discrimination for refusal to provide assisted suicide.

Title II: Role of Public Programs

The sections addressed within the role of public programs that impact older adults and people with disabilities include the following highlights

- Improved access to Medicaid
- Improvement to Medicaid insurance
- Medicaid prescription drug coverage
- Medicaid improvement of quality for patients and providers
- Protection for American Indians and Alaskan Natives

Title II of the ACA addresses the role of public programs and improving access to healthcare, especially preventive healthcare. It specifically addressed access to Medicaid, CHIP, Medicaid prescription drug access, Indian healthcare access, and access for mothers and children through the Maternal and Child Health Programs.

Improved access to Medicaid includes the expansion of coverage for people through grants to states for the purpose of healthcare coverage. Some states, such as Kentucky and Mississippi, opted into these opportunities to expand the range of people who could be covered by Medicaid. Under this program, states would be reimbursed through the federal government for a portion of the funding that they invested into Medicaid expansion.

Enhanced support for CHIP is also addressed within Title II. These programs are not necessarily identified as CHIP programs from state to state, but most states have expanded the number of children who receive a medical card and medical access within this program. Authorization for this enhanced funding for this program actually expired on September 30, 2017, although reauthorization for funding was extended until September 30, 2018. A part of this process also includes the simplification of enrollments for Medicaid and CHIP coverage. This will definitely benefit people with disabilities across the life span including children living with disabilities.

This title also provides the consumer with enhanced prescription drug coverage and improvements through Medicaid for patients and providers. This portion of the ACA will provide for low-income older adults and low-income people with disabilities. It also enables the medical provider to offer more comprehensive care to the consumer.

Title III: Improving the Quality and Efficiency of Healthcare

The sections of Title III addressing the improvement of quality and efficiency of healthcare that impact older adults and people with disabilities include as the following

- Improving Medicare for patients and providers
- Rural protections
- Improving payment accuracy
- Medicare Part D improvements for prescription drug plans
- Ensuring Medicare sustainability

Although a number of areas are covered under Title III that address the quality and efficiency of how healthcare is delivered, a few sections specifically address or have an impact upon the needs of people growing older and people with disabilities. Specifically, the approach to develop new patient care models and to improve Medicare for patients and providers, impacts our target group of interest.

Improving Medicare for Patients and Providers

Part I of this title addresses linking payments to quality outcomes under the Medicare program. This provision includes quality reporting for people who are residing or are patients in long-term care hospitals, inpatient rehabilitation hospitals, and hospice programs. This creates new benchmarks for quality and outcomes to address accountability that should be of lasting benefit for older adults and people with disabilities. Under this segment of the legislation, if a person is readmitted into a hospital for the same health condition before 30 days postdischarge, the fee for service is either readjusted or a fine is levied on the facility. Prior to the ACA, limited public accountability was expected on the part of the healthcare industry. However, part of the ACA, requires data collection and public reporting of data related to patient care and outcomes. Part II of this title also supports an interagency working group to improve healthcare quality, the development of quality measures, and a national strategy with the goal of consistency in reporting.

The concept of new patient care models to address the needs of older adults and people with disabilities is addressed in Title III of the legislation. Under Title III is the establishment of a Center for Medicare and Medicaid Innovation within the Centers for Medicare and Medicaid Services (CMS). The development of innovative patient care models to improve patient outcomes occurs through this center. Demonstration funds are also available for innovations that help enhance the "person in environment" or "aging in place" models of care. This segment of the ACA drives innovations for patient care to help them stay as independent and community based as possible. Similarly, the legislation also addressed the need for new community-based care models that facilitate transitions from varying levels of independence and care.

Title III also targets improving Medicare for patients and their providers. This improvement is achieved through a variety of strategies to include increasing the payment schedule for physicians through both general payments and geographical appropriations. For example, less densely populated areas such as rural communities may see a higher level of payments because of the travel time and patient mix. Some of the capitations for specific Medicare therapies that would be covered under part B were also lifted, based upon the situation. Pathologies are also included and under consideration. Mental health services under some conditions could also be expanded as are situational needs for expansion of payment for long-term care and hospital services. These provisions benefit older adults and people with disabilities particularly in rural communities, where options for care and treatment can be limited. Under this title, physician assistants can also bill Medicare/Medicaid for care to offer and order home-health services and extended care services for posthospital care services. Other areas addressed include pharmaceutical care exemptions for people impacted by certain accreditation rules that may hinder care in smaller centers and rural communities. Other areas that have been expanded to improve care include the provision of bone density tests, and the ability to have some complex laboratory tests covered for Medicare and Medicaid eligible patients.

Rural Protections

Under Title III, Rural communities and healthcare providers are somewhat protected. For example, given that many tests for patients in certain rural hospitals may be costly, the ACA provides for an extension of Medicare reasonable costs for certain clinical diagnostic laboratory tests furnished to hospital patients in certain rural areas. Hospitals that experience a low volume of patients who utilize services also benefit from the ACA through the adjustment to Medicare payments. Studies have also been in the works as a result of this legislation to ensure that Medicare payments for healthcare providers are both accurate and cover the cost of carrying out business.

Improving Payment Accuracy

Medicare Advantage (MA; Part C) is also addressed in Title III. MA payments are based on the average of the bids submitted by insurance plans in each market. Bonus payments are available to improve the quality of care and are based on an insurer's level of care coordination and care management, as well as achievement on quality rankings. New payments will be implemented over a 4-year transition period. MA plans are prohibited from charging beneficiaries cost sharing for covered services greater than what is charged under fee-for-service. Plans providing extra benefits must give priority to cost-sharing reductions, wellness, and preventive care prior to covering benefits not currently covered by Medicare.

Medicare Part D

Medicare Prescription Drug Plan Improvements (Part D) is another area that benefits older adults and people with disabilities. As of July 1, 2010, drug manufacturers who want to have their drugs covered under the Medicare Part D program must provide a 50% discount to Part D beneficiaries for brand-name drugs and biologics purchased during the coverage gap. The initial coverage limit in the standard Part D benefit is now $3,750 for 2018, compared to $2,250 at the program's start in 2006 and $2,930 in 2010.

Medicare Sustainability

Ensuring Medicare sustainability is an area of concern under the ACA and is addressed in Title III. A productivity adjustment is added to the market basket update for inpatient hospitals, home-health providers, nursing homes, hospice providers, inpatient psychiatric facilities, long-term care hospitals, and inpatient rehabilitation facilities. The Act creates a 15-member Independent Payment Advisory Board to present Congress with proposals to reduce costs and improve quality for beneficiaries. When Medicare costs are projected to exceed certain targets, the Board's proposals will take effect unless Congress passes an alternative measure to achieve the same level of savings. The Board will not make proposals that ration care; raise taxes or beneficiary premiums; or change Medicare benefit, eligibility, or cost-sharing standards.

Healthcare quality improvements are also a focus of Title III. The ACA creates a new program to develop community health teams supporting medical homes to increase access to community-based, coordinated care. A *medical home*, known in full as a *patient-centered medical home* (PCMH), is a primary care model that delivers comprehensive healthcare via a team of practitioners, including physicians, nurses, social workers, nutritionists, and other health professionals (Agency for Healthcare Research and Quality [AHRQ], 2018).

It supports a health delivery system research center to conduct research on health delivery systems and best practices that improve the quality, safety, and efficiency of healthcare. It also supports medication management services by local health providers to help patients better manage chronic disease and promotes the permanency of demonstration model community-based, long-term care programs. Patient navigator programs to improve the health of older adults are also addressed in this title of the ACA.

Title IV: Prevention of Chronic Disease and Improving Public Health

- The sections of Title IV that impact older adults and people with disabilities include the following highlights: Modernizing disease prevention and public health systems.
- Improving access to clinical prevention and public health systems.
- Increasing access to clinical preventive services such as oral health.
- Creating healthier communities.
- Supporting prevention and public health innovation.

Improving Access to Clinical Prevention and Public Health Systems

The focus of Title IV of the ACA is toward the prevention of chronic disease and the improvement of public health. Both of these areas are of prime interest and importance to older adults and people with disabilities. The main idea is that prevention will address chronic health conditions and prevent ongoing disease and healthcare costs. To this end, a focus is on clinical and community preventive services along with community health promotion activities. A new interagency prevention council has been supported by the Prevention and Public Health Investment Fund initiative established by the ACA.

A number of initiatives through the use of Medicare were also proposed in the ACA, although they have been implemented to varying degrees. For example, the ACA proposed that barriers to accessing preventive services in Medicare be removed, and all fees for service for Part B services in Medicare be eliminated (ACA, Section 4104). While this would be fantastic for older adults and people with disabilities, it would not be realistic because of the costs involved. However, the initial Medicare coverage of the Welcome to Medicare visit is covered for older adults and people with disabilities, and people do receive an annual wellness visit and personalized prevention plan. Incentives for the prevention of chronic diseases for those enrolled in Medicaid have also been addressed through Title IV (Section 4108).

Creating Healthier Communities

The creation of healthier communities across the life span, including older adults, is also a focus of Title IV. Community transformation grants have been made available to older nongovernmental organizations (NGOs) and community-based organizations for the purpose of transforming communities to take on a wellness approach (Section 4201). Areas that focus upon these details include healthy aging, living well, and the evaluation of community-based prevention and wellness programs for Medicare beneficiaries (Section 4202). The removal of barriers and improving access to wellness for people living with disabilities is also a focus of the ACA (Section 4203). An example of one such wellness strategy is nutrition labeling of standard menu items at chain restaurants. But most Americans are familiar with this concept, since it was designed to help promote wellness across all segments of the population, not only for older adults or people with disabilities (Section 4205). Demonstration projects that seek to avoid cuts in services by controlling costs through improvement and integration of medical care and support services is another initiative of the ACA that impacts older adults and people with disabilities.

This titles support for prevention and public health innovation, offers significant benefits for older adults and people with disabilities, especially given that these groups have otherwise been largely ignored in this regard. Support for the Centers for Disease Control and Prevention (CDC) and the public health infrastructure are a part of this set of subtitles in the legislation intended to understand health disparities, carry out data collection, and expand epidemiological investigations. The investigation of strategies for pain management that are not medication oriented (i.e., not relying on opioids) is also addressed within this title. This is very important because, as Chapter 14 discusses, older adults and people with disabilities are very vulnerable to opioid and medication misuse. Other provisions of the ACA seek to ensure that wellness programs that are developed also prove to be effective.

Title V: Healthcare Workforce

The sections within Title V, The Health Care Workforce, that impact older adults and people with disabilities include the following highlights

- Innovations in the healthcare workforce
- Increasing the supply of the healthcare workforce
- Enhancing healthcare workforce education and training
- Supporting the existing healthcare workforce
- Strengthening primary care and other workforce improvements
- Improving access to healthcare services

This aspect of the ACA was written to address the importance of developing a competent workforce prepared to address the challenges that the healthcare industry was presenting. It was designed to address and foster innovative strategies within training, recruitment, and retention as well as to increase the pool of available healthcare workers. Overall, the goal is to build a new workforce training model and educational infrastructure through a host of strategies.

Innovations in the Healthcare Workforce

The ACA established the National Health Care Workforce Commission to analyze the state of workforce needs and to ensure that the ACA's administration is aligned with federal policies to meet the needs identified at the national level. It also established a number of grant mechanisms to enable states to conduct their own workforce needs assessments and to build workforce development training strategies.

Increasing the Supply of Healthcare Workers

A number of strategies were proposed within the ACA to increase the supply of the healthcare workforce. These included modifications to the federal student loan program, such as adjusting the payback period to make loans more attractive. Nursing student loans were expanded to help build a pool of nurses. Loan repayments were offered to public health students and workers in exchange for working at least 3 years at a federal, state, local, or tribal public health agency. Loan repayment programs were also established to be offered to allied health professionals employed at public health agencies or in healthcare settings located in health professional shortage areas, medically underserved areas, or with medically underserved populations. Social workers and others typically found working within interdisciplinary teams with older adults and people with disabilities were included. A mandatory fund for the National Health Service Corps scholarship and loan repayment program was created to help build financial opportunities for these up-and-coming professionals. A $50 million grant program was also established to support nurse-managed health clinics, which also impacts older adults and people with disabilities, especially those in rural community areas.

Enhancing Healthcare Workforce Education and Training

New support for workforce training programs was established by ACA in a number of key areas that impact older adults and people with disabilities such as

- Family medicine, general internal medicine, and physician assistantship.
- Rural physicians.
- Direct care workers providing long-term care services and supports.
- General and public health dentistry.
- Alternative dental healthcare providers.
- Geriatric education and training for faculty in health professions schools and family caregivers.
- Cultural competency, prevention, and public health and individuals with disabilities training.
- Nurse education, practice, and retention grants to nursing schools to strengthen nurse education and training programs and to improve nurse retention.
- Nurse practitioner training programs in community health centers and nurse-managed health centers.
- Nurse faculty loan program for nurses who pursue careers in nurse education.
- Grants to the community health workforce to promote positive health behaviors and outcomes in medically underserved areas through use of community health workers.
- Fellowship training in public health to address workforce shortages in state and local health departments in applied public health epidemiology and public health laboratory science and informatics.
- A U.S. Public Health Sciences Track to train physicians, dentists, nurses, physician assistants, mental and behavior health specialists, and public health professionals emphasizing team-based service, public health, epidemiology, and emergency preparedness and response in affiliated institutions.

Many state-based education centers such as Geriatrics Workforce Enhancement Programs (GWEPs) have become visible across the nation and are a direct outgrowth of this subtitle of the ACA. The GWEPs have replaced the geriatric education training centers. In addition, there has been an increase in interdisciplinary professional educational initiatives to help professional groups work more cohesively as teams, and team-based services are a frequent requirement when working with older adults and people with disabilities.

Supporting the Existing Healthcare Workforce

The Patient Protection and ACA reauthorized the Centers of Excellence program for minority applicants for health professions, expanded scholarships for disadvantaged students who committed to work in medically underserved areas, and authorized funding for the Area Health Education Centers (AHECs) program. A Primary Care Extension program was established to educate and provide technical assistance to primary care providers about evidence-based therapies, preventive medicine, health promotion, chronic disease management, and mental health. The result of this portion of the ACA was improved healthcare delivery and outcomes to areas where strong health disparities among older adults and people with disabilities were apparent and evident. The evidence-based approach to therapeutic interventions is also key to working with older adults and people with disabilities to ensure that they are receiving treatments that have a clinical record of being effective and work to improve patient health outcomes.

Strengthening Primary Care and Other Workforce Improvements

Beginning in 2011, the Secretary of Health and Human Services (HHS) may redistribute unfilled residency positions, redirecting those slots for training of primary care physicians. A demonstration grant program was also established to serve low-income persons to develop core training competencies and certification programs for personal and home care aides. Also, a grant program was established to provide grant funding and payments to teaching health centers that focus on training primary care providers in the community. This initiative brought about the concept of the community health worker, primarily a peer oriented "boots on the ground" worker who serves a community as a liaison between the consumer and the health professional. Medicare was also directed to test new models for improving the training of advance practice nurses, which had a direct impact for people such as older adults and people with disabilities who are receiving Medicare oriented treatments.

Improving Access to Healthcare Services

The ACA authorized new and expanded funding for federally qualified health centers and reauthorized a program to award grants to states and medical schools to support the improvement and expansion of emergency medical services for individuals impacted by trauma and in need of critical care treatment. While this provision primarily impacts children, it does help deal with premature disability and protect people from long-term injury and disability. Also supported are grants for coordinated and integrated services through the colocation of primary and specialty care in community-based mental and behavioral health settings.

Title VI: Transparency and Program Integrity

New support for transparency and program integrity addressed within Title VI was established by ACA in a number of key areas that impact older adults and people with disabilities, including

- Physician ownership and other transparency
- Nursing home transparency and improvement
- Improving transparency of information
- Targeting enforcement
- Improving staff training
- Patient-centered outcomes research
- Elder Justice Act

To help address and ensure the integrity of federally financed and sponsored health programs, this title created new requirements to provide information to the public on the health system and promoted a newly invigorated set of requirements to address fraud and abuse within publicly and privately funded and run programs.

Physician Ownership and Other Transparency

Physician-owned hospitals that did not have a provider agreement prior to August 2010 were not eligible to participate in Medicare. Drug, device, biological, and medical supply manufacturers must report gifts and other transfers of value made to a physician, a physician medical practice, a physician group practice, and/or a teaching hospital. Referring physicians for imaging services must inform patients in writing that the individual may obtain such service from a person other than the referring physician, a physician who is a member of the same group practice, or an individual who is supervised by the physician or by another physician in the group. Prescription drug makers and distributors must report to the HHS Secretary information pertaining to drug samples currently being collected internally. Pharmacy benefit managers (PBMs) or health benefits plans that provide pharmacy benefit management services that contract with health plans under Medicare or the ACA Exchanges must report information regarding the generic dispensing rate; rebates, discounts, or price concessions negotiated by the PBM. All of these areas have a direct impact on older adults or people with disabilities who receive Medicare benefits.

Nursing Home Transparency and Improvement

The Act requires that skilled nursing facilities (SNFs) under Medicare and nursing facilities (NFs) under Medicaid make available information on ownership. SNFs and NFs are now required to implement a compliance and ethics program, as a result of ACA. The secretary of HHS also now publishes new information on the Nursing Home Compare pages on the Medicare website (www.medicare.gov/what-medicare-covers/part-a/report-problems-in-snf.html) such as standardized staffing data, links to state Internet websites regarding state survey and certification programs, a model standardized complaint form, a summary of complaints, and the number of instances of criminal violations by a facility or its employees. The secretary also has developed a standardized complaint form for use by residents in filing complaints with a state survey and certification agency or a state long-term care ombudsman. All of these areas have direct impact on the quality of care and assurance of care for people residing in nursing homes, particularly older adults and people with disabilities.

Targeting Enforcement

Under this subtitle of the ACA, the secretary for HHS may reduce civil monetary penalties for facilities that self-report and correct deficiencies. The secretary will establish a 2-year demonstration project to test and implement a national independent monitoring program to oversee interstate and large intrastate chains. (This has not happened yet.) The administrator of a facility preparing to close must provide written notice to residents, legal representatives of residents, the state, the Secretary, and the long-term care ombudsman program in advance of the closure.

Improving Staff Training

Facilities must now include dementia management and abuse prevention training as part of preemployment training for staff. The ACA requires, the Secretary of HHS to establish a Nationwide Program for Background Checks on Direct Patient Access Employees of Long Term Care Facilities and Providers as part of the ACA. This program establishes a framework through which states can conduct national and state background checks of all prospective direct patient access employees of nursing homes and long-term care providers.

Patient-Centered Outcomes Research

The ACA established a private, nonprofit entity (the Patient-Centered Outcomes Research Institute) governed by a public/private board appointed by the comptroller general to provide for comparative clinical outcomes research. No findings may be construed as mandates on practice guidelines or coverage decisions, and important patient safeguards protect against discriminatory coverage decisions by HHS based on age, disability, terminal illness, or an individual's quality of life preference.

Additional Program Integrity Provisions

Employees and agents of multiple employer welfare arrangements (MEWAs) are subject to criminal penalties if they provide false statements in marketing materials regarding a plan's financial solvency, benefits, or regulatory status. A model uniform reporting form was developed by the National Association of Insurance Commissioners, under the direction of the HHS Secretary. The Department of Labor adopted regulatory standards and/or issue orders to prevent fraudulent MEWAs from escaping liability for their actions under state law by claiming that state law enforcement is preempted by federal law. The Department of Labor is authorized to issue "cease and desist" orders to temporarily shut down operations of plans conducting fraudulent activities or posing a serious threat to the public, until hearings can be completed. MEWAs are required to file their federal registration forms, and thereby be subject to government verification of their legitimacy, before enrolling anyone.

Elder Justice Act

The Elder Justice Act, enacted as part of the ACA, was designed to help prevent and eliminate elder abuse, neglect, and exploitation. Owners, operators, and employees would be required to report suspected crimes committed at long-term care facilities. Chapter 12 addresses the Elder Justice Act in more detail.

Sense of the Senate Regarding Medical Malpractice

The ACA expresses the sense of the Senate that health reform presents an opportunity to address issues related to medical malpractice and medical liability insurance. Consequently, states are encouraged to develop and test alternative models to the existing civil litigation system, and Congress has been given the opportunity to consider state demonstration projects to evaluate such alternatives. Ultimately these provisions impact older adults and people with disabilities.

Title VII: Improving Access to Innovative Medical Therapies

New support for improving medical therapies was established by ACA in key areas that impact older adults and people with disabilities such as

- Biologics
- Affordable medicines
- Underserved communities

A key goal of Title VII is to ensure access to medication and therapeutic interventions for the population, with a specific interest in making affordable medications available and reaching underserved communities. This benefits older adults and people with disabilities who reside in areas where there are pockets of consumers living in medically designated shortage areas.

Title VIII: Class Act

Establishment of a National Voluntary Insurance Program for the Purchase of Community Living Assistance Services and Support

The ACA established a new, voluntary, self-funded long-term care insurance program, the Community Living Assistance Services and Supports (CLASS) Independence Benefit Plan, for the purchase of CLASS by individuals with functional limitations.

Title IX: Revenue Provisions

Title IX addresses how money will be raised to address the programs and services provided in the preceding titles. Many of the provisions outlined in the ACA within this title are subject to change based upon the current administration in the White House; thus, the specific details within this title will be discussed at a minimum. Since this appears to be a moving target under the Trump administration, the details are changing and evolving. Hence, the specific details are not addressed in this section because they are likely to be quickly outdated. Outlined in the original ACA was how insurance companies would work with addressing insurance premiums for their consumers. This provision included the additional fee structure for people at increased risk of disease and illness, that is people 55 years of age and older. It also addressed how and when people needed to apply for Medicare and penalties to consumers if these rules were not followed.

Title X: Strengthening Quality, Affordable Healthcare for All Americans

Title X made many improvements to the preceding nine titles, and descriptions of those changes are included in the descriptions of the first nine titles. This section discusses the details of Title X amendments that are pertinent to older adults and people with disabilities and to the healthcare professionals and institutions that cater to the needs of these groups that were not covered under the earlier titles.

Improvements in the Role of Public Programs

Title X creates some financial incentives, including federal medical assistance percentage (FMAP) increases, for states to shift Medicaid beneficiaries out of nursing homes and into home- and community-based services (HCBS). This provision would lead to higher functioning older adults moving out of nursing home situations and back into the community. The major impact has been seen by people with disabilities who may have been living in long-term care nursing situations but eligible to live in community home-based settings with support services.

Indian Healthcare Improvement

Title X authorized appropriations for the Indian Health Care Improvement Act, which has included programs to increase the Indian healthcare workforce, new programs for innovative care delivery models, behavioral healthcare services, new services for health promotion and disease prevention, efforts to improve access to healthcare services, and construction of Indian health facilities. This aspect provides definite improvements for programs and services to both older adults and people with disabilities living in areas covered by the National Indian Health Act. Both of these target populations have been largely ignored or lack development. In addition, the Older American's Act, although it outlines specific criteria for jurisdictions governed by the Indian Health Act, has been under-funded and not consistent with areas governed by the Administration on Aging.

Medicare Improvements

Title X calls attention to improvements to Medicare beneficiary services, including coverage for individuals exposed to environment health hazards; prescription drug review through medication therapy management programs; development of a "Physician Compare" website to help beneficiaries learn more about their doctors; and a study on beneficiary access to dialysis services. Medicare payment changes include financial protections for states in which at least 50% of counties are frontier. Other changes in this section include grants to develop networks of providers to deliver coordinated care to low-income populations.

Public Health Program Improvements

Title X of the ACA enables the Secretary of HHS to develop a national report card on diabetes to be updated every 2 years, and to work with states to improve data collection related to diabetes and other chronic diseases. This process should help both older adults and people with disabilities since the risk of acquiring diabetes increases with age.

Workforce Improvements

Title X authorized grants for medical schools to establish programs that recruit students from underserved rural areas who have a desire to practice in their hometowns. Since many older adults want to age in place and live within their home community, especially people living in rural communities, this provision helps support a medical infrastructure within underserved rural and frontier communities.

SUMMARY

The Patient Protection and ACA was a landmark piece of healthcare legislation intended to provide universal access to care to people throughout the United States. Along with access to medical care and health insurance were many other important provisions, which addressed how to build a health and public health infrastructure and improve the quality and outcomes of healthcare delivery. This chapter deals with specific aspects of the legislation that impact older adults and people with disabilities. The reader may be familiar with some elements (e.g., remaining on one's parents' health insurance until age 26) that have not been addressed within this chapter because they do not have an impact on people growing older or people with disabilities who benefit from Medicare and Medicaid coverage. Many of the provisions related to financing the ACA have faced criticism by the Republican Party. There have been various modifications to provisions of the ACA (Mach & Kinzer, 2018). In 2017, various amendments to the ACA were proposed under the Republican-backed American Health Care Act (AHCA), in an effort to repeal parts of the ACA. However, AHCA failed to pass after a 49–51 vote in the Senate.

DISCUSSION QUESTIONS

1. How would the cases studies (Lorraine and Joan) presented at the beginning of the chapter benefit from provisions and resources of the ACA?
2. What types of training initiative can you and your colleagues benefit from as a result of Title V, Geriatric Workforce Training and Development? What areas are still needed to improve the geriatric workforce or the workforce dedicated to working with people who have disabilities?
3. If revisions are made to the Patient Protection and Affordable Care Act (ACA), what elements do you believe should be protected, and what elements could be eliminated or revised? Why do you feel the way you do? How would you lobby your local congressional representative and senator to endorse these changes?

DISCUSSION QUESTIONS *(continued)*

4. How can you go about designing a fact sheet and advocacy campaign to help educate local consumers about their rights under the current ACA and/or proposed changes to the ACA? You may also want to consider how to prepare consumers to address these same areas with local legislators.

ADDITIONAL RESOURCES

YouTube Videos

The ACA: Explained: www.youtube.com/watch?v=Dqabs9xysYA

This YouTube video provides the viewer with easy to understand facts that explain the various titles of the Patient Protection and ACA. The video has been created in a humorous manner to make the points easily to digest and understand.

Obamacare versus the ACA: www.youtube.com/watch?v=N6m7pWEMPlA

This entertaining video provides an overview of the layperson's understanding of the ACA. It showcases the general lack of understanding and literacy that people demonstrate in relation to the ACA.

What is Medicare Wellness Visit: www.youtube.com/watch?v=RLhKuYG3mlI

This video provides an overview of what to expect in the Medicare Wellness visit for first time users.

Websites

Catch on for Community Health: www.catch-on.org

This website provides a range of training information for a variety of healthcare professionals. It was designed by a specific GWEP funded under Title V of the ACA.

Welcome to Medicare Preventative Visit: www.medicare.gov/people-like-me/new-to-medicare/welcome-to-medicare-visit.html

This website provides an overview of the tests and process one would encounter during the "Welcome to Medicare" initial visit.

A checklist for your Annual Medicare Visit: www.acponline.org/system/files/documents/running_practice/payment_coding/medicare/hra.pdf

This website provides the consumer a checklist of specific items to discuss with his or her healthcare provider upon the initial Medicare Wellness visit.

Podcasts

Bob Blancato on the Affordable Care Act and advocacy. **Listen now:** https://bcove.video/2DzabHl

Robyn Golden, Dr. Erin Emery, and Michelle Newman discuss Catch-On and the Geriatric Workforce Enhancement Program through the Affordable Care Act's Title V. **Listen now:** https://bcove.video/2DABTUd

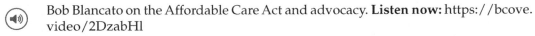

REFERENCES

Agency for Healthcare Research and Quality. (2018). *Defining the PCMH*. Retrieved from http://pcmh.ahrq.gov/page/defining-pcmh

Mach, A. L., & Kinzer, J. (2018). *Legislative actions to modify the Affordable Care Act in the 111th-115th Congresses* (Congressional Research Service, Report R45244). Washington, DC: Congressional Research Service. Retrieved from http://fas.org/sgp/crs/misc/R45244.pdf

Patient Protection and Affordable Care Act, 42 U.S.C. § 18001 et seq. (2010).

11

Caregivers/The Caregiver Support Act

LEARNING OBJECTIVES

At the end of this chapter, readers will:

1. *Understand the history of the Caregiver Support Act.*
2. *Understand specific components of the Caregiver Support Act.*
3. *Understand how the Caregiver Support Act provides resources to older adults and people with disabilities.*

Caregiving is an often understated and underrepresented area for discussion. Erica and Theresa fond that many people they met within their focus groups and discussions indicated that caregivers were often unsung heroes. A couple of cases worth noting included Nora and Susan.

Susan: *Susan is a 57-year-old woman who has sustained a work-related injury that has impacted her knees and mobility. In addition to her own mobility impairment, she lives with her older parents, Irma and Gus. Gus was diagnosed with early stages of Alzheimer's disease about 10 years ago, and this has progressed to the point where he is mobility impaired and needs constant supervision. Irma is a brittle diabetic and cannot handle the care needs of her husband, and relies mostly on Susan for help. They lived on a farm, but now have moved to a metropolitan area with their daughter Susan. They have five other adult children. Despite the other siblings in the family, Susan was resigned to looking after her father following her work injury and limitations to her mobility. Erica and Theresa were interested in how Susan's caregiving role was impacted and how community resources and supports help the family unit.*

Nora: *Nora is both a caregiver to her 87-year-old father and disabled due to an orthopedic injury while riding a bicycle. Her recent knee replacement surgery has left her with less mobility in her right knee, than prior to her surgery. Caregiver to her father leaves her with limited emotional resources at the end of a day. Nora's father is legally blind suffers from Crone's disease and has had a series of mini strokes. They live together in the three-bedroom family home and receive in home services to support Nora in her caregiving role. Nora's father also attends a day program 3 days per week. Nora's mother passed away 10 years ago, and she also* *helps in the caregiving role for her two grandsons. Nora's father was emotionally distant to her while growing up and she is an only child. Erica and Theresa were curious to learn how Nora's caregiving role would be impacted by the fractured relationship she had with her father. How did existing programs and services help Nora with her caregiving duties and provide for her emotional support?*

CAREGIVERS AND THE CAREGIVER SUPPORT ACT

The Caregiver and the Caregiver Support Act was established in 2000 and the National Family Caregiver Support Program (NFCSP) provides grants to states and territories, based on their share of the population as a result of Section 371 (Title IIIe) of the Older Americans Act (OAA) Amendments of 2000. This is an important component of the OAA because it enables people to remain in their home as long as possible, whether they are living with a disability or are aging. The National Family Caregiving Support Program provides five types of services

- Information to caregivers about available services
- Assistance to caregivers in gaining access to the services
- Individual counseling, organization of support groups, and caregiver training
- Respite care
- Supplemental services, on a limited basis

These services work in conjunction with other state and community-based services to provide a coordinated set of supports. Studies have shown that these services can reduce caregiver depression, anxiety, and stress as well as enable caregivers to provide care longer, thereby avoiding or delaying the need for costly institutional care.

The Aging Services network has long been an advocate for caregivers and the needs that caregiving presents for both those being cared for and the caregiver. As of the 2016 Reauthorization of the OAA, the following specific populations of caregivers are now eligible to receive services

- Adult family members or other informal caregivers age 18 and older providing care to individuals 60 years of age and older.
- Adult family members or other informal caregivers age 18 and older providing care to individuals of any age with Alzheimer's disease and related disorders.
- Older relatives (not parents) age 55 and older providing care to children under the age of 18.
- Older relatives, including parents, age 55 and older, providing care to adults ages 18 to 59 with disabilities.

Family caregivers present their unique needs and preferences for the types of programs and services they wish to receive at any given time. Further, available programs and services vary among states and communities. Fortunately, a number of national organizations and programs exist to inform and support program development and innovation. (See resources and links at the end of this chapter for additional information on research, technical assistance, and support for program development).

In 2014, the most recent year for which service data is available, more than 700,000 caregivers received services through the NFCSP (Administration for Community Living [ACL], 2017). These services helped them to better manage caregiving responsibilities while ensuring their loved ones remained in the community for as long as possible. Service highlights include

- **Access Assistance Services** provided more than 1.3 million contacts to caregivers, helping them to locate services from a variety of private and voluntary agencies.
- **Counseling and Training Services** provided more than 100,000 caregivers with counseling, peer support groups, and training to help them cope with the stresses of caregiving.
- **Respite Care Services** were provided to more than 604,000 caregivers through nearly 6 million hours of temporary relief from caregiving responsibilities—at home or in an adult day care or institutional setting.

Data from the ACL's 2017 national survey of caregivers of older adult clients shows the following

- OAA services, including those provided through the NFCSP, are effective in helping caregivers keep their loved ones at home.
- Nearly 42% of caregivers report they have been providing care for 2 to 5 years, while approximately 27% of family caregivers have been providing care for 5 to 10 years.
- Seventy-four percent of caregivers of program clients report that services enabled them to provide care longer than would have been possible otherwise.
- Eighty-eight percent of caregivers reported that services helped them to be a better caregiver.
- Nearly 62% of caregivers indicated that without the services they received, the care recipient would be living in a nursing home.

The Lifespan Respite Care Program was authorized by Congress in 2006 under Title XXIX of the Public Health Service Act (42 U.S.C 201). Lifespan Respite Care programs are coordinated systems of accessible, community-based respite care services for family caregivers of children and adults of all ages with special needs. Such programs reduce duplication of effort and assist in the development of respite care infrastructures at the state and local levels.

Lifespan Respite Care Programs work to improve the delivery and quality of respite services available through the following objectives

- Expand and enhance respite services in the states.
- Improve coordination and dissemination of respite services.
- Streamline access to programs.
- Fill gaps in service where necessary.
- Improve the overall quality of the respite services currently available.

Since 2009, Congress has appropriated approximately $2.5 million per year to implement Lifespan Respite Programs. As of 2016, competitive grants of up to $200,000 each were awarded to eligible agencies in 35 states and the District of Columbia.

Eligible agencies are those administering the state's program under the OAA of 1965 or Title XIX of the Social Security Act (Medicaid), or those designated by a governor to administer the state's program under this title. The eligible state agency must be an aging and disability resource center and work in collaboration with a public or private nonprofit statewide respite care coalition or organization.

A number of initiatives have been developed that address the caregivers' needs and the infrastructure that supports these needs and services. Grants and supports to aid these initiatives through the Caregiver Support Act include the following

- Environmental scanning to understand available respite programs and family caregiver needs.
- Marketing and outreach campaigns to educate family caregivers about respite and how to access services.
- Training of volunteer and paid respite providers to increase the availability of respite services.
- Partnering with communities of faith to develop respite programs.
- Developing or enhancing statewide databases of respite care programs, services, and information to improve access for family caregivers.
- Developing and implementing person-centered respite service options, such as vouchers.

ACL has since funded states to build upon and expand the efforts started during their previous 3 years of work. Grantees are focusing on more fully integrating Lifespan Respite Care Programs into state systems of long-term services and supports. New grant initiatives also support family caregivers and to develop strategies which address program performance and outcome assessment measures.

RAISE FAMILY CAREGIVERS ACT—PUBLIC LAW 115–119

In January 2018, the U.S. Senate passed the Recognize, Assist, Include, Support, and Engage (RAISE) Family Caregivers Act. The House of Representatives had passed this House Bill in December 2017 (S 1719/HR 3099), and it was signed into law (Pub. L. No. 115–119) by President Donald Trump. Some of the hallmark features of this legislation will be instructions to the Secretary of Health and Human Services (HHS) to develop a strategy to support family caregivers through the establishment of an advisory body to bring together representatives from private and public sectors for advice and recommendations. These recommendations will include recommended actions for communities, providers, and government representatives in efforts to support family caregivers. The RAISE Family Caregivers Act supports the millions of family caregivers in the United States, the individuals who rely on them, as well as the economy and workplaces who benefit from their contributions.

The law directs the Department of HHS to develop, maintain, and periodically update a national family caregiving strategy. As a result of the RAISE Family Caregivers Act, HHS will convene a Family Caregiving Advisory Council to develop the national family caregiving strategy. The advisory council will include at least one family caregiver, an older adult with long-term support needs, a person with a disability, a healthcare provider, a long-term service and support provider, an employer, a veteran, state and local officials, and the heads of other relevant federal agencies.

Importance of Family Caregivers

Family caregivers provide an average of 18 hours a week caring for their loved one, with almost one third of family caregivers providing an average of 62 hours of care a week. They help with an array of activities including eating, bathing, dressing, managing finances, performing medical/nursing tasks, managing multiple and complex medications, coordinating care among multiple providers and settings, and paying for services to help their loved ones such as home modifications, transportation, or a home care aide. The assistance family caregivers provide saves taxpayer dollars, helps delay or prevent loved ones from needing more costly care, and prevents unnecessary hospital readmissions.

In 2013, about 40 million caregivers provided unpaid care valued at $470 billion to loved ones who need help with daily activities (AARP, 2017). That sum was more than the total Medicaid spending in the same year. According to Caregiving in the US 2015, about 3.7 million family caregivers provided care to a child under age 18 because of a medical, behavioral, or other condition or disability, and 6.5 million family caregivers assisted both adults and children. Estimates show 3.5 million individuals with intellectual or developmental disabilities (I/DD) live with family caregivers, of whom over 850,000 are age 60+.

Although well intentioned, the writer is dubious of the impact and reach this legislation may have because of its unfunded mandate. On the positive side, however, the legislation does raise the importance and value of caregiving and caregiving issues.

Caregivers typically are spouses or daughters, followed by other relatives and sons (National Study on Caregiving, 2011). Transportation is by far the greatest aid provided by caregivers, followed by mobility (i.e., help getting out of one's bed moving about in their home.) Medical or healthcare-related aid accounts for a little more than half of caregiver activities, followed by self-care, as illustrated in Figure 11.1 (National Study on Caregiving, 2011). Most caregivers are typically women, and they fall within the 55 to 64 age group (National Study on Caregiving, 2011). Figure 11.2 (National Study on Caregiving, 2011) provides an overview of the age categories and gender breakdown of caregiving duties. Caregiving involves both people growing older and people with disabilities.

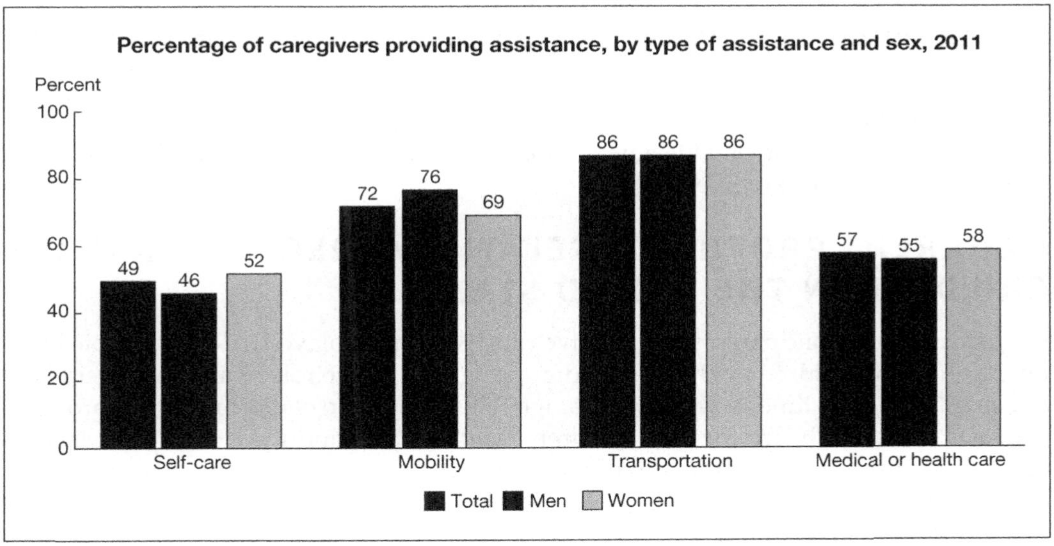

Figure 11.1 Type of caregiving assistance by caregiver type.

Note: Respondents reported whether they helped with different types of activities. Self-care activities include bathing, dressing, eating, and toileting. Mobility-related activities include getting out of bed, getting around inside one's home or building, and leaving one's home or building. Health or medical care tasks were assistance with diet, foot care, giving injections, and managing medical tasks, such as ostomy care, IV therapy assistance, or blood tests.

Reference population: People of all ages who, in the last month, helped with one or more self-care, household, or medical activities for a Medicare enrollee age 65 or over who had a chronic disability.

Source: National Center for Health Statistics (2011). *National Study on Caregiving*. Hyattsville, Md: Author; Federal Interagency Forum on Aging Related Statistics (2016). *2016 Older Americans: Key indicators of well-being*. Hyattsville, MD: Government Printing Office.

Percentage distribution of informal caregivers and number of caregiving hours provided, by relationship to care recipient, 2011

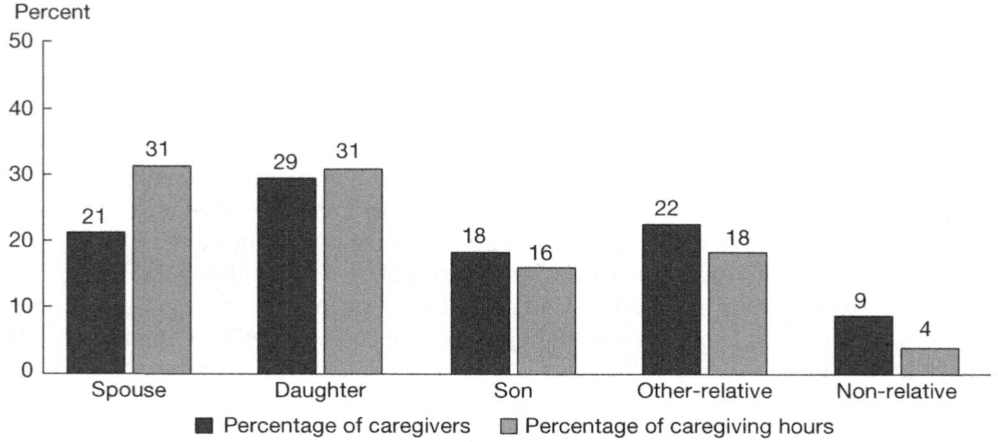

Reference population: People of all ages who, in the last month, helped with one or more self-care, household, or medical activities for a Medicare enrollee age 65 or over who had a chronic disability.

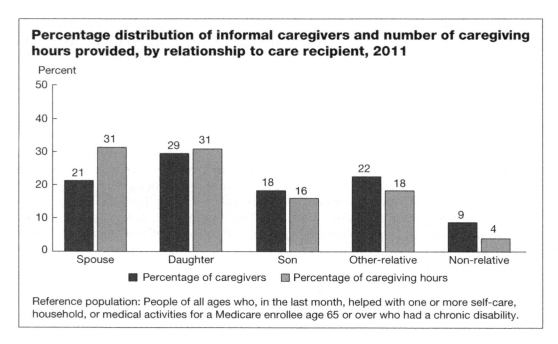

Figure 11.2 Overview of informal caregivers and hours provided by caregiver type.

Source: National Center on Health Statistics.(2011). *National Study on Caregiving*. Hyattsville, MD: Author.

The definition of caregiver also extends to relative caregivers of children who are younger than the age of 18. This next section addresses some of these unique needs and situations of relative caregivers.

A CURRENT PROFILE OF RELATIVE CAREGIVERS RAISING CHILDREN IN THE UNITED STATES

For generations, grandparents and relative caregivers have played a definitive role in the raising of grandchildren or children under the age of 18. The role of a grandparent is an esteemed accomplishment—a rite of passage. The parent role of disciplinarian, provider, taxi, and sounding board for their children has dwindled, and the fruit of their labor is becoming a grandparent. To many older adults, this rite of passage is an exciting time and a spectacular event that can be savored and enjoyed without feeling the strain of responsibility that raising children produces.

Unfortunately, for many older adults, this rite of passage is met with many cumbersome details and unexpected twists and turns, including the movement into a role of grandparents raising grandchildren. According to the U.S. Census Bureau (2016a), 7,271,261 grandparents reported living in a household with one of more of their own grandchildren under 18 years of age. Of this number, 35% were solely responsible for their grandchildren. Within this framework, American Indian and Alaskan Native children were the most prevalent (21.0%), followed by Native Hawaiian and Pacific Islander children (17.9%), African American children (13.3%), Hispanic children (9.3%), White children (6.3%), and Asian children (4.7%; U.S. Census Bureau, 2016c). The national demographic breakdown of grandparents raising grandchildren is: 20% African American, 20% Hispanic/Latino, 2% American Indian or Alaskan Native, 3% Asian, and 53% White (U.S. Census Bureau, 2016d).

Where are these grandparents who are raising their grandchildren? According to the U.S. Census Bureau (2016b), the top 10 states with the highest number of grandparent-raised grandchildren include: California (831,793), Texas (674,531), Florida (373,692), New York (345,528), Georgia (235,194), Illinois (210,685), Pennsylvania (195,405), Ohio (188,920), North Carolina (177,173), and Arizona (158,528). Throughout the United States, nearly 6million children were living in a grandparent-headed household; this statistic represented a 21% increase from the years 2006 to 2016 (U.S. Census Bureau, 2016c). In Illinois alone, the 210,685 children living in grandparent-headed households represented 7.2% of the children in that state.

Nationwide, of the 6 million children living in a grandparent-headed household, just over 1 million were there with no parent present. Although the trend may be slowing, with a Census Bureau report of only slight increases in the number of children living in this arrangement (5.5 million in 2011 to 6.0 million in 2016), it has not abated.

Grandparents raising grandchildren face a broad range of issues that come with this responsibility. Some of the issues are financial, legal, health (physical and mental health, insurance), housing, education, respite care, supportive services, child rearing (special needs of grandchildren), social isolation, and access to information/education (AARP, 2005). The research from an AARP study and others, learned that agencies' outreach services have not adequately provided opportunity for education and services for this target population. Grandparents tend to be highly uninformed about existing supports and services, and all too often are misinformed by the professionals or primary care providers who seek to help them (AARP, 2006; Holliamn, Giddings, & Closson, 2001; Smith, Beltran, Butts, & Kingson, 2001; Wallace, 2001).

More than 1 in 10 grandparents (10.9%) at some point raise a grandchild for at least 6 months, and usually for far longer periods of time. The median age of grandparent caregivers is 59.3 and more than half are age 60 and older (Fuller-Thomson, Minkler, & Driver, 1997). Now that we have a profile of our grandparent caregivers, let's consider why this phenomenon is on the increase,

REASONS FOR THE INCREASE IN RELATIVE CAREGIVING

What turn of events or circumstances have led to the increases in relative caregiving? A part of the increase in kinship care beginning in the 1980s is attributed to legal mandates and changes in child welfare reimbursement policies and practices that encouraged placement with relatives over nonrelative foster care. Federal and state laws and policies promoting formal kinship care, however, do not explain the sizable concomitant growth in the number of children who informally have been "going to Grandma's"—to stay (Cox, 1999). It has also been suggested that for each grandchild in the formal foster care system, another six were informally being raised by relatives (Harden, Clark, & Maguire, 1997).

Key among the social factors contributing to the increase in this phenomenon of grandparents raising grandchildren include alcohol and drug abuse, unemployment, child abuse and/or neglect, incarceration, abandonment, divorce, teenage pregnancy, mental health problems, family violence, death of a parent, HIV/AIDS, and poverty.

Substance abuse, one of the leading contributing factor to grandparents raising grandchildren, has included the cocaine epidemic (Burnette, 1997) and more recently, the methamphetamine and opioid epidemics. The facts that an estimated 15% of women ages 15 to 44 are substance abusers, and that almost 40% of these women have children living with them (Administration for Community Living [ACL], 2018), suggest that drug and alcohol abuse are likely to remain important contributing factors. It has been more recently identified that drug and substance abuse is one of the leading factors for grandparents to raise their grandchildren (ACL, 2018).

Divorce, teen pregnancy, and the rapid growth in single-parent households also are major factors responsible for the rise in intergenerational households headed by grandparents. Such trends have contributed to the dramatic drop in the number of children living in two-parent households (from more than 86% in 1950 to about 70% by the mid-1990s)—a factor that appears to increase the likelihood of children entering relative care (Harden et al., 1997).

Grandparents also are primary caregivers to well over half of the children of imprisoned mothers in the United States. Dramatic increases in the number of incarcerated women, which grew sixfold over a 15-year period in the early part of this century (AoA, 2002; Glass & Huneycut, 2002), suggested that this trend will likely continue to contribute to the growth of intergenerational households headed by grandparents. In 2017, the Bureau of Justice found that about half of the children of incarcerated mothers were in the care of grandparents (Adcox, 2017). Substance abuse also contributed to grandparents raising grandchildren (ACL, 2018).

ISSUES FACING GRANDPARENTS RAISING GRANDCHILDREN

A number of issues face grandparents raising grandchildren, including financial burdens or poverty, role expectations and realities, changes in social support, and health conditions. This section explores these issues in greater detail.

Poverty

First, many of the factors discussed in the previous section are tied in fundamental ways to the continued problem of poverty in our nation, which itself remains a significant vulnerability factor for grandparent caregiving (Burnette, 1997; Minkler, 1999). Grandparent-headed households are more likely to be raising their grandchildren in poverty, and over 20% of households were living in poverty in at least 18 states in the United States, according to the U.S. Census Bureau (2003, 2014), while in at least 33 states at least 15% of their grandparents were raising grandchildren in poverty. According to the Children's Defense Fund, children in kinship foster placements are more likely to live with a family that must spend half of its income on rent, has difficulty with getting adequate food, and does not own a car. For older working relatives, the assumption of caregiving frequently means quitting a job, cutting back on hours, or making other job-related sacrifices that may put their own future economic well-being in jeopardy. Retired or unemployed caregivers also frequently suffer financially and sometimes report spending their life savings, selling the car, or cashing in life insurance policies to cope financially with the new role (Fuller-Thompson & Minkler, 2000b; Hayslip, Fruhauf, & Dolbin-McNab, 2017; Minkler, Driver, Roe, & Bedein, 1993).

Social/Role Issues

A number of social/role issues also challenge grandparents in their role as caregivers. In a qualitative study of 26 grandparent caregivers, a number of themes emerged related to the grandparents' perception of their roles. These included the grandparent caregiver role being off-time or unexpected, role conflict, and role ambiguity (U.S. Department of Health and Human Services, Administration on Aging, 2002). In terms of role timing, grandparents felt that parenting skills were not as much an issue as attempting to raise a child within contemporary society—that is the timing of the parenting role did not fit with their life stage, and they had lost touch with the current trends, music, and expectations of an up-and-coming generation. Role conflicts were expressed by grandparents who struggle between wanting to be the grandparent but sliding into the role of the parent attempting to provide discipline and establish clear boundaries (Gerard, Landry-Meyer, & Guzell-Roe, 2006).

Socialization

An online assessment of grandmothers raising their grandchildren (McGowen, Ladd, & Strom, 2006) revealed that grandmothers' health played a role in their ability to care for their grandchildren. Many stated that they tired more easily, were not physically capable of doing some of the activities that they would like with their grandchildren and felt an impact on their private time. Private time and social relationships with their spouses and friends were impacted by their caregiving role. In addition, the focus for grandmothers also changed from homemaking and careers to caregiving.

These issues have also been found previously by researchers and have been documented in the literature. Decreased socialization with friends and/or family and an inability to continue participation in senior centers and church activities as a consequence of caregiving responsibilities have been widely reported among caregiving grandparents (Burton, 1992; Hayslip & Patrick, 2003; Hayslip, Shore, Henderson, & Lambert, 1998; Jendrenk, 1994; Minkler et al., 1993; Shore & Hayslip, 1994). Reduction in marital satisfaction also has been noted (Jendrenk, 1994).

Healthcare

High rates of depression, poor self-rated health, and/or the frequent presence of multiple chronic health problems have been reported in both national and smaller-scale studies of grandparents raising grandchildren (Chen, Mair, Bao, & Yang, 2015; Clottey, Scott, & Alfonso, 2015; Mignon & Holmes, 2013; Minkler, Fuller-Thomson, Miller, & Driver, 1997; Samuel et al., 2017). Such problems appear particularly prevalent among caregiving grandmothers. One national study found that 32% of caregiving grandmothers met the clinical criteria for depression, compared to 19% of noncaregiving grandmothers. Similarly, grandmothers raising grandchildren were significantly more likely to have limitations in activities of daily living (ADLs) such as caring for personal needs, climbing a flight of stairs, or walking six blocks, with fully 56% reporting at least one ADL limitation (Fuller-Thomson & Minkler, 2000a).

In addition to the grandparents having health problems, children also share in a host of health issues and problems, although Solomon and Marx (1995) found that children in relative-headed households may have better health overall than children living with a single parent. Some of the significant health and health-associated problems that have been observed, particularly among those children who came into their grandparents' care, include prenatal exposure to drugs or alcohol, and/or parental abuse or neglect. High rates of asthma and other respiratory problems, weakened immune systems, poor eating and sleeping patterns, physical disabilities, and attention deficit hyperactivity disorder (ADHD) are among the problems grandchildren have experienced, which in turn may impact the caregiver's physical and mental health (Dowdell, 1995; Lin, 2018; McDonald & Hayes, 2018; Minkler & Roe, 1996; Shore & Hayslip, 1994; Whitley & Fuller-Thomson, 2018).

Several studies have documented the tendency for caregivers to delay or fail to seek formal help for themselves, particularly with mental or emotional health problems (Burnette, 1999; Condon, Luszcz, & McKee, 2018; Minkler et al., 1993; Shore & Hayslip, 1994). Coping strategies had been greatly impacted by the acceptance of responsibility, confrontive coping, self-control, positive reappraisal, and distancing from specific

Table 11.1 Length of Time Grandparents Were Responsible for Raising Grandchildren

Length of Time	30–59 years of age	60 years and older
Not responsible for grandchild	50%	69%
Less than 1 year	13%	5%
1–2 years	13%	5%
3–4 years	8%	4%
Responsible for 5 years or more	16%	17%

Source: U.S. Census Bureau (2001). *Grandparents living with grandchildren* (C2KBR-31). Retrieved from https://www.census.gov/prod/2003pubs/c2kbr-31.pdf

issues for which limited coping strategies are available (Ross & Aday, 2006). Strategies to improve coping, identified by 50 African American grandparents (mean age = 63.12) included seeking social support and developing a series of adaptive coping strategies, particularly when confronted with a difficult child or parents who were dysfunctional. Length of time as a grandparent raising a grandchild also led to a variety of adaptation techniques and improved coping strategies (Harper & Hardesty, 2001; Henderson & Cook, 2005; Noriega, Musil, Zauszniewski & Warner, 2018). These adaptation techniques are important over the long term for grandparents. Table 11.1 provides an overview of the length of time grandparents were responsible for grandchildren.

Policy and Legislation

The policies that dictate how programs and services for grandparents raising grandchildren will be developed and delivered fall under the OAA. The OAA originated in 1965 and contains different titles that address aging issues. The act created the AoA. It also "authorizes grants to states for community planning and services, programs, as well as for research, demonstration and training projects in the field of aging" (Pub. L. No. 89–73). Under Title IV, grants are available for discretionary programs for the aging population. This is where many of the services for grandparents raising grandchildren are covered (See Chapter 7).

Another policy affecting grandparents raising grandchildren falls under the NFCSP. Under this program "state agencies on aging work with area agencies on aging and community service provider organizations to provide support services including information and assistance to caregivers, counseling, support groups, respite, and other home- and community-based services to families" (USDHHS AoA, 2006). The Illinois Family Caregiver Support Program, for example, offers services to older adults who are 60 and older. This program contains supplemental services that aim to address caregiver emergencies, such as providing school supplies and other assistance where there are gaps in services (Illinois Department on Aging [IDoA], 2007).

PROGRAMS AVAILABLE TO MEET THE NEEDS OF RELATIVE CAREGIVERS AND GRANDPARENTS RAISING GRANDCHILDREN

Medicare

Medicare does not provide any services for individual grandparents raising grandchildren. However, some limited support is available for mental health counseling for people who may benefit from supportive counseling to buffer the stress of "parenting" as a grandparent.

Medicaid

Medicaid in most states supports healthcare coverage for grandchildren who otherwise may not have health insurance. The Children's Health Insurance Program (CHIP), although federally mandated, operates at a state level, with different eligibility criteria for each state. Health insurance can be a tremendous asset for families where healthcare coverage would be prohibitive due to the cost factor. Many insurance companies refuse to allow grandparents to include grandchildren as dependents on their insurance policies unless the children are in legal custody of the policy holder. In 1996, one in three children in grandparent-headed households were without health insurance, compared to one in seven in the overall child population (Casper & Bryson, 1998).

Area Agencies on Aging

According to PL. No. 109–365, the OAA Amendments of 2006, Title IV, there is an allotment for funding in the planning of activities to prepare communities for the aging of the population, which includes grandparents who are 55 years of age and older and are raising children. Previously the cut off was 60 years of age. This allotment can include those caring for a child by blood, marriage, or adoption.

Child Welfare

Child welfare authorities can provide a wealth of information to grandparents raising grandchildren on a range of issues from child care/day care to custody and legal issues. Custody options can range from physical custody, legal custody, and private guardianship to kinship foster care and finally adoption. Each one of these categories provides a different level of responsibility and legal mandate, which can be identified on a state-by-state level through the state's child welfare programs. Support programs for special needs children and adoption assistance are also available within most states to grandparents raising grandchildren.

Finally, assistance to grandparents serving as foster care parents is currently available through some states. Grandparents raising grandchildren can qualify as foster parents and may be able to access funds for after school programs, respite care, day care, and assistance with board and care.

MODEL PROGRAMS AND PROACTIVE APPROACHES TO ADDRESSING THE NEEDS OF GRANDPARENTS SERVING AS CAREGIVERS FOR GRANDCHILDREN

A number of programs and interventions have shown promise to be helpful to grandparents raising grandchildren. This section outlines some of these programs, including strengths-based case management, a satellite video program, a "Let's Talk" tape series program, and a cooperative extension program.

Whitley, White, and Yorke (1999) explored the use of a strengths-based case management approach with grandparents raising grandchildren through a project known as "Project Healthy Grandparents." This strengths-based case management method embraces the strengths of individuals and utilized these strengths as a strategy to build resilience and resolve current problems and issues. Although there is a lack of empirical evidence on the impact of using a strengths-based approach to case management, it is clear that this approach garners the resources of the individual, enables a positive approach to problem solving, and makes a qualitative difference in the lives of grandparents raising grandchildren. Success was also measured through the expanded choices and opportunities that the grandparents believed that they had acquired and the measure of empowerment and control reported by grandparents.

In the hopes of raising awareness of the issues related to grandparents raising grandchildren, a national satellite video program was developed and broadcast to a national audience in January of 1999 (Targ & Brintnall-Peterson, 2001). The video conference, known as "Grandparents Raising Grandchildren: Implications for Professionals and Agencies," was designed to provide information, skills, resources, and supports to better serve the population of grandparents raising grandchildren. Although nationally based, each site had a local facilitator who was able to tailor the information and intervention to meet local needs and concerns. Activities immediately before and after the video conference broadcast series was designed to encourage local agencies and organizations to share information and identify service gaps and barriers within their home-based communities in efforts to promote issues of grandparents raising their grandchildren. Outcomes suggest that this approach has provided communities with a better understanding of the issues, programs, and resources and facilitated the expansion of services within organizations. The video conference also served as a springboard to start local support groups, address local needs, and expand services within individual organizations. A follow-up to this session indicated that the video conference approach also improves awareness, encourages the need for support groups, encourages new groups to join forces with existing coalitions to develop resources for grandparents raising grandchildren (67% increase), and encourages the development and/or expansion of new groups (61% expansion). In addition to the actual improvement in knowledge, skills, and awareness, this approach also facilitated an awareness of the benefits of a distance education approach to skills development with grandparents raising grandchildren (Targ & Brintnall-Peterson, 2001).

The "Let's Talk" tape series is an audiotape series of eight tapes that deals with a different topic valued by grandparents (Kropf & Wilks, 2003). The tapes are presented in an easy listening format that provides a conversation between a grandparent and commentator in a question and answer format and runs in length between 11 and 23 minutes. The topics attempt to bridge the needs for materials related to parenting/grandparenting and caregiver stress and have been designed for busy people so that they can be inserted into a tape player during convenient times of day and listened to during those spare moments. Topics include: (a) taking care of your health; (b) being involved in relationships with family and friends; (c) addressing your legal questions and concerns related to custody, guardianship, and wills; (d) community resources; (e) building relationships with one's grandchildren; (f) raising one's grandchildren, joys and challenges; (g) taking care of oneself; and (h) making the most of the experience and taking care of oneself again. Each tape follows a set structure; grandparents review basic information about a topic, identify risk situations, and make a behavioral plan. The series was evaluated with a pre-/post-test design on 60 grandparents using a variety of instruments such as the Grandparent Burden and Satisfaction Questionnaire, the General Health Questionnaire, Center for Epidemiological Studies-Depression (CES-D) scale, Ways of Coping, and Parental Locus of Control Index. The intent behind this series is to minimize potential crises that one may experience as a grandparent, help in raising a grandchild, enhance coping strategies, reduce behavioral issues on the part of the child, and avert any negative or adverse situations.

Cooperative extension programs have built a network of resources throughout at least 10 states throughout the country known as the Relatives as Parents Program (RAPP). While the cooperative extension program is the lead organizer, they have created partnerships with other agency entities such as area agencies on aging, AARP, Health Start, Tribal Partners, and others to create programs and resources that are helpful to grandparents raising grandchildren (Crocoll, 2004). With these programs, grandparents learn about resources within their community and can take advantage of local support groups and other supportive services, and agencies can become part of a statewide network of service providers.

CHALLENGES FOR RELATIVE CAREGIVERS AND GRANDPARENTS RAISING GRANDCHILDREN IN THE FUTURE

A number of challenges face, and will continue to face, grandparents raising grandchildren. The rate and number of grandparents raising grandchildren will continue to grow in the future, especially within smaller and rural communities. Grandparents will also face the same review and audit by child welfare agencies licensed for foster parenting. This interface with the child welfare system will pose its own unique challenges for both the aging and child welfare systems.

Grandparents under age 60 raising grandchildren will also face their own set of challenges, since resources mandated for grandparents through the OAA exclude grandparents younger than 60. Thus, these individuals will be left to deal with an existing limit to resources, through a resource-poor child welfare system. Dealing with the child welfare system, kinship and guardianship rights will also present its own myriad challenges for grandparents, regardless of age.

Another challenge worth noting is the interruption of one's life stage and the boomerang back to an earlier stage of development, which many grandparents have long passed. This challenges the roles of both the individuals raising and those being raised. Challenges also result from generational differences and generation gaps both in communication and in socializing a child from an age cohort different from that of the grandparents' own children.

Grandparents over the age of 60 also face challenges when dealing with rules and regulations facing housing, finances, and so on. Many senior housing settings do not allow children to live or stay for prolonged periods of time on the premises. For some grandparents, this has meant moving to a family-friendly setting in order to accommodate their grandchildren.

Finally, a major challenge is health and associated health issues. Stressors related to the burden of caregiving can contribute adversely to one's health, and this situation requires both consideration and address by local programs and respite services for grandparents raising grandchildren.

SUMMARY

This chapter provides an overview of the current status of family members serving as caregivers, with special attention to grandparents raising grandchildren. It also provides some background into the literature and promotes an awareness of issues that grandparents face as primary caregivers. A literature review examines some of the current issues and services needed. Resources and services designed to meet the needs of grandparents raising grandchildren are discussed, and programmatic responses are identified through the national resources. Finally, some best practice interventions are outlined for review in the text.

ADDITIONAL RESOURCES

Websites

Grandparenting: www.aarp.org/families/grandparents/

The AARP grandparents' resource center provides the grandparent with useful information ranging from parenting skills, and caregiver stress, to legal advice. The site also provides for fact sheets that are state-specific and provide state-based information.

Grandparents Raising Grandchildren: Aging Internet Information Notes: https://acl.gov/news-and-events/news/trump-signs-supporting-grandparents-raising-grandchildren-act-law

This site provides a range of helpful information spanning statistics to best practice resources.

Grandparents Raising Grandchildren: Benefits and Assistance: www.firstgov.gov/Topics/Grandparents.shtml

This government website provides a range of topics of interest to grandparent caregivers including benefits and assistance, health and safety information, reports and publications, and state-based contacts for grandparents to locate resources within their own state.

YouTube Videos

A Day in the Life of the Caregiver: www.youtube.com/watch?v=bs_7jWqSeIM

This beautiful video captures a number of caregiving situations and brings them to life for the viewer in terms of the joys and practices of caregiving. Produced by AARP, this YouTube video provides a well-rounded series of caregiving situations related to people with disabilities and older adults.

Caring for the Caregiver TED Talk. www.youtube.com/watch?v=duhJHedj82g

This TED Talk provides an opportunity for the viewer to understand some of the specific challenges that a caregiver faces and how the caregiver can be better equipped to deal with the role of caregiver.

How to Manage Compassion Fatigue in Caregiving: Navigating the Road to Wellness: www.youtube.com/watch?v=7keppA8XRas

This TED Talk provides a summary of the concept of compassion fatigue and how to address the pain and suffering that a caregiver assumes through secondary trauma that one takes on as a result of assuming the caregiving function.

Podcasts

Dr. Elaine Esbach discusses caregiving challenges. **Listen now:** https://bcove.video/2DzKtT6

Cinda Page discusses the joys and challenges of caregiving from a caregiver's perspective. **Listen now:** https://bcove.video/2OUs2uh

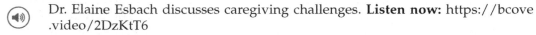

DISCUSSION QUESTIONS

1. What resources are available within your community to assist caregivers in their joys and challenges with caregiving? What gaps exist that could be addressed?
2. Interview a caregiver dealing with a chronic health condition of a loved one, and interview a caregiver of a loved one living with Alzheimer's Disease or a related dementia. What are the differences and what are the similarities between these caregiving experiences?
3. What roadblocks exist for caregivers trying to secure more resources in their caregiving efforts? What policy or program-related issues currently limit the availability of caregiving resources?
4. Consider the issues for Susan and Nora in the case studies at the beginning of the chapter. What resources would be important to them in their journeys as caregivers?

REFERENCES

AARP. (2005). *AARP Illinois state fact sheet: A resource for grandparents and other relatives raising children*. Retrieved from https://assets.aarp.org/rgcenter/general/kinship_care_2005_il.pdf

AARP. (2018). *RAISE family caregivers act now law*. Retrieved from www.aarp.org

Adcox, S. (2017). Demographic information about grandparents today: Everything you wanted to know about modern grandparents. Retrieved from www.liveabout.com

Administration for Community Living. (2017). *National caregiver support program*. Retrieved from http://www.acl.gov/programs/support-caregivers/national-family-caregiver-support-program

Administration for Community Living. (2018, June 3). *Grandparents stepping in to care for grandchildren amid opioid epidemic*. Retrieved from https://acl.gov/news-and-events/news/grandparents-stepping-care-grandchildren-amid-opioid-epidemic

Burnette, D. (1997). Grandparents raising grandchildren in the inner city. *Families in Society, 78*, 489–499. doi:10.1606/1044-3894.818

Burnette, D. (1999). Physical and emotional well-being of custodial grandparents in Latino families. *American Journal of Orthopsychiatry, 69*, 305–318. doi:10.1037/h0080405

Burton, L. M. (1992). Black grandparents rearing grandchildren of drug addicted parents: Stressors, outcomes and social service needs. *Gerontologist, 32*, 744–751. doi:10.1093/geront/32.6.744

Casper, L. M., & Bryson, K. R. (1998). *Co-resident grandparents and their grandchildren: Grandparent maintained families*. (Working Paper No. 26). Washington, DC: U.S. Census Bureau Population Division. Retrieved from https://www.census.gov/content/dam/Census/library/working-papers/1998/demo/twps0026.pdf

Chen, F., Mair, C. A., Bao, L., & Yang, Y. C. (2015). Race/ethnic differentials in the health consequences of caring for grandchildren for grandparents. *The Journals of Gerontology. Series B, Psychological Sciences and Social Sciences, 70*(5), 793–803. doi:10.1093/geronb/gbu160

Clottey, E. N., Scott, A. J., & Alfonso, M. L. (2015). Grandparent caregiving among rural African Americans in a community in the American South: Challenges to health and wellbeing. *Rural and Remote Health, 15*(3), 3313.

Condon, J., Luszcz, M., & McKee, I. (2018). The transition to grandparenthood: A prospective study of mental health implications. *Aging & Mental Health, 22*(3), 336–343. doi 10.1080/13607863.2016.1248897

Cox, C. B. (1999). *Group leaders: Springer series on lifestyles and issues in aging*. New York, NY: Springer Publishing Company.

Crocoll, C. E. (2004). Grandparents raising grandchildren: Help from cooperative extension. *Journal of Family and Consumer Sciences, 96*(4), 59–60.

Dowdell, E. (1995). Caregiver burden: Grandmothers raising their high risk grandchildren. *Journal of Psychosocial Nursing Mental Health Services, 33*(3), 27–30.

Federal Interagency Forum on Aging-Related Statistics. (2016). *2016 Older Americans: Key indicators of well-being.* North Charleston, SC: CreateSpace.

Fuller-Thomson, E., & Minkler, M. (2000a). African American grandparents raising grandchildren: A national profile of demographic and health characteristics. *Health & Social Work, 25*(2), 109. doi:10.1093/hsw/25.2.109

Fuller-Thomson, E., and Minkler, M. (2000b). America's Grandparent Caregivers: Who are they? In B. Hayslip Jr. and R. Goldberg-Glen (Eds.), *Grandparents raising grandchildren: Theoretical, Empirical and Clinical perspectives* (pp. 3–21). New York, NY: Springer Publishing.

Fuller-Thomson, E., Minkler, M., & Driver, D. (1997). A profile of grandparents raising grandchildren in the United States. *Gerontologist, 37*, 406–411. doi:10.1093/geront/37.3.406

Gerard, J. M., Landry-Meyer, L., & Guzell Roe, J. (2006). Grandparents raising grandchildren: The role of social support in coping with caregiving challenges. *International Journal of Aging & Human Development, 62*(4), 359–383. doi:10.2190/3796-DMB2-546Q-Y4AQ

Glass, J. C., & Huneycut, T. L. (2002). Grandparents raising grandchildren: The courts, custody, and educational implications. *Educational Gerontology, 28*(3), 237–251. doi:10.1080/036012702753542535

Harden, A. W., Clark, R., & Maguire, K. (1997). *Formal and informal kinship care* (Report for the Office of the Assistant Secretary for Planning and Evaluation, Task Order HHS 100–95–0021). Washington, DC: U.S. Department of Health and Human Services. Retrieved from http://aspe.hhs.gov/hsp/cyp/xskincar.htm

Harper, W. J., & Hardesty, P. H. (2001). Differentiating characteristics and needs of minority grandparent caregivers. *Journal of Ethnic & Cultural Diversity in Social Work, 9*(3/4), 133–150. doi:10.1300/J051v09n03_07

Hayslip, B., & Patrick, J. H. (2003). *Working with custodial grandparents.* New York, NY: Springer Publishing.

Hayslip, B., Shore, R. J., Henderson, C. E., & Lambert, PL. No. (1998). Custodial grandparenting and the impact of grandchildren with problems on role satisfaction and role meaning. *Journals of Gerontology, 53*, S164–S173. doi:10.1093/geronb/53B.3.S164

Hayslip, B., Jr., Fruhauf, C. A., & Dolbin-MacNab, M. (2017). Grandparents raising aGrandchildren: What have we learned over the past decade? The Gerontologist. 57(6), 1196. doi:10.1093/geront/gnx124

Henderson, T. L., & Cook, J. L. (2005). Grandma's hands: Black grandmothers speak about their experience rearing grandchildren on TANF. *International Journal of Aging & Human Development, 61*(1), 1–19. doi:10.2190/Q4A1-BG9G-XDXK-1VP0

Holliamn, D. C., Giddings, M. M., & Closson, S. (2001). Beyond the myth of collaboration: Creating genuine partnerships to support grandparents raising grandchildren. *Reflections, 1*, 88–97.

Illinois Department on Aging. (2007). *Older adult services act: 2007 report to the general assembly.* Retrieved from http://www.state.il.us/aging/1news_pubs/publications/oasa_anreprt2007.pdf

Jendrenk, M. P. (1994). Policy concerns of white grandparents who provide regular care to their grandchildren. *Journal of Gerontological Social Work, 23*(1/2), 175–199.

Kropf, N. P., & Wilks, S. (2003). Grandparents raising grandchildren. In B. Berkman & L. Harootyan (Eds.), *Social work and health care in an aging society* (pp. 177–200). New York, NY: Springer.

Lin, C. (2018). The relationships between child well-being, caregiving stress and social engagement among informal and formal kinship care families. *Children and Youth Services Review, 93*(Oct).203–216. doi:10.1016/j.childyouth.2018.07.016

MacDonald, M., & Hayes, D. (2018). Understanding informal kinship care: a critical narrative review of theory and research. *Journal of Public Finance and Public Choice. 7*(1). 71–87. doi:10.1332/204674316X14534

McGowen, M. R., Ladd, L., & Strom, R. D. (2006). On-line assessment of grandmother experience in raising grandchildren. *Educational Gerontology, 32*(8), 669–684. doi:10.1080/03601270500494048

Mignon, S. I., & Holmes, W. M. (2013). Substance abuse and mental health issues within Native American grandparenting families. *Journal of Ethnicity in Substance Abuse, 12*(3), 210–227. doi:10.1080/15332640.2013.798751

Minkler, M. (1999). Intergenerational households headed by grandparents: Contexts, realities, and implications for policy. *Journal of Aging Studies, 13*(2), 199–218. doi:10.1016/S0890-4065(99)80051-6

Minkler, M., Driver, D., Roe, K. M., & Bedein, K. (1993). Community interventions to support grandparent caregivers. *The Gerontologist, 33*(6), 807–811. doi:10.1093/geront/33.6.807

Minkler, M., Fuller-Thomson, E., Miller, D., & Driver, D. (1997). Depression in grandparents raising grandchildren: Results of a national longitudinal study. *Archives of Family Medicine, 6*, 445–452. doi:10.1001/archfami.6.5.445

Minkler, M., & Roe, K. M. (1996). *Grandmothers as caregivers: Raising children of the crack-cocaine epidemic.* Newbury Park, CA: Sage.

National Alliance for Caregiving & AARP. (2015, June). *Caregiving in the U.S.* (Research Report). Retrieved from https://www.caregiving.org/wp-content/uploads/2015/05/2015_CaregivingintheUS_Final-Report-June-4_WEB.pdf

National Center for Health Statistics. (2011). *National Study on Caregiving.* Hayattsville, MD: Government Printing Office.

Noriega, C., Musil, C., Zauszniewski, J., & Warner, C. (2018). Conflicts, concerns and family circumstances in custodial grandmothers over 8 years. *Grandfamilies: The Contemporary Journal of Research, Practice and Policy, 5*(1). Available at https://scholarworks.wmich.edu/grandfamilies/vol5/iss1/5

Ross, M., & Aday, L. (2006). Stress and coping in African American grandparents who are raising their grandchildren. *Journal of Family Issues, 27*(7), 912–932. doi:10.1177/0192513X06287167

Samuel, P. S., Marsack, C. N., Johnson, L. A., LeRoy, B. W., Lysack, C. L, & Lichtenberg, P. A. (2017). Impact of grandchild caregiving on African American grandparents. *Occupational Therapy in Health Care, 31*(1), 1–19. doi:10.1080/07380577.2016.1243821

Shore, R. J., & Hayslip, B. (1994). Custodial grandparenting: Implications for children's development. In A. E. Gottfried (Ed.), *Redefining families: Implications for children's development* (pp. 171–218). New York, NY: Plenum Press.

Smith, C. J., Beltran, A., Butts, D. M., & Kingson, E. R. (2001). Grandparents raising grandchildren: Emerging program and policy issues for the 21st century. *Journal of Gerontological Social Work, 35*(1), 33–45. doi:10.1300/J031v12n01_02

Solomon, J. C., and Marx, J. (1995). "To my grandmother's house we go": Health and school adjustment of children raised solely by grandparents. *The Gerontologist, 35*, 386–394. doi:10.1093/geront/35.3.386

Targ, D. B., & Brintnall-Peterson, M. (2001). Grandparents raising grandchildren: Impact of a national satellite video program. *Journal of Family Issues, 22*(5), 579–593. doi:10.1177/019251301022005003

U.S Census Bureau. (2001). *Grandparents living with grandchildren* (C2KBR-31). Retrieved from https://www.census.gov/prod/2003pubs/c2kbr-31.pdf

U.S. Census Bureau. (2003). *Household relationships and living arrangements of children under 18 years of age.* Retrieved from http://www.census.gov/prod/2003pubs/c2kbr-31.pdf

U.S. Census Bureau. (2014). 10 Percent of grandparents live with a grandchild, Census Bureau reports. Retrieved from http://www.census.gov/newsroom/press-releases/2014/cb14-194.html

U.S. Census Bureau. (2016a). *B10050: Grandparents living with own grandchildren under 18 years by responsibility for own grandchildren by length of time responsible for own grandchildren for the population 30 years and over. 2016 American Community Survey 1-year estimates.* Retrieved from http://factfinder.census.gov/faces/tableservices/jsf/pages/productview.xhtml?pid=ACS_16_1YR_B10050&prodType=table

U.S. Census Bureau. (2016b). B10001: *Grandchildren under 18 years living with a grandparent householder by age of grandchild. 2016 American Community Survey 1-year estimates.* Retrieved from http://factfinder.census.gov/faces/tableservices/jsf/pages/productview.xhtml?pid=ACS_16_1YR_B10001&prodType=table

U.S. Census Bureau. (2016c). *S1001: Grandchildren characteristics. 2016 American Community Survey 1-year estimates.* Retrieved from http://factfinder.census.gov/faces/tableservices/jsf/pages/productview.xhtml?pid=ACS_16_1YR_S1001&prodType=table

U.S. Census Bureau. (2016d). *B10051B, C, D, H, I: Grandparents living with own grandchildren under 18 years by responsibility for own grandchildren by presence of parent of grandchildren and age of grandparent (by race). 2016 American Community Survey 1-year estimates.* Retrieved from https://factfinder.census.gov/faces/tableservices/jsf/pages/productview.xhtml?pid=ACS_16_1YR_B10051I&prodType=table

U.S. Department of Health and Human Services, Administration on Aging. (2002). *Grandparents and other relatives raising children: Challenges of caring for the second family.* Washington, DC: Author.

U.S. Department of Health and Human Services, Administration on Aging (2006). *Grandparents raising grandchildren.* Retrieved from www.aoa.gov/press/grand/gpd.asp

U.S. Department of Health and Human Services, National Institute of Drug Abuse. (1997). *Trends in drug and other substance use.* Rockville, MD: U.S. Government Printing Office.

Wallace, G. (2001). Grandparent caregivers: Emerging issues in elder law and social work practice. *Journal of Gerontological Social Work, 34*(3) 127–136. doi:10.1300/J083v34n03_17

Whitley, K. R., White, S. J., & Yorke, B. (1999). Strengths-based case management: Application to grandparents raising grandchildren. *Families in Society, 80*(2), 110–119. doi:10.1606/1044-3894.653

Whitley, D. M. & Fuller-Thomson, E. (2018). Latino grandparents raising grandchildren. *Hispanic Health Care international. 16*(1). 11–19. doi:10.1177/1540415318757219

Zuchowski, I., Gair, S., Henderson, D., & Thorpe, R. (2018). Convenient yet neglected: The role of grandparent kinship carers. *The British Journal of Social Work.* bcy085. doi:10.1093/bjsw/bcy085

12

The Elder Justice Act

LEARNING OBJECTIVES

At the end of this chapter, readers will:

1. *Understand the history of the Elder Justice Act (EJA).*
2. *Understand specific components of the EJA and how programs and services flow for older adults and people with disabilities.*
3. *Understand limitations in programs and services within the EJA.*

Ida: *Ida, a resident of a Medicaid funded long-term care facility in Denton, Texas, has lived with symptoms of multiple sclerosis since she was 52 years old. Now 80 years of age, Ida is a widow, and her stepchildren look after her needs. Her stepchildren are spread throughout the Dallas area, while her daughter, June, and four grandchildren reside in Washington state. One stepdaughter secured Power of Attorney over Ida's body and estate and had Ida admitted into the long-term care facility. She told Ida that she would pack up Ida's lakefront property, store her treasured fossil collection at her home, and transfer the collection back to Ida once she was settled in the nursing facility. After much intervention on the part of Ida's daughter and sister, it was discovered that Ida's possessions were sold, donated, or taken to the garbage dump. June's finances were also not accounted for when the stepdaughter was pressed for these details. Ida has also requested her sister help put locks on some of her drawers because her money and her precious fossils and jewelry have slowly disappeared.*

Gerry: *Gerry was born with Cerebral Palsy and Hydrocephalus. During the first year of his life, a shunt was surgically implanted into his skull, however the shunt needs to be replaced periodically. Gerry is on Social Security Disability, and receives funding monthly. Gerry lives in a rural community, attends Master's level classes in Rehabilitation Studies at a local university, mobilizes himself with an electric wheelchair. He boasts that he is 38 years of age—1 year younger than Jack Benny! Gerry has a worker that helps him with his personal finances, banking, shopping, and money management. Despite Gerry's Social Security and Disability payments, he never has enough funds to purchase items at the end of the month and when he would like to buy books or some other items for his personal needs. Gerry's father recently found some payments made by a PayPal account, but Gerry insists that he has not used PayPal for any bill payments.*

 DOI:10.1891/9780826128393.0012

Lorraine: *Lorraine is a 96-year-old woman who has survived the Holocaust and currently lives in Fort Myers, Florida. Lorraine moved into an assisted living facility 2 years ago when she lost her driving privileges and had been reported to be falling within her home. She is renting her family home to her adult grandson. Lorraine, a divorcee lived in an abusive relationship for most of her 27 years of marriage. Lorraine's grandson consistently makes excuses up when she asked to return to the family home. Her grandson had promised her that he would maintain the property and use a joint account to deposit the monthly rent, and upkeep the property. Lorraine goes to visit the home with a nephew when he visits from out of town and discovers that her grandson has turned her perennial flower beds into a hemp garden and that the home is looking much more run down than when she left it 2 years ago. Her once manicured yard is now overgrown. When she confronts the grandson, he tells her she is hallucinating and reports her to her assisted living facility as mentally incompetent.*

Joan: *Joan currently lives in Ohio and manages independently, despite a car accident that left her with a severe head injury 36 years ago. Joan became a parent shortly after her head injury, and often suffers from aphasia. She currently lives in her own home, with her adult son. Disabled for 36 years, she struggles with money management and her aphasia leads others to think she is not capable of making sound decisions on her own. Joan's adult son would like to assume responsibility to manage her affairs and her finances.*

THE ELDER JUSTICE ACT

The Elder Justice Act (EJA) represents one set of policies nestled within the Patient Protection and Affordable Care Act (ACA; Pub. L. No. 111–148) to address the complexities of elder abuse. The EJA may best serve as a catalyst for further federal coordination and action that can bring about greater public awareness and attention to the needs of a growing, and potentially vulnerable, aging population (Coelello, 2017). According to the Government Accountability Office (GAO), the EJA "provides a vehicle for setting national priorities and establishing a comprehensive, multidisciplinary elder justice system in this country" (GAO, 2011, p. 34).

Elder justice is defined in the statute, from a societal perspective, as efforts to: (a) prevent, detect, treat, intervene in, and prosecute elder abuse, neglect, and exploitation; and (b) protect elders with diminished capacity while maximizing their autonomy (ACA, 2010). From an individual perspective, elder justice is defined as the recognition of an elder's rights, including the right to be free of abuse, neglect, and exploitation (ACA, 2010).

LEGISLATIVE PROVISIONS ADDRESSED WITHIN THE ELDER JUSTICE ACT

The EJA requires the oversight and the appropriation of federal funding to protect people growing older and people with disabilities from abuse. A number of structural initiatives were developed through the legislation since the Act lays out structural entities designed to provide safeguards against abuse. These include

- The establishment of the Elder Justice Coordinating Council.
- The establishment of an Advisory Board on Elder Abuse.

- The establishment of Elder Abuse, Neglect, and Exploitation Forensic Centers.
- The enhancement of long-term care resources for protection of residents.
- The establishment of funding to state and local adult protective service (APS) offices.
- Provision of grants for long-term care ombudsmen programs and funding to ensure the evaluation of these programs.
- The provision of funding through a small grant program available to state agencies to perform surveys of care and nursing facilities and identify pockets of abuse directed toward residents of the facility.
- A nurses' aide registry which helps identify nurses' aides who have completed training within their state with a component related to elder abuse and neglect.
- Training for multidisciplinary professionals working in the older adult arena.

These initiatives largely focus on education, research, leadership, and guidance. Ideally, they are directed toward the establishment of programs to address and help to prevent elder abuse. Prosecution of elder abusers is identified as a challenge, so the EJA tasks the Department of Justice with dedicating resources, studying and evaluating existing laws, and providing grants to local and state agencies (GAO, 2011). Some of the new initiatives of the EJA include the following

- Develop objectives, priorities, policies, and long-term plans for elder justice programs.
- Develop and conduct a study of state laws and practices relating to elder abuse, neglect, and exploitation.
- Make available grants to develop training and support programs for law enforcement and other first responders, prosecutors, judges, court personnel, and victim advocates
- Ensure that DOJ dedicates sufficient resources to the investigation and prosecution of cases relating to elder justice
- Require that any elder abuse perpetrated in a long-term care facility be reported immediately to law enforcement.

Under the EJA, grants are available to state and community agencies to create and promote awareness programs that focus on scams, online fraud, and abuse. Before the EJA was enacted, federal funding for programs and justice regulations was not available. Through the ACA, or more specifically, through the EJA, community education and awareness campaigns and training for law enforcement personnel and APS are available. Table 12.1 provides an overview of the kinds of programs that have received legislatively appropriated funding for addressing abuse and neglect among the most vulnerable in society. The very interesting nature of the EJA is that it places the importance of the issue of elder abuse at the same level as similar legislation for child abuse and domestic violence against women. Thus, the EJA is intended to have the same impact for older adults as legislation such as the Child Abuse Prevention and Treatment Act and the Violence Against Women Act have for their target groups.

Despite some of the advances that the EJA does make, one major limitation is the lack of strength within the act to create and enforce multidisciplinary teams in the development mechanisms to identify, report, and respond to elder abuse at the ground level. Although it was proposed in earlier attempts to pass an EJA, the final Public Law (passed as part of the Affordable Care Act) does not include statutes for the establishment and fostering of multidisciplinary teams.

Table 12.1 Selected Elder Justice Act Program Activities Enacted by the Affordable Care Act

ELDER JUSTICE COORDINATING COUNCIL
- Establishes within the office of the Health and Human Services Secretary an Elder Justice Coordinating Council composed of the Secretary and the Attorney General or their designees, and the head of each federal department or agency identified as having responsibilities or administering programs relating to elder abuse, neglect, and exploitation.
- Charges the Coordinating Council with making recommendations regarding coordination of Health and Human Services, Department of Justice, and other federal, state, local, and private organizations relating to elder abuse, neglect, exploitation, and other crimes against elders.
- Requires the Council to submit an annual report on its activities to the Senate Committee on Finance and the House Committees on Energy and Commerce and Ways and Means.
Advisory Board
- Establishes an Advisory Board of 27 members with expertise in elder issues to create short- and long-term multidisciplinary strategic plans for the development of the field of elder justice and make recommendations to the Council.
ADULT PROTECTIVE SERVICES
- Authorizes funding that the Health and Human Services Secretary shall ensure is provided to state and local services that investigate reports of abuse, neglect, and exploitation of elders.
- Defines adult protective services to include case planning, monitoring, evaluation, and other case work and/or providing medical, social service, economic, legal, housing, law enforcement, or other protective, emergency, or support services.
- Stipulates that each state or local unit of government must use these funds to supplement, not supplant, other federal, state, and local funds expended to provide APS services in the state, and that funds are distributed in proportion to each state's share of residents age 60 and over that are resident in all 50 states.
Demonstration Grants
- Establishes that the Health and Human Services Secretary shall award grants to states to conduct demonstration programs that test: training modules developed to detect or prevent abuse; methods to detect or prevent financial exploitation of elders or detect elder abuse; whether training on elder abuse forensics enhances detection of elder abuse by employees of the state or local unit of government.
- Requires states to provide reports in a manner and containing such information as the Secretary requests on the results of such demonstration programs conducted by the state.

(continued)

Table 12.1 Selected Elder Justice Act Program Activities Enacted by the Affordable Care Act (*continued*)

LONG-TERM CARE FACILITIES
- Authorizes the Health and Human Services Secretary to make grants to long-term care facilities to assist in offsetting the costs related to purchasing, leasing, developing, and implementing certified electronic health records technology designed to improve patient safety and reduce adverse events and healthcare complications resulting from medication errors.
- Stipulates that these grants are to be used in updating and improving existing computer software and hardware, enabling e-prescriptions, and providing education and training to eligible long-term care facility staff on the use of such technology.
Long-Term Care Ombudsman Programs
- Charges the Secretary to make grants to eligible entities with relevant expertise and experience in abuse and neglect in long-term care facilities or Long-Term Care Ombudsman programs and responsibilities to: improve the capacity of state Long-Term Care Ombudsman programs to respond to and resolve complaints about abuse and neglect; conduct pilot programs with state Long-Term Care Ombudsman offices or local Ombudsman entities; and provide support for such Long-term Care Ombudsman programs and pilot programs (such as establishing a national Long-Term Care Ombudsman Resource Center).
- Requires applicants for a grant to provide the Health and Human Services Secretary with such information as may be required to conduct an evaluation or audit and to reserve a portion of funds (not less than 2% of the funds appropriated) to be used to provide assistance to eligible entities to conduct evaluations of the activities funded under each program.
National Training Institute
- Charges the Health and Human Services Secretary to enter into a contract with an entity to establish and operate a National Training Institute for federal and state surveyors with the aim of improving the training of surveyors with respect to investigating allegations of abuse, neglect, and misappropriation of property in programs and long-term care facilities.
- Requires the Institute with: providing a national program of training, tools, and technical assistance to federal and state surveyors; developing and disseminating information on best practices; assessing the performance of state complaint systems; analyzing and reporting annually on the total number and sources of complaints of abuse, neglect, and misappropriation of property; and providing a national 24/7 (including holidays) back-up system to state complaint intake systems in order to ensure optimum national responsiveness to complaints of abuse, neglect and misappropriation of property.

(*continued*)

Table 12.1 Selected Elder Justice Act Program Activities Enacted by the Affordable Care Act (*continued*)

Nursing Facilities
- Stipulates a national study of the cost to state agencies of conducting complaint investigations of skilled nursing facilities and nursing facilities and make recommendations to the Health and Human Services Secretary on options to increase the efficiency of those investigations.
- Requires the Health and Human Services Secretary to make grants to state agencies that survey skilled nursing facilities and nursing facilities in order to prioritize complaints, respond quickly and efficiently, and optimize collaboration between local authorities, consumers, and providers.
Elder Abuse, Neglect, and Exploitation Forensic Centers
- Requires the Health and Human Services Secretary, in consultation with the Attorney General, to make grants to eligible entities to establish and operate stationary and mobile forensic centers to develop forensic expertise regarding, and provide services relating to, elder abuse, neglect, and exploitation.
- Authorized activities include development of markers and methodologies to assist in determining whether abuse, neglect, or exploitation occurred and whether a crime was committed and to conduct research to describe and disseminate information on forensic markers and determining how healthcare, emergency, social, and protective service providers should report a case to law enforcement.
- Charges the Health and Human Services Secretary, in coordination with the Attorney General, with using data made available by grant recipients to develop the capacity of geriatric health care professionals and law enforcement to collect forensic evidence, including forensic evidence relating to a determination of elder abuse, neglect, or exploitation.
Reporting Requirements
- Requires owners, operators, and personnel of long-term care facilities receiving at least $10,000 of federal support to comply with required reporting of any suspicion of crimes against residents. These reports are to be made to the Health and Human Services Secretary and one or more law enforcement agencies. If the events that cause the suspicion result in bodily injury the report must be made immediately or within 2 hours.
- Stipulates that a long-term care facility cannot discharge, demote, suspend, threaten, harass, deny promotion to any employee, or file a complaint against a nurse as retaliation for filing a report of abuse, neglect or misappropriation of property.

(*continued*)

Table 12.1 Selected Elder Justice Act Program Activities Enacted by the Affordable Care Act (*continued*)

Direct Care Workers
- Charges the Health and Human Services Secretary to coordinate with the Secretary of Labor to provide incentives for individuals to train for, seek, and retain employment providing direct care in long-term care facilities.
- Authorizes grants for continuous training and varying levels of certification for workers providing direct care to elder adults.
- Requires entities that receive grants to improve management practices using methods to promote retention of direct care workers and establish motivational and thoughtful work organization practices that foster a workplace culture that respects the rights of residents and results in improved care of residents.

Source: U.S. Congress. (2010). Subtitle H—Elder Justice Act. In *Public Law 111-148, the Patient Protection and Affordable Care Act*. Retrieved fromhttps://www.gpo.gov/fdsys/pkg/PLAW-111publ148/pdf/PLAW-111publ148.pdf

A CURRENT PROFILE OF ELDER ABUSE FACING OLDER ADULTS IN THE UNITED STATES

Is elder abuse a grave issue in the United States? Do we have a profile of the prevalence of elder abuse in the United States? According to a study conducted in 2004 by the Survey of State APS, findings show that there was an increase of 19.7 % in the combined total of reports of elder and vulnerable adult abuse and neglect and an increase of 15.6% in substantiated cases since the reports were conducted in the year 2000. In 2003, APS reported that their agencies nationwide had received 565,747 reports of suspected elder and vulnerable adult abuse as compared with 482,913 reports identified in the 2000 study. In 2016, these figures were updated and once again on the rise (Acierno et al., 2010; Laumann et al., 2008; Williams, Racette, Hernandez-Tejda, & Acierno, 2017) and reported to be at 19.2%.

Within the APS survey, nationwide, 253,426 incidents were reported. These included a low of 85 reports in Guam to a high of 66,805 in California. On average, this resulted in 8.3 reports of abuse per 1,000 older Americans in 2006 and rose to 11.2 reports per 1,000 older Americans in 2016 (NCEA, 2006).

The 2004 survey of APS resources found that older women were far more likely than older men to suffer from abuse or neglect. In fact, it was found that nearly two out of every three victims (65.7%) of elder abuse were women. Abused victims were also older, and nearly half of victims (42.8%) were age 80 or older (NCEA, 2006). Although victims are represented by some diversity, the majority of victims (77.1%) were White. These figures remained stable when rereviewed in 2016.

Although each state is mandated to host an APS registry, not all respond to the reporting of their data. Hence, according to the NCEA Protection's recent survey, not all states reported to survey calls for information regarding elder abuse statistics. Thus, we have some profile of alleged perpetrators, but it is somewhat incomplete. What we do know, however, is that more than half of the alleged perpetrators of elder abuse or neglect were female (52.7%) and three quarters of the alleged offenders (75.1%) were less than 60 years of age. The majority of perpetrators in 2003 were adult children of the victims (32.6%) or other family members (21.5%). Only 11.3% of perpetrators were identified as spouses or intimate partners (National Center for Injury Prevention and Control, 2016).

As of 2017 less than half of the states in the United States maintained an abuse registry or database to identify alleged perpetrators. This has made it difficult to glean a clear picture of the abuse profile; 40.4% of the states (21 states) maintain an abuse registry, but 31 states/territories or 59.6% do not (National Center for Injury Prevention and Control, 2016),

When examining types of specific maltreatment that has been substantiated, it appears that self-neglect occurs most frequently (37.2%), followed by caregiver neglect (20.4 %), financial exploitation (14.7%), emotional/psychological/verbal abuse (14.8%), physical abuse (10.7%), sexual abuse (1.0 %), and other (1.2%). Despite these statistics, it is estimated that only 10% of all cases of neglect or abuse are ever reported, and an even smaller percentage of substantiated reports are available.

WHO REPORTS ELDER ABUSE?

In the final analysis, whom do we find who reports abuse? Although there are a variety of sources, the most common source of reports of elder abuse and neglect allegations appeared to be first family members (17% of cases), followed by human and social service workers (10.6%) and followed by friends and neighbors (8%). Although these data are reported from only 11 states, when compared to some specific states, such as Illinois, it appears to be an average (Illinois Department on Aging [IDOA], 2007).

PROGRAMS AND SERVICES AVAILABLE TO ADDRESS ISSUES OF ELDER ABUSE

Medicare

Although Medicare does not have any specific mandate for elder abuse services, funds are available for counseling resulting from the trauma related to abuse, through the mental health provisions (see Chapter 9). Providers can use *International Classification of Disease, Tenth Revision, Clinical Modification (ICD-10-CM)* codes for "elder abuse" to denote that the hospitalization or treatment was as a result of abuse. However, since these codes are not used as often as they should be, it is difficult to determine to what extent elder abuse is represented in Medicare claims cases.

State-Based Services Offered Through Departments on Aging

Each state, through the Older Americans Act and Administration on Aging (AoA), is mandated to provide APS, for people over the age of 60 years. APS oversees cases of complaints related to financial, emotional, sexual, and physical exploitation, and neglect. Most states have a confidential reporting hotline, which allows those concerned to confidentially report cases of concern, which are then followed up by APS workers for substantiation and potential charges. While APS concerns itself for the most part with adults over the age of 60 years of age living in the community, people who are living within long-term care settings are followed by a state-based ombudsman program.

The Centers for Disease Control and Prevention

The Centers for Disease Control and Prevention (CDC) do not offer specific services to address abuse and neglect; however, they do sponsor several data collection systems that have variables that address issues of abuse, neglect, and violence. Some of these specific databases include the following

- National Home and Hospice Survey (NHHS): asks questions regarding recognizing elder abuse.
- National Electronic Injury Surveillance System (NEISS): contains information on the assaults of elders; perpetrator data not always noted in the medical record and not coded.
- Chronic Disease Behavioral Risk Factor Surveillance System (BRFSS): has some questions on elder abuse in the caregiver survey being implemented as part of BRFSS.

Area Agencies on Aging

A program designed to protect the rights of older persons who live in long-term care facilities is overseen through local Area Agencies on Aging. It received its mandate through the Older Americans Act, known as the Long-Term Care Ombudsman Program. It protects and promotes the rights and quality of life for people who reside in long-term care facilities (specifically nursing homes and skilled care facilities). This service is offered through regional ombudsmen who have hands-on working relationships with the residents and staff of the facilities within their program areas.

The Long-Term Care Ombudsman Program works in conjunction with long-term care facilities to ensure that residents and their families are aware of their rights; to resolve complaints; to provide information on residents' needs and concerns to their families, facility staff, and communities; and to advocate for quality institutionalized care. Although the program is limited to facility residents over the age of 60, the program does provide for current residents, prospective residents, or former residents of a long-term care facility. The program generally will act upon resident or family concerns or long-term care facility staff members and administrators with resident-related concerns. The program is also responsive to individuals and families who are considering nursing home placement as a long-term care option, the community at large, and other interested groups concerned about the welfare of residents of long-term care facilities.

Essentially, ombudsmen listen to resident and family concerns through a confidential approach. They will generally involve the resident and/or family in the investigation and resolution plan and try to resolve problems within the facility, prior to seeking outside counsel. The Long-Term Care Ombudsman Program can be of assistance to individual residents or prospective residents, and/or family members when these parties are seeking information about long-term care facilities, or answers about issues such as facility services or standards, medical coverage, resident rights, and/or transfer or discharge.

Although concern about elder abuse and neglect is mandated in the Older Americans Act, state departments on aging choose how they will administer this type of community program. The 2006 amendments to the Older Americans Act (Pub. L. No. 109–365) incorporated self-neglect into the definitions associated with elder abuse and neglect. In addition, Title VII expanded elder abuse prevention to include financial literacy, grants to expand best practices, and data collection efforts. This version of the OAA updates amended Section 721 authorizing the use of Title VII funds to carry out public education and outreach to promote financial literacy and prevent identity theft and financial exploitation of older individuals. Other innovations in these amendments include the creation of a new Section 752, entitled "State and Tribal Grants to Strengthen Long-Term Care and Provide Assistance for Elder Justice Programs." This new section authorizes grants to states and Indian tribes to strengthen long-term care and provide assistance for elder justice programs. It also provides for the use of funds for a number of elder justice activities, including elder abuse prevention and detection, safe haven models, case review and assistance, volunteer programs, multidisciplinary elder justice activities, programs to address underserved populations of elders, and others. The amendment also creates a new Section 753, authorizing grants to improve, streamline, and promote the uniform collection of national data on elder abuse, neglect, and exploitation.

TYPES OF ELDER ABUSE AND NEGLECT

Elder abuse is an umbrella term referring to any knowing, intentional, or negligent act by a caregiver or any other person that causes harm or a serious risk of harm to a vulnerable adult. Definitions of specific types of abuse and neglect as follows

- Physical abuse is inflicting, or threatening to inflict, physical pain or injury on a vulnerable elder, or depriving that person of a basic need.
- Sexual abuse is the infliction of nonconsensual sexual contact of any kind.
- Emotional or psychological abuse is the infliction of mental or emotional anguish or distress on an elder person through verbal or nonverbal acts.
- Financial or material exploitation is the illegal taking, misuse, or concealment of funds, property, or assets of a vulnerable elder.
- Neglect is the refusal or failure by those responsible to provide food, shelter, health-care, or protection for a vulnerable elder.
- Self-neglect is characterized as the behavior of an elderly person that threatens his or her own health or safety.
- Abandonment is the desertion of a vulnerable elder by anyone who has assumed the responsibility for care or custody of that person.

MODEL PROGRAMS AND BEST-PRACTICE APPROACHES TO ADDRESSING THE LEGAL NEEDS OF OLDER ADULTS

Some model programs do exist within law enforcement that address issues of abuse and neglect. Although the examples showcased are not exhaustive, they do provide for some guidance for innovative interventions for the future. It should be noted that the programs showcased have been identified as best-practice programs by the AoA.

Breaking the Silence—Media Campaign (Illinois Department on Aging)

The IDOA Office of Elder Rights offers an Elder Abuse Awareness Campaign Tool Kit to elder care provider agencies and Area Agencies on Aging throughout the State of Illinois in its attempt to educate providers on elder abuse and promote prevention efforts. The kit includes news releases that can be used with television stations, radio station news editors, and local newspapers to promote events or provide some background to the issue of elder abuse.

The B*SAFE Program

B*SAFE is an acronym for *Bankers and Seniors Against Financial Exploitation*. This program was developed through support from the IDOA. The B*SAFE program is a partnership that helps train bank personnel on the detection, prevention, and reporting of financial exploitation. The program is supported by the following

- IDOA
- Illinois Bankers Association
- Illinois Community Bankers Association
- Office of the Attorney General
- TRIAD, an organization comprising law enforcement, government entities, and advocacy groups committed to the prevention of crimes against the elderly.

This program was developed in 2001 through a collaboration of law enforcement and state agencies, to address the growing problem of financial exploitation. B*SAFE is a public education program that targets bank personnel as the first line of defense against financial exploitation. A senior often sees the same teller who routinely handles his or her financial transactions each time the senior visits the banking facility. That teller is in a prime position to be able to detect any changes from the senior's normal transactions.

The B*SAFE program educates the teller on potential signs of financial exploitation. The program also encourages networking between the bank, local law enforcement, and the Elder Abuse Prevention & Awareness (EAPA) State Clearinghouse. The teller training is handled through the EAPA. Each EAPA has a staff member who has been through the B*SAFE train-the-trainer program, who will be able to provide training to bank personnel.

In 2005, the IDOA received a grant from the Illinois Criminal Justice Information Authority (ICJIA) to develop and print inserts to be distributed to bank customers via their monthly bank statements. The grant also included the development and printing of a financial exploitation brochure targeted at senior customers, to be made available at banking facilities, as well as posters that financial institutions can display in their lobbies. The materials are available in English and Spanish. Publications are available on the website for the IDOA.

CHALLENGES FOR ELDER ABUSE AND NEGLECT PROGRAMS IN THE FUTURE

Cultural values, beliefs, and traditions significantly affect family life. They dictate family members' roles and responsibilities toward one another, how family members relate to one another, how decisions are made within families, how resources are distributed, and how problems are defined (Kosberg & Garcia, 1995; Tatara, 1999). Culture further influences how families cope with stress and determines if and when families will seek help from outsiders. Understanding these factors can significantly increase professionals' effectiveness. Colleagues, coworkers, clients themselves, and members of the community are workers' most valuable resource in understanding the role of culture. Although it is not possible to achieve an understanding of all the diverse cultures workers are likely to encounter, learning the questions and framing the role of culture and elder abuse using the health belief model set the stage as a critical first step to understand this dilemma. Questions to consider include the following

- What role do seniors play in the family? In the community?
- Who, within the family, are expected to provide care to frail members? What happens when they fail to do so?
- Who makes decisions about how family resources are expended? About other aspects of family life?

- Who, within the family, do members turn to in times of conflict or strife?
- What conduct is considered abusive? Is it considered abusive to use an elder's resources for the benefit of other family members? To ignore a family member?
- (With immigrant seniors) When did they come to the United States and under what circumstances? Did they come alone or with family members? Did other family members sponsor them and, if so, what resources did those family members agree to provide? What is the seniors' legal status?
- What religious beliefs, past experiences, attitudes about social service agencies or law enforcement, or social stigmas may affect community members' decisions to accept or refuse help from outsiders?
- Under what circumstances will families seek help from outsiders? To whom will they turn for help (e.g., members of the extended family, respected members of the community, religious leaders, physicians)?
- What are the trusted sources of information in the community? What television and radio stations, shows, and personalities are considered reliable? What newspapers and magazines do people read?
- How do persons with limited English speaking or reading skills get their information about resources?

The answers to these questions can provide guidance to professionals in working with members of diverse ethnic and cultural communities. They help workers understand expectations and dynamics within families and determine what services will be most appropriate and acceptable. They help workers identify trusted persons who can be called upon for help. Finally, they can provide insight into promising approaches and vehicles for spreading the word about available services.

CHALLENGES FOR LEGAL ISSUES IN AGING FOR THE FUTURE

A number of challenges are apparent within the field of elder abuse. These include some of the following

- There need to be consistent definitions and measures for reporting that are used across every state to ensure that elder abuse trends can be tracked and studied nationwide (Dulop, Rothman, Condon, & Martinez, 2000).
- Data are currently not consistently reported on the race and ethnicity of both the victims and alleged perpetrators. This information is an important dimension as communities attempt to understand how ethnic variation plays a role in the face of the perpetrators and victims of elder abuse. Some states do collect this data routinely, while others do not (National Committee for the Prevention of Elder Abuse, n.d.).
- There needs to be training in the detection and reporting of elder abuse for non-traditional "gatekeepers" in the community who are in contact with older adults. These gatekeepers include the postal service workers, bank employees, and utility workers who may witness signs of elder abuse but not know how to report or what to report (Anetzberger et al., 2000).
- Outcome data that documents substantiation of cases following reports are not consistently collected by state-based agencies. This data collection would be extremely helpful in developing an understanding of the process of the investigation and barriers that impede any further investigation or intervention.
- State APA and ombudsman programs are largely underfunded, making it difficult to follow up on cases or substantiate abuse within cases reported.

- Older adults themselves may feel vulnerable or at risk for being abused; however, they may not believe that options are available to them for recourse should they report abusive family members or want to ensure that their family members do not continue to abuse them. This reluctance may be an impediment for resolving cases effectively and efficiently or even reporting cases at all.
- The concept of self-neglect will become increasingly important and controversial. Many professional groups and their codes of ethics for practice may value self-determinism and autonomy; however, the concept of self-neglect may receive more attention as larger cities face building code and fire regulation violations due to individual self-neglect and hoarding. Dealing with the balancing act between community safety, public health concerns, and individual rights will be a challenge in the future.

LEGAL ISSUES AND OLDER ADULTS

The United States has been touted by some experts to be one of the most litigious countries in the world. It should come as no surprise that families, long-term care facilities, and nursing homes are riddled with anxieties with respect to legal issues and the aging segment of the population (Kapp, 2003). One can hardly be admitted into a hospital currently without some aspect of legal issues cropping up—especially related to one's living will or healthcare advance directive. These issues cover respect of one's choices through informed consent and decision-making capacity and also include life-sustaining treatment concerns. Major items of concern with life-sustaining treatments include do-not-resuscitate orders, withdrawing treatment, tube feeding, active euthanasia, and assisted suicide.

Legal issues, especially issues related to informed decision making, generally identified through documents such as a power of attorney or medical power of attorney, are important and critical documents to ensure that one's wishes are carried out in business and personal transactions. The following section of this chapter addresses legal issues with a special emphasis on the concept of a power of attorney.

POWER OF ATTORNEY

A power of attorney is a legal instrument that is used to delegate legal authority to another. The person who signs (executes) a power of attorney is called the principal. The power of attorney gives legal authority to another person (called an agent or attorney-in-fact) to make property, financial, and other legal decisions for the principal.

A principal can give an agent broad legal authority or very limited authority. The power of attorney is frequently used to help in the event of a principal's illness or disability, or in legal transactions where the principal cannot be present to sign necessary legal documents.

Types of Powers of Attorney

Three types of powers of attorney exist regardless of the state within which one resides: nondurable, durable, and springing powers of attorney.

A nondurable power of attorney takes effect immediately. It remains in effect until it is revoked by the principal or until the principal becomes mentally incompetent or dies. A nondurable power of attorney is often used for a specific transaction, like the closing on the sale of a residence or the handling of the principal's financial affairs while the principal is traveling outside of the country.

Durable power of attorney enables the agent to act for the principal even after the principal is not mentally competent or physically able to make decisions. The durable power of attorney may be used immediately and is effective until it is revoked by the principal, or until the principal's death.

Springing power of attorney becomes effective at a future time. That is, it "springs up" upon the happenings of a specific event chosen by the power of attorney when the principal is no longer capable of making decisions or has become incapacitated due to illness or injury. Often that event that is the catalyst in the shift of decision-making power is the illness or disability of the principal. Springing power of attorney will frequently provide that the principal's physician will determine whether the principal is competent to handle his or her financial affairs. A springing power of attorney remains in effect until the principal's death or until revoked by a court.

Durable and springing powers of attorney are frequently used to plan for a principal's future incapacity or disability and loss of competence resulting, for example, from Alzheimer's disease or a catastrophic accident. By appointing an agent under a durable or springing power of attorney, the principal is setting up a procedure for the management of his or her financial affairs in the event of incompetence or disability.

A nondurable power of attorney enables a principal to decide in advance who will make important financial and business decisions in the future. It is also helpful in avoiding the expense of having a court appoint a guardian to handle the principal's affairs in the event of incompetence or disability.

Legal Authority Granted via a Power of Attorney

Whether nondurable, durable, or springing, a power of attorney can be used to grant any or all of the following legal powers to an agent

- Buy or sell one's real estate.
- Manage one's property.
- Conduct one's banking transactions.
- Invest, or not invest, one's money.
- Make legal claims and conduct litigation.
- Attend to tax and retirement matters.
- Make gifts on the principal's behalf.

Selecting an Agent for a Power of Attorney

One should choose a trusted family member, a proven friend, or a professional with an outstanding reputation for honesty. Signing a power of attorney that grants broad authority to an agent is very much like signing a blank check. Certainly, one should never give a power of attorney to someone he or she does not trust fully, nor should anyone be forced into signing a power of attorney.

Multiple agents may also be appointed. If two or more agents are appointed, the principal must decide whether they must act together in making decisions involving one's affairs, or whether each may act separately. There are advantages and disadvantages to both forms of appointment. Requiring one's agents to act jointly can safeguard the soundness of their decisions. On the other hand, requiring agreement of all agents can result in delay or inaction in the event of a disagreement among them or the unavailability of one of them to sign legal documents.

Allowing agents to act separately may ensure that an agent is always available to act for the best interests of one's affairs. However, it may also result in confusion and disagreements if the agents do not communicate with one another, or if one of them believes that the other is not acting in the principal's best interests.

In some states, a statutory short-form power of attorney provides space to appoint an alternate or substitute agent. A substitute agent can act if the first agent is unable or unwilling to act for the benefit of the principal. It is generally a good idea to appoint a substitute agent.

Powers of attorney are only as good as the agents who are appointed. Appointing a trustworthy person as an agent is critical. Without a trustworthy agent, a power of attorney becomes a dangerous legal instrument and a threat to the principal's best interests (Georgas, 1998).

A common concern for individuals, especially older adults, is that once a power of attorney is signed, is it possible for the principal to make legal and financial decisions for oneself? An agent named in a power of attorney is only a representative, not one's boss. As long as principals have the legal capacity to make decisions, they can direct their agents to do only those things that they want done.

Obligations of an Agent

The agent is obligated to act in the best interests of the principal and to avoid any "self-dealing." Self-dealing is acting to further the selfish interests of the agent rather than the best interest of the principal.

An agent appointed in a power of attorney is a fiduciary, with strict standards of honesty, loyalty, and candor to the principal. An agent must safeguard the principal's property, and keep it separate from the agent's own personal property. Money should be kept in a separate bank account for the benefit of the principal. Agents must also keep accurate financial records of their activities and provide complete and periodic accountings for all money and property coming into their possession.

It should be made clear to one's agent that an accurate accounting of records of all transactions completed is expected, and periodic accountings are also expected. An agent can also be directed to provide an accounting to a third party—a member of one's family or trusted friend—in the event that the principal is unable to review the accounting personally.

Potential Abuses by Agents

A power of attorney can be abused, and dishonest agents have used powers of attorney to transfer the principal's assets to themselves and others. Hence, it is important to appoint an agent who is completely trustworthy, and to require the agent to provide complete and periodic accountings to the principal or to a third party.

Transfer of Assets

Another common concern that may face older adults, their children, or people with chronic disabilities relates to the transfer of assets and weighing out whether the transfer of a principal's assets to other people is positive and advantageous. A principal may want to authorize transfers or gifts of property for estate planning and other valid purposes. In some states, it is possible for powers of attorney to permit agents to make gifts to members of the principal's family if the principal so authorizes in the power of attorney. The principal can also customize a power of attorney to permit the agent to make gifts to nonfamily members.

Monitoring and Oversight

There is no official or government monitoring of agents acting pursuant to power of attorney. That is the responsibility of the principal. It is therefore important to insist that an agent keep accurate records of all transactions completed and provide periodic accountings. Should a principal, a member of the principal's family, or a friend have grounds to believe that an agent is misusing a power of attorney, the suspected abuse should be reported to the police or other law enforcement authority to protect the principal from the loss of his or her property. Consider asking a lawyer for help and advice.

The power of attorney may be revoked at any time. This revocation should be in writing, and the principal should inform their agent that their powers are being revoked, and a request made to return all copies of their power of attorney. In addition, one should notify their bank or other financial institution where one's agent has used the power of attorney that it has been revoked. A copy of the revocation should also be filed with the county clerk if your power of attorney has been filed in the clerk's office. Generally speaking, if one should decide to revoke a power of attorney, it is probably in their best interests to consult a lawyer and arrange to have a new power of attorney executed.

A power of attorney is not necessarily filed within a specific government office unless it is used in a real estate transaction. In that case, it must be filed in the county clerk's office. And when it is filed in the county clerk's office, the power of attorney is a public record open to inspection by the public. A writing that revokes a filed power of attorney should also be filed in the county clerk's office.

If one should file a power of attorney in the county clerk's office, generally they should be able to get additional certified copies from the county clerk for a small fee. A certified copy is legally equivalent to the original document. It is often convenient to have certified copies of one's power of attorney on hand. One's signature on the power of attorney must be witnessed by a notary public. Although one is not required to hire a lawyer in order to prepare a power of attorney, since a power of attorney is such an important legal instrument, the careful consumer will consult a lawyer who can

- Provide legal and other advice about the powers that are appropriate to be delegated.
- Provide counsel on the choice of an agent.
- Outline the agent's legal and fiduciary obligations while acting under a power of attorney.
- Ensure that the power of attorney is properly executed and meets all legal requirements.

The typical fee for preparing a power of attorney is modest. Before engaging a lawyer to prepare a power of attorney, one should inquire about the fee and feel free to get prices from other lawyers and law firms. Local Area Agencies on Aging often fund legal clinics or resources that handle legal documents such as powers of attorney for seniors 60 years of age and older.

HEALTHCARE POWER OF ATTORNEY

A healthcare power of attorney grants an agent the power to make medical decisions for the principal when the principal cannot make that decision for themselves. This might occur when the principal slips into a coma after a motor vehicle accident, for example. With a properly drafted healthcare power of attorney, the agent has authority to consult with the principal's physician, evaluate the risks of certain medical procedures, and give or withhold consent for the physician to perform the procedure. The healthcare power of attorney only becomes effective when the principal is unable to make medical decisions for himself or herself because of mental incapacity.

Living Wills and Advance Directives

A living will, which is also known as an advanced healthcare directive, is a signed document that instructs an attending physician not to keep one alive with artificial measures if they become permanently unconscious. In other words, if one suffers from a terminal illness or catastrophic physical trauma that permanently reduces brain activity to a vegetative state, with no possibility of recovery, the living will expresses one's desire not to be kept alive under such circumstances.

Although these documents are called living "wills" they have nothing to do with a person's last will and testament. The last will and testament is for passing of one's property to the people chosen after one's death. The living will, on the other hand, expresses one's desires about their medical care near the end of their life (Carter, 1998).

PROGRAMS AND SERVICES AVAILABLE TO ADDRESS LEGAL ISSUES FOR OLDER ADULTS

Medicare

While Medicare does not offer legal assistance per se, a dimension of Medicare that does impact legal issues is the whole arena of fraud. Overbilling, and charges for services that may have never been performed, are often issues that can be cause for legal concern.

State-Based Departments on Aging

Departments on Aging in every state have a legal assistance developer. The role of this individual is to provide leadership and technical assistance in the development and enhancement of quality legal and advocacy assistance for older persons in greatest economic or social need. Developers often have other roles and responsibilities, including coordinating their states' elder rights efforts and promoting alternative legal assistance delivery systems. Legal assistance developers often refer persons in need of assistance to the appropriate legal providers for the elderly and help with outreach and public education. In addition, their role leads them to direct the design and implementation of programmatic systems to improve the quality and quantity of legal assistance for the elderly in their individual states.

The Older Americans Act and Area Agencies on Aging

The Older Americans Act (Sec. 306(a)(15)(A-E): & Sec 731 (a) (b)) incorporates language that provides funding for legal services through local Area Agencies on Aging. These financial provisions are found in Titles III and VII of the Older American's Act. Some of the specific services that can be provided include

- Last will and testament.
- Durable power of attorney.
- Healthcare power of attorney.
- Assistance with securing public benefits.
- Social Security, SSI, Medicare, Medicaid, and veteran's benefits.
- Family law: divorce and related matters.
- Consumer problems: dishonest vendors, fraud.
- Guardianship for those no longer able to care for self or property.
- Public and educational forums for senior citizens on legal issues.
- Elder abuse and related issues.

Despite this long list of services, there are some types of services not provided, which include

- Legal services for criminal cases.
- Representation in the probate of estates.
- Commercial or business matters.
- Contingency fee cases.

Although each state can set the requirements for compensation for services, generally the services are without costs to the clients. Filing fees and services fees may be required in some cases or required if the client is able to afford the payments. No clients will be refused services for lack of financial means in the majority of states.

MODEL PROGRAMS AND BEST PRACTICES TO ADDRESS THE LEGAL NEEDS OF OLDER ADULTS

American Association of Retired Persons

AARP has developed a range of resources on end of life, living wills, and dying and death, which are very helpful. These were developed following the Terri Schiavo tragedy, in the hopes that people will have a resource on making decisions for themselves and their family related to end-of-life issues. In addition, to these resources, materials have also been developed and are available for distribution to members on dealing with managed care organizations and the end-of-life issues (Fox, 1999).

American Society on Aging

The American Society on Aging (ASA) provides a comprehensive package of webinars on the legal and ethical issues of aging. The webinars provide continuing education credits and are available to professionals 24 hours per day. Topics include "Liability and Risk Management Issues in Aging Services," and "Legal and Ethical Aspects of Decision Making by and for Older Persons, Part I and II."

CHALLENGES FOR LEGAL ISSUES IN THE AGING ARENA FOR THE FUTURE

A number of challenges will continue to grow in the future with regard to power of attorney, healthcare power of attorney, and legal issues in general. One of the most significant will be the importance of choosing and preparing agents to truly act on one's behalf. The future may hold some planning venues or "individualized legal action plans" developed by the principal in order to provide a guide for agents. This can be more critical in cases where the principal sees a decline in his or her overall health and cognitive function.

A second challenge is to enable individuals to plan for their future while they are of sound mind and cognitively intact, especially in cases where people will lose their cognitive function over time. Issues related to capacity, decision making, and informed consent will also be paramount as we move into the future. Kapp (2001, 2002) raises these issues very eloquently and makes the case that planning by individuals and with individuals prior to diminished capacity is essential as a step to preserving the rights of individuals as they grow older.

A third challenge will include the availability of hospice and end-of-life care experts who are culturally competent. Duffy, Jackson, Schim, Ronis, and Fowler (2006) showcase the differences in racial/ethnic preferences in end-of-life care between Whites and Blacks. In addition, they suggest that there are gender preferences that will illuminate the need for specific intervention options for men and women as well as strategies that take into account one's racial and ethnic background.

The healthcare market will also drive medical or healthcare power of attorney decisions in the future. The notion of purchasing services for one's healthcare in light of diminished cognitive capacity and the ethics associated with this idea has been raised eloquently by Kapp (1999). In addition, skyrocketing healthcare costs, and declines in the overall availability of medical resources for the increasingly graying population could call attention to the need to consider a process to "ration" resources for older adults. This rationing concept can lead to situations within which assisted suicide becomes an option for people that is legal in the majority of states. Currently, physician-assisted death is legal in California, Colorado, District of Columbia, Hawaii, Montana, Oregon, Vermont, and Washington. In 2008, when the first edition of this book was written, Oregon was the only state in the United States in which physician-assisted suicide was a legal option (State of Oregon, n.d.), but debates on either side of this issue, especially econometric debates, led to the legalization of physician-assisted suicide options.

Finally, the debates around end-of-life care, physician-assisted suicide, and right to life will continue to be challenges that will face us, especially as we move into a "booming" graying society. This discussion may require input from bioethicists and members of various religious communities, in concert with older adults, and is the scope of a more extensive discussion. Foley and Hendin (2002) and Quill and Battin (2004) have prepared a series of debates that provide a comprehensive perspective on both sides of this set of issues, which are well worth informed discussion and deliberation.

SUMMARY

This chapter explores several legal issues that face older adults. Elder abuse, power of attorney, (durable, nondurable, and springing) are also addressed in this chapter, and a differentiation made between the types of power of attorney and the healthcare power of attorney. In addition, legal services provided to older adults as a result of the Older Americans Act are explored, and challenges within the realm of legal issues outlined.

The incidence and prevalence of elder abuse is probably largely underreported. While efforts are being made to understand the magnitude of the problem, limited resources hamper progress. The Older Americans Act has some resources in place to deal with the education of providers and screening/detection of individuals who have been at risk of abuse; however, APS plays a key role in this intervention process. The role of one's cultural beliefs and help-seeking behavior also plays a significant role. Challenges in uncovering this silent epidemic face the healthcare provider, programs, and services.

ADDITIONAL RESOURCES

Websites

The International Network for the Prevention of Elder Abuse (INPEA): www.inpea.net

INPEA has produced the *Community Guide to Raise World Awareness on Adult Abuse Tool Kit.* The tool kit provides sample ideas and templates for activities and examples of materials, resources, proclamations, and messages. The tool kit is available for free download at the website.

The National Center on Elder Abuse: https: ncea.acl.gov
This website provides data, fact sheets, and other information on elder abuse, neglect, and exploitation in the United States.

The National Clearinghouse on Abuse in Later Life: www.ncall.us
This clearinghouse is responsible for information on coordinating elder abuse prevention efforts with domestic violence and sexual assault programs.

Eldercare Locator: www.eldercare.gov
This site enables one to contact a local area agency on aging about volunteering to call or visit an isolated senior.

The National Committee for the Prevention of Elder Abuse: www.preventelderabuse.org
This site provides researchers, practitioners, educators, and advocates dedicated to protecting the safety, security, and dignity of America's most vulnerable citizens. The committee was established in 1988 to achieve a clearer understanding of abuse and provide direction and leadership to prevent it. The committee is one of six partners that make up the NCEA, which is funded by Congress to serve as the nation's clearinghouse on information and materials on abuse and neglect.

AARP: www.aarp.org/caregiving
This site provides a host of resources to individuals and their families on end-of-life issues, estate planning, living wills, powers of attorney, and self-help guides for the creation of these materials.

The Center for Social Gerontology, Legal Assistance Developers: http://www.tcsg.org/lsdlist.pdf
This site provides a listing of individuals who are available through the state departments on aging to provide oversight for legal assistance through the Older Americans Act. The site provides a registry of experts for each state in the United States. Every state has a legal assistance developer who provides leadership and technical assistance in the development and enhancement of quality legal and advocacy assistance for older persons in greatest economic or social need. Developers often have other roles and responsibilities, including coordinating their states' elder rights efforts and promoting alternative legal assistance delivery systems.

American Geriatrics Society, Health in Aging, Making Your Wishes Known: www.healthinaging.org/making-your-wishes-known
This site provides a plethora of information for the reader on issues that relate to legal concerns of older adults. They include segments to enable individuals to assess competency and informed consent, as well as a host of legal issues for consideration.

State of Oregon, Death with Dignity Act: http://www.oregon.gov/oha/PH/PROVIDERPARTNERRESOURCES/EVALUATIONRESEARCH/DEATHWITHDIGNITYACT/Pages/index.aspx
This site provides an overview of links related to Oregon's Death with Dignity Act. Oregon initially was the first state in the United States state to legalize a physician-assisted

suicide option for residents of its state. This site provides an overview of the protocol, statistics, and responses to frequently asked questions.

YouTube Videos

Elder Abuse: The crime of the 21st century: www.youtube.com/watch?v=1JoUapRfjZw

This video showcases a prosecutor who has worked with elder abuse and showcases the context of elder abuse rights and context within the United States. Mr. Paul Greenwood, a reputable attorney who has had much experience in the area of elder abuse, is featured in this video.

Abuse of people with disabilities: A silent epidemic: www.youtube.com/watch?v=yhLsATwO0o4

This YouTube video addresses the issue of abuse among people with disabilities. It showcases how people with disabilities are subject to abuse of various types and also addresses how people with disabilities can take action to protect and help themselves.

Power of Attorney: Types and Powers: www.m.youtube.com/watch?v=41XgOg5jlhQ

This YouTube video goes through the various types of power of attorney and showcases the specific dynamics of each. It also helps the viewer to understand the differences between among these various types of instruments and the role each plays.

DISCUSSION QUESTIONS

1. What are some of the issues presented in the cases that set the stage for this chapter? How would you, as part of an interdisciplinary team, begin to develop strategies for detection, reporting, and intervention?
2. Are there resources within your community and region adequate to address the training, detection, investigation, and reporting of elder abuse and deal with the legal issues to protect older adults? Why or why not? What do you think should be done to address the resource allocation issue?
3. Are the interdisciplinary efforts within your region or community to address the legal needs, and elder abuse/neglect needs in your community? If not, what can be done to develop these resources? If they do exist, how functional are they? What can be done to strengthen these resources?

REFERENCES

Acierno, R., Hernandez, M. A., Amstadter, A. B., Resnick, H. S., Steve, K., Muzzy, W., & Kilpatrick, D. G. (2010). Prevalence and correlates of emotional, physical, sexual, and financial abuse and potential neglect in the United States: The National Elder Mistreatment Study. *American Journal of Public Health, 100*, 292–297. doi:10.2105/AJPH.2009.163089

Anetzberger, G. J., Palmisano, B. R., Sanders, M., Bass, D., Dayton, C., Eckert, S., & Schimer, M. R. (2000). A model intervention for elder abuse and dementia. *The Gerontologist, 40*, 492–497.

Carter, T. (1998). *Your personal directive: More than a living will. Self-counsel legal series.* Bellingham, WA: Self-counsel Press.

Colello, K. J. (2017). The Elder Justice Act: Background and issues (CRS Report No. R43707). Retrieved from Congressional Research Service website: https://fas.org/sgp/crs/misc/R43707.pdf

Duffy, S., Jackson, F. C., Schim, S. M., Ronis D. L., & Fowler, K. E. (2006). Racial/ethnic preferences, sex preferences, and perceived discrimination related to end-of-life care. *Journal of the American Geriatrics Society*, *54*(1), 150–157. doi:10.1111/j.1532-5415.2005.00526.x

Dulop, B. D., Rothman, M. B., Condon, K. M., & Martinez, I. L. (2000). Elder abuse: Risk factors and use of case data to improve policy and practice. *Journal of Elder Abuse & Neglect*, *12*(3–4), 95–122. doi:10.1300/J084v12n03_05

Foley, K., & Hendin, H. (2002). *The case against assisted suicide for the right to end-of-life care*. Baltimore, MD: Johns Hopkins University Press.

Fox, P. (1999). *End of life in managed care organizations*. Washington, DC: AARP.

Georgas, S. (1998). *Power of attorney kit: A do it yourself kit. Self-counsel legal series*. Bellingham, WA: Self-counsel Press.

Government Accountability Organization. (2011). *Elder Justice: Stronger federal leadership could enhance national response to elder abuse* (GAI-11-201). Wasington, DC: Author

Illinois Department on Aging. (2007). *Older Adult Services Act: 2007 report to the general assembly* (P.A. 093–1031). Retrieved from http://www.state.il.us/aging/1news_pubs/publications/oasa_anreprt2007.pdf

Kapp, M. (1999). From medical patients to health care consumers: Decisional capacity and choices to purchase coverage and services. *Aging and Mental Health*, *3*(4), 294–300. doi:10.1080/13607869956064

Kapp, M. (2001). Legal interventions for persons with dementia in the USA: Ethical, policy and practical aspects. *Aging and Mental Health*, *4*, 312–315. doi:10.1080/13607860120080242

Kapp, M. (2002). Decisional capacity in theory and practice: Legal process versus "bumbling through." *Aging and Mental Health*, *6*(4), 413–417. doi:10.1080/1360786021000007054

Kapp, M. (2003). Legal anxieties and end-of-life care in nursing homes. *Issues in Law and Medicine*, *19*(2), 111–134.

Kosberg, J. I., & Garcia, J. L. (Eds.). (1995). *Elder abuse: International and cross-cultural perspectives*. Binghamton, NY: Haworth Press.

Laumann, E. O., Leitsch, S. A., & Waite, L. J. (2008). Elder mistreatment in the United States: Prevalence estimates from a nationally representative study. *The Journals of Gerontology, Series B: Psychological and Social Sciences*, *63*, S248–S254. doi:10.1093/geronb/63.4.s248

National Center on Elder Abuse. (2006). *Statistics on elder abuse*. Retrieved from https://www.ncea.acl.gov

National Center for Injury Prevention and Control. (2016). *Understanding elder abuse* (Fact Sheet). Retrieved from http://www.cdc.gov/violenceprevention/pdf/em-factsheet-a.pdf

National Committee for the Prevention of Elder Abuse. (n.d.). *The role of culture in elder abuse*. Retrieved from http://www.preventelderabuse.org/issues/culture.html

Patient Protection and Affordable Care Act, Pub. L. No. 111–148, 124 Stat. 119 (2010).

Quill, T. E., & Battin, M. P. (2004). *Physician assisted dying: The case of palliative care and patient choice*. Baltimore, MD: Johns Hopkins University Press.

SSA §2011 as amended by §6703(a) of ACA [42 U.S.C. §1397j]

State of Oregon. (n.d.). *Death with Dignity Act*. Retrieved from http://www.oregon.gov/DHS/ph/pas/index.shtml

Tatara, T. (1999). *Understanding elder abuse in minority populations*. Philadelphia, PA: Taylor & Francis.

U.S. Congress. (2010). Subtitle H—Elder Justice Act. In *Public Law 111–148, the Patient Protection and Affordable Care Act*. Retrieved from https://www.gpo.gov/fdsys/pkg/PLAW-111publ148/pdf/PLAW-111publ148.pdf

U.S. Government Accountability Office. (2011). *Elder justice: Stronger federal leadership could enhance national response to elder abuse*. Report to the Chairman, Special Committee on Aging (GAO 11-208). Retrieved from http://www.gao.gov/assets/320/316224.pdf

Williams, J. L., Racette, E. H., Hernandez-Tejada, M. A., & Acierno, R. (2017). Prevalence of elder polyvictimization in the United States: Data from the Elder Mistreatment Study. Journal of Interpersonal Violence. doi: 10.1177/0886260517715604

13

Housing and Long-Term Care

LEARNING OBJECTIVES

At the end of this chapter, readers will:

1. *Understand the history of housing and long-term care for older adults and people with disabilities.*
2. *Understand specific components of the Long-Term Care Reconciliation Act.*
3. *Understand how legislation related to housing and long-term care provides resources to older adults and people with disabilities.*

After looking at various other aspects of one's being affected by programs for older adults and people with disabilities, Erica realized that housing was also an area that needed exploration. The options for older adults seemed clear cut for Erica because she had worked in long-term care previously. However, options for people with disabilities were not as clear to her since her experiences with this group were limited. Theresa had worked with people living in institutions within her career but did not agree with institutional settings, so both wondered what types of provisions and policies covered community living options and long-term care opportunities for both people with disabilities and people growing older. Read through this chapter to see what the pair identified as opportunities for living within community-based settings. They interviewed Ida, Gerry, and Lorraine to get ideas of different types of living settings and opportunities.

***Ida**: Ida, a resident of a Medicaid-funded long-term care facility in Denton, Texas, has lived with symptoms of multiple sclerosis since she was 52 years of age. Ida, now 80 years of age, is a widow, and her stepchildren look after her needs. Her stepchildren are spread throughout the Dallas area, while her daughter June and four grandchildren reside in Washington state. The facility provides her with a semiprivate room and shared bathroom. All her meals and medical needs are covered by the facility.*

***Gerry**: Gerry was born with Cerebral Palsy and Hydrocephalus. During the first year of his life, a shunt was surgically implanted into his skull; however, the shunt needs to be replaced periodically. Gerry is on Social Security Disability and receives funding monthly.*

(*continued*)

Gerry lives in a rural community within a supported living setting in an individual apartment. His roommate, John, also serves as his attendant and provides help to Gerry with both activities of daily living (ADLs such as bathing, dressing, and toileting) and instrumental activities of daily living (IADLs such as shopping, cooking, appointments, and laundry).

***Lorraine:** Lorraine is a 96-year-old woman who has survived the Holocaust and currently lives in Fort Myers, Florida. Lorraine moved into an assisted living facility 2 years ago, when she lost her driving privileges and had been reported to be falling within her home. Lorraine manages her own breakfast within her suite, but receives soup/sandwich items for lunch and a hot dinner from the facility. She is manages her own laundry within her suite. A facility van helps our by providing transportation to a local shopping mall for groceries and sundries.*

A HISTORICAL OVERVIEW OF HOUSING POLICY AND OPTIONS FOR PEOPLE GROWING OLDER AND PEOPLE WITH DISABILITIES

Historically speaking, people who fall into the categories of disability have probably had a longer history of public housing options than older adults. Some of this stemmed back to the concept of benevolence and community/charity care. It can be speculated that one of the main reasons that people with disabilities have a much longer history than people growing older. Partially this disparity is due to the limited life span for people who are growing older and partially to the culturally accepted norms, which integrated the extended family concept and embraced older adults into the nuclear extended family in North American history. It was very common for an older adult to live with family members in the 1800s and early 1900s. In contrast, a person with a disability may have been stigmatized and shunned from family life, thus necessitating housing or long-term care and/or home- and community-based care. An example of this stigma can be seen in Paris's Institution for Blind Children. After seeing a group of blind boys being cruelly exhibited as part of a "freak show" in Paris, Valentin Haüy, known as the "father and apostle of the blind," took it upon himself as early as 1767 to establish the Institution for Blind Children to help make life for the blind more tolerable. (NCLD, 2017). People with mental illness were known also to have been institutionalized as early as the late 1700s. In 1793, Philip Pinel, a physician at La Bicetre, an asylum in Paris, removed the chains attached to people with mental illnesses. Some had been noted to have been chained to walls for more than 30 years (NCLD, 2017). Thus, we have some evidence that people with severe persistent mental illness were subject to being seen as a threat to society, and the housing options available to these people were limited to public asylums. Although these scenarios date back to European roots, the same practices and attitudes that led to the development of institutional care existed in both the United States and Canada. Stories of people chained to the walls or floors are not unusual and were often the norm in institutional care for people with mental illness, especially prior to the practice of lobotomies, psychotropic medications, and electroconvulsive therapies (Szaz, 1967).

On an American front, the first related legislation that has been noted to address the housing needs of people with disabilities can be traced to President John Adams, in the late 1700s. The first military disability law signed by Adams on July 16, 1798, known as the Act for the Relief of Sick and Disabled Seamen. This public law ensured the provision of care for men impacted by their service at sea and provided for housing and care to meet their healthcare needs.

Public land grants were provided through federal legislation to address the needs of people with mental illness in the United States in 1818. The McLean Asylum for the Insane was developed as a result of public land grant provision, and the first patient was admitted to the Charlestown branch of the Massachusetts General Hospital, which is later named the McLean Asylum for the Insane, in 1818. (The hospital later became one of the best-known mental health facilities in the country, with services attracting such modern artists as Sylvia Plath, Anne Sexton, James Taylor, and Susanna Kaysen [NCLD, 2017].) Although the American Civil War (1861–1865) did not leverage legislation for housing of disabled war amputees, the issues that surfaced for these individuals brought disability issues to the minds and consciousness of Americans.

Although it took nearly 100 years to begin to see federal legislation related to housing, President John F. Kennedy's White House Commission for People with Disabilities led to The Mental Retardation Facilities and Community Mental Health Centers Construction Act of 1963. Along with setting aside money for developing State Developmental Disabilities Councils, Protection and Advocacy Systems, and University Centers, the legislation addressed housing and long-term care. In 1984, it was amended and renamed the Developmental Disabilities Assistance and Bill of Rights Act. In addition to President Kennedy's contribution to legislation impacting housing, one of the next most significant contributions to legislation that advanced community-based care options for people with mobility impairments, was The Architectural Barriers Act of 1968, which mandated the removal of obstacles for people with disabilities. The Act required that all buildings designed, constructed, altered, or leased with federal funds to be made accessible in order to accommodate people with disabilities and mobility limitations.

The Civil Rights Act of 1968 mandated accessible housing in new projects, and the Fair Housing Amendments Act of 1988 (Pub L 90–480) expands on the Civil Rights Act of 1968 to require that a certain number of accessible housing units be created in all new multifamily housing. The act covers both public and private homes, not only those in receipt of federal funding. It also addresses the needs of people with disabilities, while the Civil Rights Act of 1968 addressed minorities but did not give attention to people with disabilities.

In contrast, The Hospital Survey and Reconstruction Act of 1946 (also known as the Hill–Burton Act) paved the way for funding the construction of state-of-the-art community hospitals. Despite this legislation, the Great Depression and World War II created a tremendous backlog of facilities that needed to be upgraded, including community hospitals. This backlog resulted in a diminished priority for long-term facilities for people growing older or who were infirm (Jurkowski, 2013). The Medical Facilities Survey and Construction Act of 1954 saw to the development of nursing facilities and tried to improve the care older adults received by facilitating the construction of long-term care facilities in conjunction with hospitals. This legislation was a landmark within the history of long-term care facilities because it directed nursing home facilities to be built alongside hospital facilities. Consequently, nursing home facilities came to be built and fashioned after hospital facilities, rather than being homelike. In addition, the Medical Facilities Survey and Construction Act of 1954 moved nursing home care and provision from the welfare state/human service system into the healthcare arena. Prior to this piece of legislation, nursing care for older adults had followed the pathway charged by the Elizabethan Poor Laws and almshouses, which had historically been a part of the welfare state rather than that defined by health and the healthcare arena (Jurkowski, 2013).

Although not a public policy or public law enacted by Congress, in a landmark court case in 1999, *Olmstead v. L.C.*, the U.S. Supreme Court ruled that unnecessary institutionalization of people with disabilities constitutes discrimination and violates the Americans with Disabilities Act of 1990. Within this landmark court case, "individuals have a right to receive benefits in the most integrated setting appropriate to their needs," and that failure to find community-based placements for qualifying people with disabilities is illegal discrimination. This court case has turned the long-term care movement around for people with disabilities, and many people who had been institutionalized in nursing home care settings moved into community-based settings. It also set the stage for "least restrictive environment," which meant that people should live within settings that do not restrict their actions and abilities, and care should be centered upon what is best for the person (i.e., person-centered care) as opposed to what is most efficient and expedient for the facility.

A CURRENT PROFILE OF LONG-TERM CARE AND COMMUNITY-BASED CARE NEEDS

A continuum of services exists within the long-term care and community care settings. Within each of these settings, the standards of care may differ, the expectations of consumer functional status differs, and payment schemes may differ. In this chapter, we will discuss community-based care options such as home health, seniors congregate living, assisted living options, skilled nursing facilities, and long-term care facilities. Although differences may exist from state to state relative to who qualifies for these options and when they qualify, these will be discussed in some detail specifically providing an overview of these as options for care management of older adults (Table 13.1).

Table 13.1 Need for Help With ADLs Within Care Facilities

Year	Gender	No ADLs	1–3 ADLs	4–6 ADLs
1985	Male	8.8	28.8	62.5
	Female	3.8	25.3	70.9
1995	Male	3.0	25	72
	Female	3.8	25.3	70.9
1997	Male	5.0	25.7	74.4
	Female	1.8	20.4	77.8
1999	Male	5.0	20.7	74.3
	Female	2.4	19.6	78.0

Notes: Numbers represent percentages. The six activities of daily living (ADLs) included are bathing, dressing, eating, toileting, and transferring in and out of bed or chairs. Requiring assistance refers to assistance from nursing home facility staff. Help received from family member or friends is not included. Data refer to individuals living in long-term care facilities, rather than personal care, foster care, or domiciliary care homes.

Source: Centers for Disease Control and Prevention, National Center for Health Statistics. (2004). *National Nursing Home Survey.* Bethesda, MD: Government Printing Office.

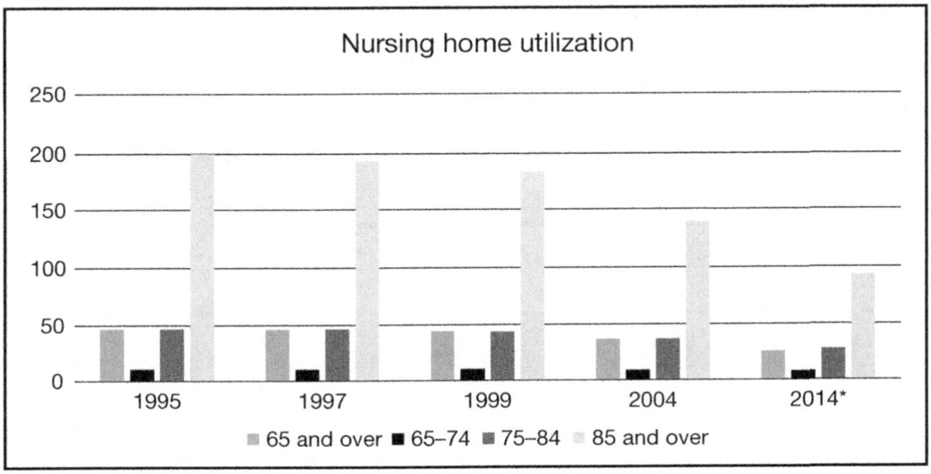

Figure 13.1 Nursing home utilization.

Notes: Data refer to rate per 1,000 of nursing home residence, age 65 and older, by age group, 1995, 1997, 1999, 2004, and 2014. Data refer to individuals living in long-term care facilities, rather than personal care, foster care, or domiciliary care homes.

Source: Centers for Disease Control and Prevention, National Center for Health Statistics. (2004). *National Nursing Home Survey*. Bethesda, MD: Government Printing Office; National Study of Long-Term Care Providers.

A common misconception about nursing home care is that the majority of older people will end up living in a nursing home. In fact, only about 4% of older adults actually reside in a nursing home setting. In addition, the rate of individuals residing in nursing homes between 1995 and 2014 is on the decline overall (46 per 1,000 in 1995 as compared to 25 per 1,000 in 2014). The oldest old, people 85 years of age and older, have also dramatically decreased in terms of nursing home census. In 1995, nearly 200 per 1,000 people of this age group resided in nursing homes, while in 2014, this same figure dropped to 93 per 1,000. Figure 13.1 provides an overview of these data and a comparison between age groups and between 1995 and 2014 (CDC, NCHS, 2004; Federal Interagency Forum on Aging-Related Statistics [FIFARS], 2016).

While fewer than 5% of Medicare enrollees age 65 and older lived in long-term care settings (as of 2016), as people age they are more inclined to live in long-term care facilities and less likely to remain in traditional community-based settings. According to the Medicare Beneficiary Survey (2016) nearly all adults 65 to 74 years of age (98%) still remained active in traditional community settings, and 93% remained in traditional community settings between ages 75 and 84 years of age. Conversely, the oldest old, 85 years of age or older, have more healthcare needs, and only 75% remain in traditional community settings, while 8% remain in community housing with services, and 17% reside in long-term care facilities. This is a dramatic difference since we see 17% of the oldest old living in long-term care facilities as compared to 5% of people in the 75 to 84 age group category. Table 13.2 illustrates these trends.

Despite the fact that older adults today have greater care needs, more people with needs for help with instrumental activities of daily living (IADLs) or ADLs are remaining in the community with supports. Although it appears that community-based residential options may be cost-effective (Hebert et al., 1999; Levine, 1999), many of these options have also led to an industry geared toward assistive care and home-health supports

Table 13.2 Medicare Enrollees Living in Residential Services, by percantage (2016)

	Age Group			
Type of facility	65 and over	65–74	75–84	85 and over
Long-term care facility	4.4	1.0	3.0	10
Community housing	2.5	0.9	2.6	8
Traditional community	93.1	98.1	92.9	75

Notes: Numbers are reported as percentages. Community housing with services applies to respondents who reported they lived in retirement communities or apartments, senior citizen housing, continuing care retirement facilities, assisted living facilities, staged living communities, board and care facilities/home, and other similar situations and who reported that they had access to one or more of the following services through their place of residence; meal preparation, cleaning or housekeeping services, laundry services, and help with medications. Respondents were asked about access to these services but not whether they actually used the services. Long-term care facilities were defined as those that were certified by Medicare or Medicaid; or has three or more beds, and is licensed as a nursing home or other long-term care facility and will provide at least one personal care service, or 24 hour, 7 day per week supervision by a caregiver. Data refer to Medicare enrollees.

Sources: Centers for Medicare and Medicaid Services, Medicare Current Beneficiary Survey.

(Albrecht, 1992; Callahan, 1998; Coughlin, 1999; Gottlieb & Caro, 1999; Kane, 1999). These supports can include home healthcare (Bishop, 1999). Although only 59% of older adults who have no activity limitations currently reside in the community, the remaining 41% reside in the community with some sort of supports, including 9% with three or more ADL limitations, 21% with one to two limitations, and 12% with an IADL limitation only. Just over one-third of people (36%) who remain in their homes with some housing services have no problems with ADLs or IADLs. Fewer than a sixth of all people living in a community-based setting (15%) have problems with IADLs only, and 32% have problems with one to two ADL functions who live in the community with supports. Despite impairment, 17% of people with three or more ADL limitations still live in the community with some supports. Figure 13.2 illustrates residential services and showcases that individuals living in long-term care facilities are the most debilitated with two thirds (67%) having three or more ADL limitations (FIFARS, 2016). Hence, it should be noted that people with activity limitations are remaining in the community longer, and home-health supports have been instrumental in enabling people to remain in the community.

Given that many people require supports to remain in their homes, it seems essential to examine what supports are available federally through the Older Americans Act, and what services are available through state-based sources. In addition, it also seems prudent to examine what options are available for housing.

Thus, although as a society, we are living longer and placing demands on the community by remaining in the community, it becomes apparent that there is a current need to ensure that programs are available within communities to meet the housing needs of older adults. In addition, it is imperative to understand the current opportunities and options for community-based living. This next section outlines some specific options for community-based living, which include part of the continuum of care.

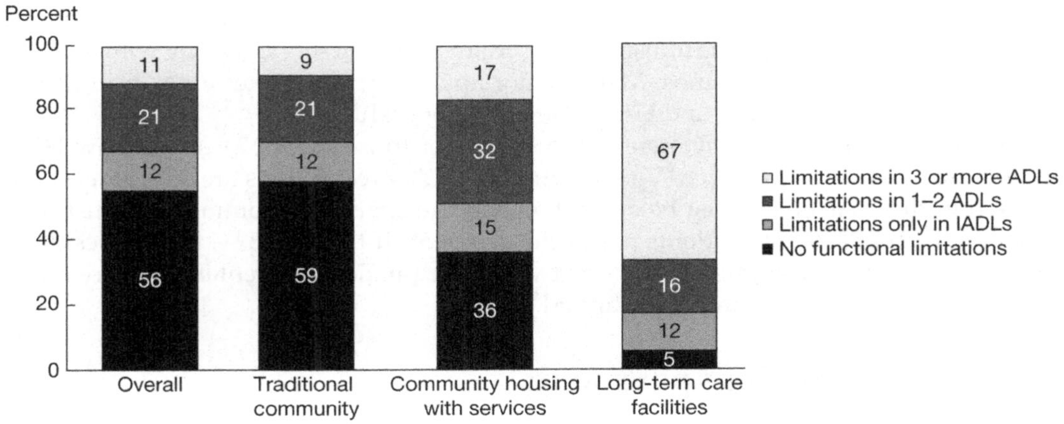

Figure 13.2 Percentage distribution of Medicare beneficiaries age 65 and over with limitations performing ADLs and IADLs, by residential setting, 2013.

Notes: Community housing with services applies to respondents who reported they lived in retirement communities or apartments, senior citizen housing, continuing care retirement facilities, assisted living facilities, staged living communities, board and care facilities/homes, and similar situations, and who reported they had access to one or more of the following services through their place of residence: meal preparation, cleaning or housekeeping services, laundry services, or help with medications. Respondents were asked about access to these services, but not whether they actually used the services. A residence (or unit) is considered a long-term care facility if it is certified by Medicare or Medicaid; or has three or more beds, is licensed as a nursing home or other long-term care facility, and provides at least one personal care service; or provides 24-hour, 7-day-a-week supervision by a non-family, paid caregiver. Long-term care facility residents with no limitations may include individuals with limitations in performing certain IADLs, such as doing light or heavy housework or meal preparation. These questions were not asked of facility residents.

Reference population: These data refer to Medicare beneficiaries.

ADLs, activities of daily living; IADLs, instrumental activities of daily living.

Source: Centers for Medicare and Medicaid Services, Medicare Current Beneficiary Survey, Access to Care; Federal Interagency Forum on Aging-Related Statistics. (2016). *Older Americans: Key factors of well-being.* Washington, DC: U.S. Government Printing Office.

AN OVERVIEW OF THE PROGRAMS TO MEET HOUSING NEEDS OF OLDER ADULTS

Senior Apartments

Senior apartments are a good choice for older adults who can take care of themselves. Usually, these apartments are developed like standard apartments but differ in that they have an age restriction. Some apartments are also equipped with assistive technology such as hand rails and pull cords. Overall, these apartments are great if one needs a community of elderly neighbors without the hassles of a larger home to manage.

Senior apartments are found in many communities; some are under federal housing guidelines and will only accept low-income seniors, but most are privately owned. They can vary in terms of services but typically offer apartment living and services designed specifically for independent active seniors 55 and older. Since many of these residences are designed for active seniors, most do not offer meal service, housekeeping, or medical assistance.

Senior apartment complexes are usually located near senior centers, parks, shopping malls, golf courses, and public transportation. Many offer van services along with monthly road trips to shows and casinos. Many senior apartment complexes are subsidized by the Department of Housing and Urban Development (HUD).

Senior age-restricted apartments are usually for those 55 or 62+ and follow HUD regulations that allow for such "age discrimination." If restrictions are 55+, at least one person in the apartment must be at least 55 and the apartment community must have no more than 20% of all residents under the age of 55. If they are 62+, then *all* residents must be at least 62. Exceptions are made by HUD regulations for renters who are under the minimum age if they are handicapped.

Categories of Senior Apartments

The three pricing categories of apartments (although not all may be available in any one market) are

- Market rate
- Above market rate, luxury rentals
- Affordable

Market-rate units are just that. They offer unit size and numbers of bedrooms and baths as nonage-restricted rentals in the area at a competitive monthly rate, or occasionally 10% to 15% under general occupancy market-rate rents. The senior orientation of the age-restricted community may, however, offer different amenities and other advantages geared to the needs and preferences of seniors.

Above market rate, luxury rentals are a relatively new phenomenon for the age-restricted market. We see them appealing to the affluent senior wanting a home in a second city, or wanting to be free of maintenance without giving up luxuries. Some high-end age-restricted properties definitely offer "snob" appeal.

Affordable apartments for seniors (sometimes 55+, more often 62+) are in high demand and short supply. Social, cultural, and medical changes have certainly contributed to the need. Contributing factors are

- Predominance of women among the 65+ population and their lower retirement income.
- High divorce rates among women now 55 to 80.
- Women outliving husbands resulting in lowered retirement income.
- Unplanned longevity leading to outliving one's financial resources.

Affordable apartments have been created by government programs since the 1930s. What is defined as affordable in one community may not match the definition of affordable in another community. Housing is "affordable" if one pays no more than 30% of monthly income for rent and utilities. The government relates affordability to the county median income.

Programs that provide opportunities for affordable housing are structured or defined by regulations from federal, county, or city government legislation.

- "Vouchers" enable a qualified recipient to rent a market-rate home or apartment, and the voucher assures the landlord that the renter will pay 30% of his or her monthly income toward the rent and the difference between that portion and the market-rate rent will come from the government entity granting the voucher.

- Bonds may be through city or county redevelopment programs and use the money raised from the bond sale to fund and subsidize specific development of housing for lower-income people. Bonds may specify what percent of the median income someone must have to qualify to rent in their building. A person may be restricted to making no more than 50% of the median income in the county. Perhaps the funding of the complex specifies that a person can make no more than 120% of median income. The funding is specifically tied to the complex, or specific units that are "affordable."
- Funding can also come from grants that are community, government, or federally based. The grant money functions similarly to bond money, designating percent of county median income at the time of the grant.
- Tax credits are another way that the federal government may encourage development of affordable housing, by awarding tax credits (money deducted from a company's federal tax obligation) in exchange for developing apartments within restrictive guidelines. Recently, properties have been developed to offer affordable apartments that combine tax credits, grants, and bond measures.

The most commonly known rental vouchers are Section 8 vouchers, which can provide benefits to a qualified renter. They provide rent subsidies so tenants who hold them do not pay more than 30% of their adjusted gross income for rent.

Congregate housing and multilevel campuses offer what they call independent living. They offer services for those in their own apartments. These services may be optional and charged separately above rent. Shared meals, transportation, and housekeeping are among the most common services provided. This housing type differs from the conventional notion of an apartment and therefore is defined separately as congregate housing or assisted living since that is the one common element for multilevel offerings. The independent living offering is most appropriate for those not able or willing to continue living alone. Recently senior apartment buildings have added services to retain their frail and aging residents.

Assisted Living

Assisted living is an industry term for multifamily housing with congregate and personal care services. Assisted living goes by many names, including personal care, residential care, congregate care, and, in some areas, board and care. The services offered vary widely but frequently include as core services meals, housekeeping, transportation, and often some assistance with laundry, grooming, medications management, and other functions of daily living (Jurkowski, Kemp, & Patterson, 2004). Special care units in some facilities care for individuals with cognitive impairment and respiratory assistance needs. Unless an assisted living facility is a component of a continuing care or "life-care" community, it does not offer the healthcare services of a nursing facility. For safety reasons most states require residents to self-evacuate their personal living quarters (with or without ambulatory equipment) in the event of an emergency.

The federal government does not establish standards for assisted living as it does for nursing homes that participate in the federal Medicare program. Most states license and regulate assisted living residences, and an increasing number of states place Medicaid-eligible adults in assisted living residences as an alternative to traditional placement in a nursing home. This trend leads many to speculate that the federal government will become increasingly involved in setting minimum standards of care in residences electing to participate in the federal-state Medicaid program. National associations representing selective areas of the industry have increased self-regulation efforts, motivated in part to delay federal oversight and regulation. The number of older adults living in assisted living is estimated to be between 600,000 and 1 million, with as many as 50,000 receiving Medicaid support, compared with 1.6 million older adults in nursing home beds including 1 million with Medicaid assistance.

Board and Care

Board and care homes are smaller in scale than assisted living facilities. They provide a room, meals, and help with daily activities. Some states will allow some nursing services to be provided, but these homes are not medical facilities. These homes may be unlicensed, and even licensed homes are infrequently monitored by the state.

Board and care is offered in a homelike setting with medical care for two to 10 residents. Some are converted/adapted single-family homes. The number of residents is a function of zoning regulations, which limit the number of unrelated occupants that can live in a single residence.

Foster Care

Foster care is sometimes limited to only two residents. Most designated converted homes offering care are allowed only five or six residents. Those that appear to be converted homes, but offer more beds, are usually licensed as assisted living residences.

A Comparison of Board and Care, Residential Care, and Foster Care

A board and care, residential care, or foster care home may be able to provide residents the services found in an assisted living facility, a skilled nursing home, or, in some cases, an Alzheimer's facility, depending on the goal and licensing of the individual facility. Many board and care facilities have their own specialty or emphasis, and the intensity or type of care needed by residents within a home may be similar. For instance, some specialize in care of seniors in the middle stages of Alzheimer's. Another may take only early stage Alzheimer's residents. Another home may be licensed to accept only those mildly impaired mentally, or needing "custodial" help (reminding, meal service, laundry, housekeeping help, and driving services). In many states they would need to be licensed to hand out medications, assist with bathing, or care for patients who cannot turn themselves in bed. Since there are so many board and care homes, hundreds in a populated county, it is also unrealistic to think that licensing can monitor them all.

Continuing Care Retirement Community

A continuing care retirement community is a gate-secured campus offering residential services ranging from independent living and assisted living to nursing home care, all on one campus. It usually provides a written contract between the resident and the community that offers a continuum of housing, services, and healthcare services, commonly all on one campus. Continuing Care Accreditation Commission (CCRC) residents enjoy an independent lifestyle with the knowledge that if they become sick or frail, their needs will continue to be met. In general, residents are expected to move into the community while they are still independent and able to take care of themselves.

CCRC is the *Consumer's Report* of the CCRC world. It rates CCRC facilities based on their excellence, integrity, volunteerism, credibility, innovation, and independence.

Some states support legislation for older adults who wish to stay in their homes by restructuring the delivery of services to include home-based services as well as institutional care. Such restructuring impacts all aspects of service, including the provision of housing, health, financial, and supportive services for older people and can include a nursing home conversion program established by state departments of public health and public aid. This program approach would reduce reliance on nursing homes by Medicaid, the federal-state program that pays the healthcare costs for the poor. Savings from this effort could then be reallocated to a broader array of options for home-based or community-based services to older adults (Albrecht, 1992; Sutton & DeJong, 1998; Wheatley, DeJong, & Sutton, 1996).

STRATEGIES FOR REMAINING IN ONE'S HOME

Home Equity Conversion

Reverse mortgages are a type of home equity conversion involving payments to, rather than from, the homeowner. This special type of loan guarantees older homeowners monthly cash advances or occasional lump sums that do not require repayment until the homeowner sells the home, moves away, or dies.

Sale Leaseback

Sale leaseback occurs when the home is sold to a third party (often the adult child of the homeowner) who immediately leases it back to the seller (older homeowner) under an agreement of life tenancy. Anyone considering home equity conversion should discuss these intentions with trusted advisors who are knowledgeable about these programs.

MAINTENANCE PROGRAMS

Home Maintenance and Repair

Home maintenance and repair programs are designed to help older persons to remain in their own homes or apartments by making repairs to the home at little or no cost to the residents. "Repairs" can include yard work, painting, electrical or plumbing repairs, repairs to steps or porches, or the addition of adaptive devices for persons with disabilities. Some of these programs are supported by federal subsidies; others are private initiatives.

Illinois Home Weatherization Assistance Program

The Illinois Home Weatherization Assistance Program is designed to help low-income residents have more energy-efficient homes. Typical kinds of weatherization include sealing cracks with weather-stripping and caulk, insulating attics and walls, and repairing windows and doors. Furnace work may also be provided. Weatherization services are free to households that are eligible for the Low-Income Home Energy Assistance Program (LIHEAP); to those who have an occupant receiving Supplemental Security Income (SSI), Temporary Assistance for Needy Families (TANF), or Aid to Aged, Blind, and Disabled (AABD); or to those with specified annual incomes. Renters may be assisted if they are eligible, but a 50% landlord contribution for weatherization work is required.

ISSUES FACING LONG-TERM AND COMMUNITY-BASED CARE FOR OLDER ADULTS

A growing number of issues face long-term and community-based care facilities for older adults. These issues are discussed in brief in the next few pages. Although they address shortcomings in long-term care facilities, skilled nursing care facilities, and additional community settings, the issues are by no means exhaustive and probably only scratch the surface of issues to be faced. Such choices are vital for the healthy and productive functioning of older adults (Greenwald, 1999).

Long-Term Care Facilities

Long-term care facilities will face challenges related to the level of care required for facilities to provide to individual residents. As the population of individuals who enter into care within these facilities grows more frail and needier in terms of care because of the increased nature of functional debilitation, facilities will both need to be better equipped to meet these needs and be prepared to work within a system of financing that may compromise care. Increasingly, these facilities will also see more cases requiring specialized dementia care units and Alzheimer's care units to support the care needs of their residents. Long-term care facilities will also be challenged with culture change issues that will push them to move toward a home-based environment rather than an institutional setting. These culture changes may also include a culture that will need to accommodate people who have habitually embraced a substance-use culture (i.e., older adults who were a product of the drug subculture that began in the 1960s). Movements are afoot within nursing homes across the country to build a so-called homelike and comfortable atmosphere for residents.

Finally, the long-term care movement may be also subjected to care for people who have been discharged from penal system, or who have served life sentences but are now frail and elderly. Although many states currently have laws that deny or defer admission to these individuals, shrinking resources in the future may challenge the current system of long-term care facilities.

Assisted Living Facilities

Assisted living facilities will be on the rise over in the future and without any oversight through accreditation bodies, may run the risk of providing uneven quality of care. Moreover, it appears that an aim of the assisted living movement could be to capitalize on older adults who have resources and can afford to pay for care; hence the marketplace and business community, rather than a long-term care system, may be dictating how these facilities are operated.

Community-Based Care

Community-based care options will be called to expand and challenge traditional strategies for doing business. An increased emphasis on home modifications and repair programs will also take place as more people want to remain in their own homes with some help in home maintenance. A second challenge will be to locate and train home-health workers to meet the growing needs of older adults, especially seniors living in rural communities. Training for home-health aides will also become critical since these workers are virtually the eyes and ears for care coordinators and family members. In the future, we can expect to see an expansion of training opportunities for the home health or home support worker. These training opportunities will ultimately be helpful and beneficial to the older adult if they succeed in making home-health workers more astute and attuned to medical and social issues that older adults present and better prepared to more clearly articulate these issues in behavioral terms.

Consumer-Directed Home Help and Care Options

Consumer-directed home help and care options will be in greater demand into the 2020s and 2030s. Two factors may contribute to this: (a) people want to age in place, and (b) the philosophical perspective shaped by the disability movement will push for consumer-directed options and remaining in a community-based setting. In order to meet baby boomers' demand for these options, state departments on aging will need to look at new strategies or ways to finance and build options within their continuing care programs to meet these needs. Consumer-directed care options will also span not only older adults but will also be sought after by people with disabilities (Sutton & DeJong, 1998).

People With Disabilities Requiring Community-Based Care

Increasingly, people with disabilities will challenge the institutional model paradigm traditionally exercised by long-term care facilities. The independent living paradigm (DeJong, 1979) set the stage for people with disabilities to be functional within the least restricted environment. The cash and counseling models of consumer-directed care will become a model sought after by people with disabilities who want to have control of their care and be empowered by their ability to manage their own care (Lee, Hammill, & Wilson, 2016; McArther, Burch, Moore, & Hodges, 2016).

OPPRESSED GROUPS AND VISIBLE MINORITIES

Oppressed groups and visible minorities will pose demands upon the current systems to be culturally relevant and to assure that policies are in place within facilities to meet the needs of individuals requiring care. Examples will include the lesbian, gay, bisexual, and transgender (LGBT) groups of elders who may request opportunities for intimate expression within long-term care settings, within environments that may not necessarily be comfortable with addressing sexual orientations other than their own. A second example may include addressing the cultural needs of ethnically diverse populations, whether that may be via religion, cuisine, or meeting rooms to meet the family needs of these groups. Last, community care options to meet the needs of people with disabilities will also need to be considered as an alternative to the traditional placements in nursing home care (Mackelprang, & Salsgiver, 2015).

SUMMARY

This chapter examines the current status of the long-term care system, describes different residential models of care for people as they require community-based settings or settings with supports and examines issues that will face the long-term and community-based care settings in the future.

DISCUSSION QUESTIONS

1. Compare and contrast the different types of needs that people with disabilities and people growing older have specific to residential living (consider the cases at the outset of this chapter—Ida, Gerry, and Lorraine). What needs are similar and what needs are different between these two groups?
2. How has stigma and public perception led to differences in residential settings for people with disabilities versus people who are growing older? What differences in philosophical paradigms (see Chapter 3) can be associated with the differences in policies that impact these settings?
3. How important do you think it is to be sure that people are allowed to live in a "least restrictive environment" and to live in a setting that reflects their needs, hobbies, and personal wishes? Should individuals be more concerned with the quality of care received in a residential setting, or should personal social and emotional needs be also a critical consideration within long-term care settings? What role does "aging in place" play in the lives of people with disabilities or people growing older?
4. What types of residential care, community care, and long-term care options exist within your community for people with disabilities and people growing older? If you were to identify some specific needed options, what would these be?

ADDITIONAL RESOURCES

Websites

Long-term care: What are my options? www.medicare.gov/what-medicare-covers/part-a/other-long-term-care-choices.html

This web page, published on Medicare.gov provides a range of housing options that can be covered by Medicare. The options range from independent to those with care needs.

Long-term Care: www.nia.nih.gov/health/caregiving/long-term-care

This web page provides an opportunity for the reader to become familiar with a variety of evidence-based opportunities for long-term care. Published by the National Institute of Aging, the information is forthright and timely.

Senior Care 101: Housing types explained: www.aplaceformom.com/senior-care-resources/articles/senior-housing-options

This website provides an overview of various housing types for older adults, along with pricing associated with such options. It also provides a housing locator to enable the viewer to be able to identify which types of options would work well for the consumer and his or her loved one.

Long-term Care Services and Supports for People with Disabilities: www.thearc.org/what-we-do/public-policy/policy-issues/long-term

This site provides information about the needs and issues related to long-term care services and supports that people with disabilities will need. Published by the ARC, it provides extensive information for the reader with the view of people with disabilities.

YouTube Videos

Community Living for People with Developmental Disabilities (Part One): www.youtube.com/watch?v=UQc7geMXDJU

This YouTube video provides the viewer with the opportunity to learn about how to provide supports to people with disabilities to be able to living within a community-based setting.

Help for the Disabled to Find Housing: www.youtube.com/watch?v=UCCY2Cig-s0

This YouTube video provides the viewer with information to be able to understand the range of opportunities available for people with disabilities. It also communicates how housing can be accessible for people living with disabilities.

Tips for Senior Housing Options: www.youtube.com/watch?v=is-uTAbQy4I

This YouTube video provides the viewer with information on a range of housing options for older adults. The video also provides the viewer with the opportunity to understand the questions to ask and resources available for senior housing opportunities.

Senior Living Options: www.youtube.com/watch?v=wB2aM5cQivc

This YouTube video provides the viewer with a quick thumbnail sketch of various housing options and how they fit with the needs of a senior older adult. It showcases the various options and provides a definition of each for the viewer.

Podcast

Dr. Elaine Jurkowski discusses housing and the least restrictive environment. **Listen now:** https://bcove.video/2OTCsKP

REFERENCES

Albrecht, G. L. (1992). *The disability business: Rehabilitation in America*. Thousand Oaks, CA: Sage.

Bishop, C. (1999). Efficiency of home care: Notes from an economic approach to resource allocation. *Journal of Aging and Health*, *11*(3), 341–359. doi:10.1177/089826439901100302

Callahan, J. J. (1998). Social policy in the age of the market. *The Public Policy and Ageing Report*, *9*(2), 13–15.

Centers for Disease Control and Prevention, National Center for Health Statistics. (2004). *National nursing home study*. Bethesda, MD: Government Printing Office.

Coughlin, J. F. (1999). Setting a national policy agenda for technology and healthy ageing. *The Public Policy and Ageing Report*, *10*(1), 1–6.doi:10.1093/ppar/10.1.1

DeJong, G. (1979). Independent living: From social movements to analytic paradigm. *Archives of Physical Medicine and Rehabilitation*, *60*, 435–446.

Federal Interagency Forum on Aging-Related Statistics. (2016). *Older Americans: Key indicators of well-being*. Washington, DC: U.S. Government Printing Office.

Gottlieb, A., & Caro, F. (1999). Extending the effectiveness of home-care through low-cost adaptive equipment. *The Public Policy and Aging Report*, *10*(1), 13–15. doi:10.1093/ppar/10.1.13

Greenwald, J. (1999, August 30). Elder care: Making the right choice. *Time*, 52–56.

Hebert, R., Dubuc, N., Buteau, M., Derosiers, J., Bravo, G., Trottier, L., ... Roy, C. (1999). *Resources and costs associated with disability of elderly people living at home and in the institutions*. Presented at the American Health Services Research 16th Annual Meeting, Chicago, IL.

Jurkowski, E., Kemp, M., & Patterson, S. (2004). Assisted living, social work practice and the elderly. In M. Holosko & M. Feit (Eds.), *Social work practice and the elderly* (364–387). Toronto, ON: Canadian Scholar's Press.

Jurkowski, E. T. (2013). *Implementing culture change in long-term care: Benchmarks and strategies for management and practice*. New York, NY: Springer Publishing.

Kane, M. D. (1999). Examining the efficiency of home care. *Journal of Aging and Health, 11*(3), 322–340. doi:10.1177/089826439901100304

Lee, D., Hammill, J., & Wilson, T. (2016). A community living management program for people with disabilities who have moved out of nursing homes: A pilot study. *Journal of Disability and Rehabilitation, 38*(8), 754–760. doi:10.3109/09638288.2015.1060266

Levine, C. (1999). Home sweet hospital: The nature and limits of private responsibilities for home care. *Journal of Aging and Health, 11*(3), 341–359. doi:10.1177/089826439901100305

Mackelprang, R., & Salsgiver, R. (2015). *Disability: A diversity model approach to human service practice*. New York, NY: Oxford University Press.

McArther, P., Burch, L., Moore, K., & Hodges, M. S. (2016). Novel active learning experiences for students to identify: Barriers to independent living for people with disabilities. *Rehabilitation Nursing, 41*(4), 202–206. doi:10.1002/rnj.208

National Consortium on Leadership and Disability for Youth. (2017). *Disability history timeline: Resource and discussion guide*. Retrieved from http://www.ncld-youth.info/Downloads/disability_history_timeline.pdf

Sutton, J., & DeJong, G. (1998). Managed care and people with disabilities: Framing the issues. *Archives of Physical Medicine and Rehabilitation, 79*, 1312–1316. doi:10.1016/S0003-9993(98)90283-0

Szaz, T. (1967). The myth of mental illness. In T. J. Scheff (Ed.), *Mental illness and social processes* (pp. 242–254). New York, NY: Harper & Row.

Wheatley, B., DeJong, G., & Sutton, J. (1996). How managed care is transforming American health care: A survey of rehabilitation providers in leading markets. *The Georgetown Public Policy Review, 1*(2), 134–147.

14

Substance Use and Misuse

LEARNING OBJECTIVES

At the end of this chapter, readers will:

1. *Understand the history of the legislation related to substance use and misuse.*
2. *Understand specific components of the Controlled Substances Act.*
3. *Understand how legislation related to substance use and misuse provides resources to older adults and people with disabilities.*

Theresa and Erika had heard that an opioid epidemic was rampant and affecting many older adults and people with disabilities. They wondered though what this news really meant in terms of people's functioning and everyday activities because they had only heard about the epidemic but had not witnessed it first-hand. Was this specifically for people who had addiction issues in the first place, or did this also entail people who were older adults and people with disabilities? As a first step in trying to unravel and understand this arena, the two decided to visit with four people: Susan; Angela and her husband, Joseph; and Nora.

***Susan**: Susan is a 57-year-old woman who has sustained a work-related injury that has impacted her knees and mobility. In addition to her own mobility impairment, she lives with her older parents, Irma and Gus. Gus was diagnosed with early stages of Alzheimer's disease about 10 years ago, and this condition has progressed to the point where he is mobility impaired and needs constant supervision. Irma is a brittle diabetic and cannot handle the care needs of her husband, so she relies mostly on Susan for help. They lived on a farm, but now have moved to a metropolitan area. Irma and Gus have five other adult children; however, the responsibility for caregiving has fallen upon Susan. In an effort to deal with the initial pain that Susan experienced, she was placed on what she thought were painkillers. Little did she realize that after 7 months, she was still in pain and quite dependent upon the prescription to enable her to sleep and to maintain her functioning.*

***Angela and Joseph:** Angela (83) and Joseph (86) are currently living in Houston, Texas; however, they have worked in many corners of the world as a result of Joseph's distinguished career in the Air Force. Upon retirement from the Air Force, Joseph joined NASA and worked*

(continued)

(continued)

as an aeronautical engineer until his full retirement at 69 years of age. Angela stayed at home while their three children were in school and then worked as a jewelry clerk at a local jewelry store. Both Angela and Joseph have experienced health issues that have led to much chronic pain. Angela had a severe car accident in her mid-40s that led to spinal surgery entailing a fusion of her vertebrae and placement of a rod along her spine. Often, she finds herself in chronic pain that is so severe that it is difficult for her to be able to tend to her activities of daily living, and she is reliant upon medication and a morphine patch for relief. Her primary care physician recently died, and she is now working with a new treatment team. This team has advised her that there may be limited benefit to her medication and pain management regime because of her prolonged use and dependence. Her husband Joseph sustained an injury while in the service and has also been on pain management medications. He enjoys his happy hour routine and has recently been advised that there is an interaction effect between his medication and his adult beverage of choice. He insists that the young physician (the age of his grandson) does not have any business telling him, and old "geezer" what choices to make and is insistent on his routine medications.

Nora: *Nora is both a caregiver to her 87-year-old father and disabled from an orthopedic injury while riding a bicycle. Her recent knee replacement surgery has left her with less mobility in her right knee than prior to her surgery. Being caregiver to her father leaves her with limited emotional resources at the end of a day. Nora's father is legally blind, suffers from Crone's disease, and has had a series of ministrokes. They have lived together in the three-bedroom family home since Nora's mother passed away 10 years ago and receive in-home services to support Nora in her caregiving role. Nora, divorced for nearly 25 years from her alcoholic and abusive husband, returned to her childhood home to care for her father following her mother's passing. Nora's father also attends a day program 3 days per week. Nora also helps in the caregiving role for her two grandsons. Nora's father was emotionally distant from her while she was growing up, and she is an only child. Nora has found herself taking antidepressants for many years. She has sought help because she feels that her medications are not working effectively. She is not seeing the benefits from her current medications for pain management and wonders whether her rituals of daily martinis are interfering with the medications she has been prescribed for depression and her other medications prescribed for pain due to her knee replacement.*

LEGISLATIVE HIGHLIGHTS RELATED TO SUBSTANCE ABUSE/MISUSE

The area of substance abuse and misuse, when compared to other areas that touch the lives of people growing older and people with disabilities, is not as developed and rich in terms of legislative initiatives. One may argue that the philosophical paradigm that has guided the development of this legislation, "blaming the victim," has tended to place the burden of the responsibility for such challenges on the individual rather than on the system or environment. For this reason, one can also argue that legislation has tended to be punitive as opposed to curative.

Legislation specific to substance use/abuse at the federal level in the United States can be found as early as 1914, when the United States Congress passed the Harrison Act. This landmark legislation criminalized the nonmedical use of prescription narcotics.

This federal piece of legislation mirrored legislative initiatives that had been signed into public law within California in 1907. The Harrison Act outlawed the use of cocaine, opium, and morphine and its various derivatives but did not include amphetamines, barbiturates, marijuana, hashish, or hallucinogenic drugs of any kind.

In order to ensure proper distribution of prescribed medications between doctor and patients, a nominal tax was paid by physicians in order to obtain a stamp that permitted the prescription of narcotics, so long as the regulations included in the Harrison Act were followed. A second tax, at a much steeper cost, was required for the nonmedical distribution of narcotics, conventional wisdom being that regulations would be followed in order to avoid the higher of the two taxes. Interestingly, if an individual was found to be in possession of one of the drugs banned by the Harrison Act, the federal criminal charge would be tax evasion. In 1970, the term "war on drugs" was first used by the Nixon administration when it enacted legislation that was a continuation of the original Harrison Act.

The Comprehensive Drug Abuse and Prevention and Control Act of 1970 was signed into Public Law by President Richard Nixon. This law integrated the Harrison Act and its various amendments and consolidated over 50 drug laws into one law meant to control the legitimate drug industry and curtail importation and distribution of illicit drugs.

The Controlled Substance Act categorized drugs into two classifications: Schedule I drugs are considered to have no medicinal qualities while having a potential for abuse; Schedule II drugs are considered to be of medicinal value while also having the potential for abuse. Drugs considered Schedule I include: heroin, marijuana, and various hallucinogenic drugs; Schedule II drugs include morphine and cocaine.

As with the Harrison Act of 1914, the Controlled Substance Act of 1970 focused mainly on the supply side of narcotic distribution and the penalties involved with possession and distribution. No attention seemed to be directed to the addict or decreasing demand.

To increase awareness of the specific impacts of substance use, Congress passed the Anti-Drug Abuse Act in 1986, which increased the federal block grant program for substance abuse and addiction services and increased funding for the study of AIDS. In 1988 Congress passed the Omnibus Anti-Drug Abuse Act, which allocated funding for school-based educational programs and for drug abuse treatment, with an increased focus on intravenous drug use.

The *Comprehensive Addiction and Recovery Act* (CARA) was signed into law by President Barack Obama on July 22, 2016. The bill was introduced by Senator Sheldon Whitehouse and Representative Jim Sensenbrenner as the first major federal addiction act in 40 years (CARA, 2016; Community Anti-Drug Coalitions of America, 2016). President Donald Trump has voiced strong support for the act (Beveraly, 2016; Corasaniti, 2016).

CARA authorizes over $181 million dollars to respond to the epidemic of opioid abuse and is intended to greatly increase both prevention programs and the availability of treatment programs. However, while this bill authorizes the program, funds must still be appropriated by congress through the usual budget process (CARA, 2016).

In May 2017, the Substance Abuse and Mental Health Services Administration (SAMHSA) announced grants totaling $2.6 million for recovery community organizations to build addiction recovery networks and engage in public education as authorized under CARA (SAMHSA, 2017).

WHAT IS THE SCOPE OF SUBSTANCE MISUSE?

Misuse of prescription opioids, central nervous system (CNS) depressants, and stimulants is a serious public health problem in the United States. Although most people take prescription medications responsibly, an estimated 54 million people (more than 20% of those age 12 and older) have used such medications for nonmedical reasons at least once in their lifetime. According to results from the 2014 National Survey on Drug Use and Health, an estimated 2.1 million Americans used prescription drugs nonmedically for the first time within the previous year, averaging approximately 5,750 initiates per day. Fifty-four percent were females and about 30% were adolescents (SAMHSA, 2015)

The reasons for the high prevalence of prescription drug misuse vary by age, gender, and other factors, but likely include ease of access (Centers for Disease Control and Prevention [CDC], 2011). The number of prescriptions for some of these medications has increased dramatically since the early 1990s (Manchikanti, Fellows, Ailinani, & Pampati, 2010). Moreover, misinformation about the addictive properties of prescription opioids and the perception that prescription drugs are less harmful than illicit drugs are other possible contributors to the problem (Daniulaityte, Falck, Carlson, 2012; Webster, 2012). Although misuse of prescription drugs affects many Americans, certain populations such as youth, older adults, and women may be at particular risk (CDC, 2013; Miech, Johnston, O'Malley, Keyes, & Heard, 2015). In addition, while more men than women currently misuse prescription drugs, the rates of misuse and overdose among women are increasing faster than among men.

More than 80% of older patients (aged 57 to 85 years) use at least one prescription medication on a daily basis, with more than 50% taking more than five medications or supplements daily (CDC, 2017). This prevalence of prescription drugs can potentially lead to health issues resulting from unintentionally using a prescription medication in a manner other than how it was prescribed, or from intentional nonmedical use. The high rates of multiple (comorbid) chronic illnesses in older populations, age-related changes in drug metabolism, and the potential for drug interactions makes medication (and other substance) misuse more dangerous in older people than in younger populations. Further, a large percentage of older adults also use over-the-counter medicines and dietary supplements, which (in addition to alcohol) could compound any adverse health consequences resulting from nonmedical use of prescription drugs.

In October 2017, President Trump declared under federal law, that the used of opioids had reached crisis proportions and a state of national emergency. Under such as declaration as a national emergency, the Public Health Act can appropriate funding for this emergency.

The State of Opioid Use

Opioids have been recently identified as the sources of a national crisis in America, and our population is suffering from their use and abuse. Advancing age and limited abilities are also impacted by use and misuse. Opioids include illicit drugs such as heroin, but also include prescription pain medication such as oxycodone, hydrocodone, codeine, morphine, and fentanyl (National Institute on Drug Abuse, 2015). The Institute reported that of the 20.5 million Americans who had a substance use disorder in 2015, two million had a substance use disorder that involved the use of prescription pain relievers.

Opioids have been driving an epidemic in America, and in 2015, we witnessed 20,101 overdose deaths related to prescription pain relievers and 12,990 overdose deaths related to prescription pain relievers (National Institute on Drug Abuse, 2018; Rudd, Seth, David,

& Scholl, 2016). While an argument is sometimes made that older adults should be allowed to live their life in the manner they choose, the impact that opioid misuse may have for older adults and people with disabilities moves far beyond personal choice and can be linked to adverse medical outcomes such as falls and hip fractures (West & Dart, 2015). The substance use disorder treatment admission rate in 2009 was 6 times the 1999 rate. In 2012, 259 million prescriptions were written for opioids, which are more than enough to give every American adult his or her own bottle of pills (Qato et al., 2008; SAMHSA, 2015). The use of opioids is on the rise and has impacted older adults and people with disabilities in staggering ways.

Alcohol and Substance Abuse Disorders

Alcohol Abuse and Dependence

Although we may carry a stereotype of an older adult as being white or gray haired, jovial, meek, or frail, we seldom think of older adults as substance abusers, out-of-control drinkers, or persons at risk for these conditions. Analyses of data examining alcohol consumption practices in older men and women drawn from sources such as the National Health Interview Survey (NHIS, 2000), the Behavioral Risk Factor Surveillance System (BRFSS, 2017; U.S. Department of Health and Human Services [USDHHS], National Center for Health Statistics, 2004) and the National Household Survey on Drug Abuse (NHSDA, 2000) have shed light on the prevalence of alcohol consumption among older adults. In fact, these data suggest that older adults in the 65 and older age category found 56.8% of the population at risk for drinking in the past 30 days, when surveyed. On the days these same older adults report that they drink, 32.1% say they have two or more drinks (NHIS, 2004). Breslow, Faden, and Smothers (2003) found in their secondary analyses of these data that about one third of the U.S. elderly population consume alcohol, regardless of risk. These authors concluded that as we see our population "graying" over the upcoming decades, practitioners, and public health officials will need to be more aware of dealing with this segment of the population.

The prevalence of heavy drinking (12 to 21 drinks per week) in older adults is estimated at 3% to 9% (Liberto, Oslin, & Ruskin, 1992). One-month prevalence estimates of alcohol abuse and dependence in this group are much lower, ranging from 0.9% to 2.2% (Regier et al., 1988). Alcohol abuse and dependence are approximately four times more common among men than women ages 65 and older (1.2% vs. 0.3%; Grant, Harford, Dawson, Chou, & Pickering, 1994). Although lifetime prevalence rates for alcoholism are higher for White men and women between ages 18 and 29, African American men and women had higher rates among those 65 years and older. For Hispanics, men had rates between those of Whites and African Americans. Hispanic females had a much lower rate than that for Whites and African Americans (Helzer, Burnam, & McEvoy, 1991). Although longitudinal studies suggest variously that alcohol consumption decreases with age (Adams, Garry, Rhyne, Hunt, & Goodwin, 1990; Temple & Leino, 1989). Recent studies have shown that alcohol abuse and drug dependence have been on the increase with baby boomers. This may be as a result of this cohort having a greater history of alcohol consumption than other cohorts of older adults.

Schonfeld (1993) examined prevalence estimates of alcohol use and misuse among older adults through surveying staff providing services to older adults. He found few staff had received in-service training on substance abuse issues, but conversely saw these topics as issues of high priority in their day-to-day work. Although this study is dated and occurred primarily in urban areas, are there differences, or have these issues changed by the present day?

This issue is further illustrated by the work of Hanson and Guthiel (2004), who made the case for brief motivational interviewing as a successful intervention when working with older adults. They argue that social workers and other health professionals do not adequately address problem drinking with older adults. These authors suggest that issues such as inadequate knowledge about addictive behaviors, limited development in assessment tools, and limited evidence-based treatment options account for social work practitioners' limitations when dealing with these issues. These findings build on the work of Klein and Jess (2002) who found that staff training and education issues were identified as limited, despite a clear awareness that alcohol posed a problem for people who were residing in intermediate care facilities. They interviewed 111 directors of intermediate care facilities in the United States to learn that although alcohol use was common in facilities, comfort level on the part of the staff related to alcohol use among older adults was limited.

Emlet, Hawks, and Callahan (2001) in their retrospective chart study of 148 community-dwelling older adults found that functional status was not a predictor for alcohol use and abuse among older persons. Males were three times more likely to drink than females. Moreover, the authors illuminate the growing problem of substance abuse/use among older adults and articulate the need for intervention with this target population. Although they did not specifically examine older adults in rural areas, we can anticipate the issues are similar.

Memmet (2003) argues that older adults in general are at risk for the development of polydrug problems due to interactive effects of alcohol and prescription or over-the-counter medications. The importance of screening elderly clients for substance abuse is a critical factor in the detection and treatment of substance use issues among the elderly.

Although minimal research has been conducted in rural areas, Musnick, Blazer, and Hays (2000) examined a sample of elderly people affiliated with the Baptist religion, living in rural areas of central North Carolina. They found a strong relationship between religiosity (being Baptist) and the nonuse of alcohol. They also found that among Baptists that did not attend services regularly, there was a relationship between symptoms of depression and alcohol use.

It has been found that older adults are at risk of alcohol abuse and has been argued that treatment for older adults should be differentiated from that of other age groups. However, LaGreca, Akers, and Dwyer (1988) found in the sample of 1,410 older adults (60+) living in retirement communities that problem drinking was not linked to members of the communities or life transitions. Conversely, social support networks did not serve as mediators for the impact of life events on alcohol use. Their work extends the work of Alexander and Duff (1988) who discovered, after surveying three retirement communities, that drinking was an integral part of the leisure subculture.

Misuse of Prescription and Over-the-Counter Medications

To date, a limited amount of information is available about the actual misuse of prescription drugs among older adults. A Special Committee on Aging (1987) reported that the use of prescription drugs among older adults was approximately three times as frequent as in the general population. In addition, Kofoed (1984) found that the use of over-the-counter medications by this group was even more extensive. Annual estimated expenditures on prescription drugs by older adults in the United States are $15 billion annually, a fourfold greater per capita expenditure on medications compared with that of younger individuals (Anderson, Kerluke, Pulcins, Hertzman, & Barer, 1993; CDC, 2006: Jeste & Palmer, 1998). It should be no surprise that problems with misuse and abuse of substances among the older adult population may be attributed to problems related to aging—failing eyesight or misunderstanding the directions. Thus underuse, overuse, or erratic use can be attributable in part to a lack of health literacy, failing eyesight, or problems such as cataracts. In extreme instances, these problems then result in drug and substance abuse.

Mental health issues and substance abuse disorders often co-occur for both adults and children (Regier et al., 1990). Despite this awareness, and evidence-based practices that have been established for treating these co-occurring disorders (Drake et al., 2001), a limited amount of work and research has been done to examine both the etiology and treatment of these disorders either individually or as co-occurring within rural areas (New Freedom Commission on Mental Health. 2004). The field appears to lack an understanding of both the need and method to tailor evidence-based approaches to treat people with co-occurring disorders in rural areas (Benavides-Vaello, Strode, & Sheeran, 2013; USDHHS, 2004).

Although older adults may be at increased risk or vulnerability to experiencing mental health-related problems, they often do not seek or are not successful at linking with the necessary mental health services (Kaplan, Adamek, & Martin, 2001; USDHHS, 1999). A variety of factors can account for this outcome including stigma of mental illness; ageism; complexity and fragmentation of services; lack of coordination between medical, mental health, and aging systems of care; lack of professional staff trained in geriatric mental health; and inadequacy of health insurance coverage (USDHHS, 1999). Symptoms of depression existing and undetected within the older adult population have been noted in the literature (Bland, Newman, & Orn, 1988; Blazer, 1999; Dorfman et al., 1995; Proctor, Morrow-Howell, Rubin, & Ringenberg, 1999; Rogers & Barusch, 2000). Consequently a poorly coordinated system of care and lack of integration between systems (especially aging, mental health, and primary care) contributes to this problem (USDHHS, 1999, 2006b). This problem becomes magnified when layered with the issues of substance use and abuse for older adults, whether the use is via prescription or over-the-counter medications.

Mental Health and Older Adults

Depressive symptoms are an important indicator of general well-being and mental health among older adults. People who report many depressive symptoms often experience higher rates of physical illness, greater functional disability, and higher healthcare utilization (Center for Behavioral Health Statistics and Quality, 2016; Mehta, Yaffe, & Covinsky, 2002). Mental health issues and substance abuse disorders often co-occur for both adults and children (Regier et al., 1990). Although older adults may be at increased risk or vulnerability to experiencing mental health-related problems, they often do not seek or are not successful at linking with the necessary mental health services (USDHHS, 1999). A variety of factors can account for this outcome including stigma of mental illness; ageism; complexity and fragmentation of services; lack of coordination between medical, mental health, and aging systems of care; lack of professional staff trained in geriatric mental health; and inadequacy of health insurance coverage (Mueller, Kashinath, & Ullrich, 1997; USDHHS, 1999). Consequently, there is a poorly coordinated system of care and lack of integration among systems (especially aging, mental health, and primary healthcare).

While most older people prefer to live in the community, mental disorders have been implicated as one of the major risk factors to institutionalization (Katz & Parmelee, 1997; USDHHS, 1999). Despite this problem, community-based services to meet the needs of older adults in community-care settings have largely been provided through the general medical sector since the mental health organizations have focused primarily on persons with severe persistent mental health disorders. However, the focus of primary care is often medical and acute care; thus, mental health issues are often overlooked (George, 1992; USDHHS, 1999). Home-health agencies provide limited short-term care (Meeks & Murrell, 1997; Meeks et al., 1990; Robinson, 1990).

Substance Use/Abuse and People With Disabilities

Evidence suggests that substance use has been on the rise for the population in general among people living in the community. However, what is the status of substance use for people with disabilities? Glazier and Kling (2013) examined the prevalence of substance abuse for people with disabilities. They found that the prevalence of overall substance abuse (a composite measure) was level over time, at 34% for persons without disabilities and 40% for persons with disabilities. The substance abuse prevalence among persons with disabilities closely paralleled that of other persons over the period 2002 to 2010 for each substance examined, but at a statistically significant higher level, with the exception of alcohol abuse, which was significantly lower. They also found that over time there were trends that were relatively stable for people with disabilities and people without disabilities. Some differences were noted by Glazier and Kling (2013) and they found that people with disabilities had less cocaine use, but higher prevalence rates of both marijuana use and oxycodone abuse.

In a meta-analysis conducted by Carrol Chapman and Wu (2012) examining substance abuse with people who have intellectual disabilities, it was found that people with disabilities was a growing population that seemed to be impacted by substance use and misuse. Surprisingly, they found in their analysis of 37 peer-reviewed articles that people with intellectual disabilities suffer to a much greater extent from substance use issues. Likely this difference occurs because we lack resources for prevention and treatment efforts that can target and reach this specific population. Although these authors reported that the literature found that people with intellectual disabilities may not necessarily use substances on a routine basis, those that did use were at high risk of having problems with substance use/misuse. In addition, people with intellectual disabilities, unlike the general population, were found to be less inclined to receive treatment for the substance misuse behavior and were also less likely to remain in treatment. This finding may be due to the lack of expertise on the part of treatment specialists to deal with people who have intellectual impairments. It is likely that much more research is needed to explore the incidence and prevalence of substance use/misuse for people with intellectual disabilities.

Further, people with physical disabilities are also at much greater risk for acquiring substance use issues (Disabled World, 2018). Weiss (2017) described the situation that with a group of people with orthopedic disabilities, spinal cord injuries, amputations, or vision impairment, around 40% to 50% of cases may be classified as "heavy drinkers." He also suggests that people with disabilities experience substance abuse rates that are 2 to 4 times that of people in the general population. People with forms of disabilities to include arthritis, deafness, or multiple sclerosis experience substance abuse rates that are at least double the rate for those in the general population. Why is this the situation with people who live with disabilities? Weiss argues that "the major causes of disabilities in the United States are changing from medical to social and behaviorally-related conditions and are increasingly involving complications that include violence, substance abuse, and poor mental health" (Weiss, 2017).

In summary, people with disabilities experience many situations that increase their chances for substance abuse impacting their lives in negative ways. These include enabling, health and medication issues, and a dearth of prevention and treatment options/services. People living in rural communities may be further compromised because these resources are not available (Lambert, & Agger, 1995).

Rural Communities Versus Urban Communities

The realities that specialty mental health services for older adults have been underutilized is identified in the literature (National Institute on Aging [NIA], 2000; Proctor et al., 1999; Proctor et al., 2003; Taube, Morlock, Burns, & Santos, 1990). In addition, general health has served in fact as the mental health system of care for older adults (Regier, Goldberg, & Taube, 1978). Social services have in fact been underutilized by older adults who are in need of mental health services (Proctor et al., 1999); however, older adults with physical care needs and comorbid medical conditions were more likely to be in need of mental health services (Proctor et al., 2003). Patients living in rural areas were less likely to use certain mental health services than their urban counterparts; however, the need was documented to be similar in nature across both locations (Bird, Dempsey, & Hartley, 2001; Illinois Rural Health Association, 2006;).

SOCIAL WORK, MENTAL HEALTH, AGING, AND SERVICE UTILIZATION

Despite the dearth of research and efficacy studies on the benefits of various treatment modalities for mental health issues and older adults, *Mental Health: The Report of the Surgeon General* (USDHHS, 1999) argues for a range of services that can be an adjunct to the formal treatment setting and supports the concept of health education and health promotion strategies to create an awareness of the aging process and mental health functioning within the aging process. A range of interventions that have largely not been evaluated can be used to help improve the mental health of older adults living in the community. These may include peer support, wellness programs, life reviews, bereavement groups, health promotion, and health education programs (Cohen, 1995; Haight, Michel, & Hendrix, 1998; Rowe & Kahn, 1997; Scott-Lennox & George, 1996; Waters, 1995; USDHHS, 2005). Social workers can play a major role in this educative process if they understand mental health and older adults, as well as the role that health disparities can play in the continuum of mental health functioning (USDHHA, 2000). The intersection of disability, chronic physical conditions, and depression is not well understood or underscored often by social workers working in community-care settings. These issues may be compounded with the location of one's residence and socioeconomic status. Studies should be conducted to address these issues conceptually and lay the foundation for pilot data that can be utilized to better prepare social workers working in community-care and home-health settings.

From our previous studies, we can see that we are in need of programming to meet the mental health needs of older adults. The next section addresses programs available to meet the mental healthcare needs of older adults.

PROGRAMS AVAILABLE TO MEET THE SUBSTANCE ABUSE CARE NEEDS OF OLDER ADULTS

Medicare

Medicare has a small provision for mental healthcare in its original plan. Under the original plan, Medicare Part A, some expenses related to mental healthcare given in a hospital are covered, which include one's room, meals, nursing care, and other related services and/or supplies. Medicare Part A has a lifetime cap on the number of days one is able to have paid while in an inpatient psychiatric facility. Although there is no lifetime limit for inpatient care provided through a general hospital, Medicare will cover up to only 190 days of inpatient psychiatric hospital services care during one's lifetime.

Medicare Part B will help pay for mental health services generally given outside a hospital, including visits with a doctor, clinical psychologist, clinical social worker, clinical nurse specialist, nurse practitioner, and/or physician's assistant and lab tests. These services, however, are paid for by Medicare only when provided by a health professional who has been approved to accept Medicare reimbursement.

Medicare Part B also helps pay for outpatient mental health services or services provided for through an outpatient or mental health clinic, physician's office, therapist's office, or outpatient hospital department. In addition, services such as individual and group therapies approved by one's local state are covered, family counseling in relation to the older adult's treatment plan is covered, lab work and psychological assessments, occupational therapy related to one's treatment plan, individual patient training, and education and diagnostic tests are covered.

A number of services are not covered within the Medicare plan. Some of these include any meals and transportation to or from mental health treatment, support groups that are offered in nonmedical settings for peer support, and any testing/job training that has not been a part of the prescribed mental health plan.

Partial hospitalization programs are also funded through Medicare Part B. This type of therapeutic program provides intensive psychiatric care through active treatment but differs from counseling or outpatient care in its intensity, duration, and depth of treatment available from one's physician or therapist. Partial hospitalization treatment offers day treatment and does not require any inpatient overnight stays. Generally these partial hospitalization programs are provided through either hospital outpatient departments or local community mental health centers. Medicare can pay for partial hospitalization programs on the condition one's physician can make the case that without such a program, the consumer would require an inpatient stay for treatment. In addition, the physician and partial hospitalization program need to be provided by a recognized Medicare provider in order to receive reimbursement.

Medicare is a program available to individuals who have worked up to 40 quarters and contributed through payroll tax into a plan. In the event that one does not have this plan to qualify for, or lives below a specific income level, mental health services are still available under the Medicaid program.

Medicaid

Generally, one can qualify for resources through Medicaid or public aid mental health services if one's resources or monthly income are less than a fixed amount which is initially set by Medicare, and then established within the state in which one resides. These rates change on January 1 of each year. Alaska and Hawaii also have slightly higher income limits. Generally speaking, therapists working with older adults and receiving state public aid or Medicaid funding may be required to provide therapeutic treatment based upon an evidence-based best-practice model. These are intervention strategies that have been approved by the SAMHSA and National Institute of Mental Health (NIMH) as being interventions guided by successful clinical trials and an evidence-based approach to treatment. Not all state public aid/Medicaid sources require these intervention approaches, and some states, such as Illinois, currently allow for therapists to utilize their professional judgment as to which intervention strategies work best for a specific diagnosis and patient.

Area Agencies on Aging

Under the Older Americans Act of 2000, some funding was available to area agencies for short-term supportive counseling for mental health needs. However, these funds did not cover the areas of screening and assessment for older adults adequately and were designated for pilot initiatives rather than long-term programs. The Older Americans Act Amendments of 2006 (Pub. L. No. 109–365) expands the delivery of mental health services. "Mental health services" or "mental health screening" replace the terms "health screening" or "health services" in the act, including Section 306. The amendments of 2006 also proposed new Mental Health Multidisciplinary Centers under Title IV. The House bill amends Section 419 by adding new language requiring centers to collect information on best practices in long-term care service delivery, housing, and transportation. It also requires mental health multidisciplinary centers to provide training and technical assistance to support community-based mental health services to older people. The Senate bill S. 3570 amended Section 419 by authorizing new grants to states on a competitive basis for the development and delivery of systems for mental health screening and treatment services for older individuals. Such grants support programs that (a) increase public awareness related to benefits of prevention and treatment of mental health conditions faced by people 60 years of age and older and (b) target stigma associated with mental disorders and other barriers that impact the diagnosis and treatment of mental health disorders. State agencies that receive such funds are required to allocate the funds through area agencies on aging to carry out the programs. Succeeding amendments to the OAA have reinforced the need for substance misuse and mental health counseling, as has the current opioid epidemic.

SERVICE DELIVERY SETTINGS FOR SUBSTANCE USE/MISUSE CARE FOR OLDER ADULTS AND PEOPLE WITH DISABILITIES

Traditionally services for mental healthcare for older adults have been constrained and limited to settings designed for chronically mentally ill adults, and specialized services for treating the older adult has been limited. The *Surgeon General's Report on Mental Health* (USDHHS, 1999) provided an overview of settings within which mental health treatment occurs. This report suggests that mental health services for older adults within communities occurs within homes, group homes, retirement communities, primary care and general medical care sectors, outpatient therapy, board and care homes, assisted living facilities, and community mental health centers. Institutional settings for mental health treatment of older adults occurs within nursing homes, general hospitals with psychiatric units, general hospitals without psychiatric units, state mental hospitals, and Veterans Affairs hospitals.

Unfortunately these settings have tailored interventions to meet the needs of an adult population rather than offering any specializations for an older adult population. In addition, when state funds are limited or budgets are in need of retrenchment, the first target group to be dismissed are older adults who do not fit into the category of chronically mentally ill. This situation calls into question the need to look at alternative treatment modalities and policies that embrace the older adults and build in their unique needs and therapeutic approaches.

Increasingly, primary care settings are also beginning to address mental health needs of older adults, through screening, assessment, and educational approaches. Several model programs have incorporated social work staff to provide screening and assessment services to patients during their wait for the primary care physician (Gask, Sibbald, & Creed, 1997; Katon et al., 1996; Katon et al., 1997; Schulberg et al., 1995; Stolee, Kessler, & Le Clair, 1996). While these approaches are still in their infancy, and primary care still requires being addressed before physicians will adequately deal with the older adults' mental health needs adequately, these intervention schemes hold great promise. Such approaches minimize the potential for stigma and prejudice on the part of both the provider and the patient. Overall, models that consider the integration of mental health treatment into primary care were designed to meet the needs of people with depression, but other disorders may also be targeted within primary care settings. A set of recommendations for appropriate referrals to specialty mental healthcare is available through the American Association for Geriatric Psychiatry (AAGP, 1997).

ISSUES FACING OLDER ADULTS AND PEOPLE WITH DISABILITIES WITH SUBSTANCE ABUSE/MISUSE CARE NEEDS

A number of issues currently face older adults with substance use/abuse care needs residing in the community. These include the financing of treatment and recovery services for older adults and people with disabilities, community-based care, prevention services, screening and detection, and detoxification management. This section reviews some of these specific issues and showcases areas for further development.

Financing Mental Healthcare for Older Adults

Until the Older Americans Act Amendments of 2006, financing mental healthcare for older adults was an issue that led to a battleground between divisions of aging and mental health and substance abuse. Each group perceived that mental healthcare for older adults was not its mandate, and funding for services and resources was limited if existent. Departments on Aging perceived mental health issues and services to be the role of Departments/divisions for Mental Health (DMH). Conversely, divisions of mental health perceived their role to be one of intervention for people with chronic mental illness rather than acute, short-term issues. DMHs also perceived that issues related to service delivery for older adults was the mandate of the aging directorates, regardless of specialty area need. Consequently, financing (or lack of financing) is and remains an issue for older adult service delivery settings.

Financing also plays a critical role when delivering services, either assessment or intervention. Ultimately, one must work with an older adult with a different set of approaches than one would take when working with children, teenagers, or younger adults (Mackenzie, Gekoski, & Knox, 1999). Older adults and/or people with disabilities may require a longer time period within which to complete assessments because of the need for a slower-paced interview, and a longer period of time to develop rapport or engage the individual in the therapeutic relationship. This need becomes difficult for caseworkers who may be reimbursed per session as opposed to per case. Effective models of financing assessments may revert to using a block-funded approach to service delivery rather than a case-by-case approach.

Community-Based Care

Community-based care for substance abuse/misuse concerns has largely been delivered through local community mental health centers or drug rehabilitation centers. The community mental health centers were originally developed to meet the needs of the deinstitutionalized long-term psychiatric patients, who moved into local communities following the passage of the Community Mental Health Centers Act of 1966 (Pub. L. No. 88–164). These settings have aged along with their constituents, and now many of the young adults with chronic mental health problems and substance use issues have also aged and are in the older adult (60+) target group. Unfortunately, the funding schemes and the modus operandi are very much focused on providing community-based services to stabilize individuals with chronic mental health needs, rather than older adults with acute and short-term care needs. Inpatient community-based settings are not equipped to work with people with disabilities or people growing older. In addition, the settings are often stigmatizing, and unfavorable to older adults with short- or long-term substance use/misuse needs. Treatment groups available through partial hospitalization programs often target the younger patient, and older adults often feel out of place. These issues become compounded when considering a smaller rural community setting, where privacy is limited, and one would not be able to maintain anonymity when confronted with visiting a community mental health center for substance misuse issues—an issue that can be ameliorated by the use of technology (Benavides-Vaello, Strode, & Sheeran, 2013).

Models for Gero-Psychiatry

A number of models are beginning to develop around the United States for gero-psychiatry. These model demonstration projects hold promise for innovative ways to provide screening, detection, education, and intervention services for older adults. Such approaches will be imperative for the effective treatment of older adults. These models will also hopefully provide for a nonstigmatizing approach to dealing with older adults and will also improve the specialty areas for intervention services from older adults. These model approaches will also require some legislative base and intervention to provide a legislative mandate for individual states to create these services (a sample piece of legislation is available at http://www.ilga.gov/legislation/publicacts/pubact91/acts/91–0799.html).

Prevention Services

Currently, federal legislation does not have any provisions for prevention-oriented services. The legislative base behind Medicare and the Older Americans Act (2000 amendments) does not provide for preventative services. Individual states and funded initiatives through NIMH, NIA, and SAMHSA have provided funds to develop evidence-based prevention interventions; however, these approaches are often not funded federally; once they are deemed effective, individual states may introduce them into their systems for their constituents. The Administration for Community Living (ACL), among others, are now seeing the need for prevention resources and education on the use and misuse of substances by the disabled and aging populations, and funds are being appropriated by Congress for substance use prevention focused on these populations. The impact of these initiatives will need to be examined as they are implemented.

Screening and Detection

The ideal venue for an older adult to be assessed for substance use/misuse is during an initial assessment for home-health services or within primary care settings. Currently, not all community-care settings screen for substance use or misuse during their initial assessments or follow-ups. In addition, not all home-health caseworkers are trained to understand the behavioral symptoms associated with the *Diagnostic and Statistical Manual of Mental Disorders* (5th ed.; *DSM-5*, 2013) diagnostic groups. Without training of caseworkers or primary care health providers, many signs of substance misuse may go undetected or untreated. The screening and assessment tools also used for this population group are limited and require further development. Drug interaction effects between medications prescribed for chronic health conditions and other substance use and abuse also need further exploration as we are only beginning to understand the impacts of these interaction effects.

Medications

Medications for the treatment of substance use/misuse disorders are often tested within clinical trials on a younger adult population; hence, there is limited information about how these metabolize within an older adult's system. It is quite common for people over the age of 60 to require several attempts with different medications prior to finding the one that will best work within one's body and among the other drugs one may be taking. One may be required to pursue a variety of medications prior to finding one that will work effectively. Challenges are that we have a limited understanding of clinical trials that can be used with an older adult population. Entangled within this scheme is the fact that people may be over-medicated or overly reliant upon pain medications and opioids. Second, with Medicare Part D enrollment periods only once per year, one may have greater out-of-pocket expenses than anticipated because of different medication prescriptions required to stabilize an acute conditions.

MODEL PROGRAMS AND BEST-PRACTICE APPROACHES TO SUBSTANCE USE/MISUSE SERVICE DELIVERY

Although a range of behavioral health approaches exist to meet the mental health and substance misuse needs of older adults, the concept of evidence-based interventions is becoming widely prescribed by behavioral health service providers. Levkoff, Chen, Fisher, and McIntyre (2006) have developed a guide to the implementation of such programs. In the section to follow, some specific programs, recognized by the SAMHSA, are presented for potential intervention strategies and best-practice models for mental health service delivery.

The Center for Older Adult Recovery at Hanley Center

In 1998, the Hanley Center in West Palm Beach, Florida opened its pioneering Center for Older Adult Recovery, after developing an age-responsive model of treatment of alcohol and chemical addictions. Hanley's outcomes suggest that the older adult target group can be the most successful with recovery rates when compared to any other age group.

The program offers prevention for late onset addiction as well. Situated in lush tropical enclaves, Hanley Center offers its older adult consumers a Serenity Fountain and Garden and a homey, comfortable residence. Hanley's holistic treatment model addresses patients' physical and mental status as well as the values of this generation.

After an initial thorough evaluation, individualized treatment takes on a slower pace, due to the normal aging process, as well as chronic medical conditions, cognitive impairment, and possible dual diagnosis. Hanley's interdisciplinary team of highly skilled professionals provides holistic treatment in the areas of medicine, psychiatry, psychology, and counseling, wellness, spirituality, and expressive arts. Continuing care plans are put into place prior to patients' discharge and are specific to the individual's special needs (USDHHS, 2006b).

SUBSTANCE USE/MISUSE CARE CHALLENGES FOR THE FUTURE

Substance abuse/misuse challenges for the future are many, and although this chapter touches upon several, it is certainly not exhaustive. The biggest challenge will probably be the very nature of financing to meet the community-based noninstitutionalized population. Since substance use/misuse is often perceived as "blaming the victim," models of care and rehabilitation are often not taken into serious consideration. Prevention, screening, detection, and intervention strategies to meet the needs of baby boomers as they age will be another challenge. Models of service delivery that are innovative, preventative in nature, and nonstigmatizing will also be an important goal to strive toward. Working with this target population of older adults and people with disabilities may also require that we seek alternative programs that address substance use issues through harm reduction rather than direct abstinence. Establishing systems of care that are not fragmented and provide a seamless system of service delivery will also be an important goal for mental health, healthcare, and public health service delivery systems.

SUMMARY

This chapter takes us through a journey to examine the current status of substance use and older adults, with a particular emphasis on opioids and pain management medications. Programs and services are reviewed and issues still outstanding within the substance use and abuse arena are discussed. This chapter concludes by laying out some challenges for the future in the area of substance use and abuse among older adults and people with disabilities.

DISCUSSION QUESTIONS

1. Revisit the cases at the beginning of this chapter and identify the presenting issues. What do you think are appropriate interventions for these individuals?
2. Consider your own community where you live and work. What resources are available to deal with the opioid crisis within your community? How can you work with existing resources to develop a needs assessment and intervention to meet this growing need?

DISCUSSION QUESTIONS *(continued)*

3. What assessment and intervention resources are available to meet the needs of younger people and people with disabilities within your community area who are struggling with substance use and misuse issues?
4. To what extent in your community do you think prescription drugs pose a problem with use and abuse? What stakeholders in your community can assist you in understanding the extent of this issue among older adults and people with disabilities?
5. What do you think that you can do with existing coalitions or stakeholder groups in your community to raise awareness of the issues related to substance use and misuse? Would these solutions include community town hall meetings, fact sheets, radio and newspaper coverage, and so on?

ADDITIONAL RESOURCES

Websites

Mental Health America: www.nmha.org

This website provides consumer-oriented information on a range of mental health topics by audience, issue, disorders, treatments, and medications. It also provides links to a range of policy issues and mental health topics.

Suicide and Depression Fact Sheets: www.nimh.gov/publicat/elderlydepsuicide.cfm

This site provides an excellent set of fact sheets on older adults, depression, and suicide. It is written on a level that enables the reader to glean some behavioral signs and symptoms about suicide and identify whether they or a loved one is at risk. The fact sheets are a product of the NIMH.

NIMH: www.nimh.nih.gov

This website provides up-to-date health information on a range of disorders including anxiety disorders, posttraumatic stress disorder, depression, and eating disorders, with some vantage points for older adults.

SAMHSA: www/samhsa.gov

This website provides a matrix of services for older adults. It includes information and linkages to the Older Americans Substance Abuse and Mental Health Technical Assistance Center and campaigns for public awareness. Current campaigns include a "Do the Right Dose" campaign and an "As You Age" campaign. The site also provides links to professional resources that can be useful in gleaning current knowledge in the area and developing resources for professional development and public education.

Senior Health online Depression information: nihseniorhealth.gov/depression/toc.html

This site provides an overview of numerous health topics of interest, including depression in older adults. Since approximately two million Americans age 65 or older suffer from major depression, and another five million suffer from less severe forms, a collaborative effort between the NIA and the National Library of Medicine (NLM) worked conjointly to develop this senior-friendly medical website.

SAMHSA Fact Sheets on drugs of interest: www.oas.samhsa.gov/drugs.cfm

This website provides fact sheets on various drugs, with up-to-date medical background information.

YouTube Videos

Top Ten Facts about Prescription Drug Abuse in America: www.youtube.com/watch?v=l6yKQRqWxVQ

This YouTube video provides a series of facts related to prescription drug use and abuse. It reviews facts shared by the CDC within the top 10 areas that the general public is generally unaware of and explains how prescription drugs can silently lead to abuse.

Commonly Abused Prescription Drugs: www.youtube.com/watch?v=rIBF3lwBtA0

This YouTube video provides a list of common names of prescription drugs that can be abused. It also helps the viewer understand both the prescription and the street names for such drugs.

Signs and Symptoms of Prescription Drug use: www.youtube.com/watch?v=16YhXNIC414

This YouTube video showcases some of the specific signs and symptoms of prescription drug use and abuse. While some symptoms of abuse are obviously specifically related to alcohol and marijuana, prescription drugs may not necessarily be as obvious.

Addiction: www.youtube.com/watch?v=ao8L-0nSYzg

This YouTube video provides a new view of how to intervene with addiction and challenges the traditional paradigms related to addiction and addiction treatment. The concept of "social recovery" tries to help people see the important role social connections and one's social environment play in the intervention and recovery process.

Podcast

Dr. Michelle McLernon and Dr. Bill McCreary on the opioid crisis. **Listen now:** https://bcove.video/2Q7P8lW

REFERENCES

Adams, W. L., Garry, P. J., Rhyne, R., Hunt, W. C., & Goodwin, J. S. (1990). Alcohol intake in the healthy elderly. Changes with age in a cross-sectional and longitudinal study. *Journal of the American Geriatrics Society*, *38*, 211–216. doi:10.1111/j.1532-5415.1990.tb03493.x

Alexander, F., & Duff, R. W. (1988). Social interaction and alcohol use in retirement communities. *The Gerontologist*, *28*(5), 632–636. doi:10.1093/geront/28.5.632

American Association for Geriatric Psychiatry. (1997). *Recommendations from primary care physicians: When to refer depressed elderly patients to a geriatric psychiatrist*. Bethesda, MD: Author.

American Psychiatric Association. (2013). *Diagnostic and statistical manual of psychiatric disorders* (5th ed.). Washington, DC: Author.

Anderson, G. M., Kerluke, K. J., Pulcins, I. R., Hertzman, C., & Barer, M. L. (1993). Trends and determinants of prescription drug expenditures in the elderly: Data from the British Columbia Pharmacare Program. *Inquiry*, *30*, 199–207.

Behavioral Risk Factor Surveillance System. (2017). Retrieved from https://www.cdc.gov/brfss/annual_data/annual_2017.html

Benavides-Vaello, S., Strode, A., & Sheeran, B.(2013). Using technology in the delivery of mental health and substance abuse Treatment in rural communities: A review. *Journal of Behavioral Health Services & Research, 40* (1): 111–120.

Beveraly, K. (2016, November 9). *Addiction treatment policy under President Trump*. Retrieved from http://www.quitalcohol.com/treatment/addiction-treatment-policy-president-trump.html

Bird, D. C., Dempsey, P., & Hartley, D. (2001). *Addressing mental health workforce needs in underserved rural areas: Accomplishments and challenges*. Portland, OR: Maine Rural Health Research Center, Muskie Institute, University of Southern Maine.

Bland, R. C., Newman, S. C., & Orn, H. (1988). Prevalence of psychiatric disorders in the elderly in Edmonton. *Acta Psychiatrica Scandinavica, 338*, 57–63. doi:10.1111/j.1600-0447.1988.tb08548.x

Blazer, D. (1999). Depression in the elderly. *New England Journal of Medicine, 320*, 164–166. doi:10.1056/nejm198901193200306

Breslow, R. A., Faden, V. B., & Smothers, B. (2003). Alcohol consumption by elderly Americans. *Journal of Studies on Alcohol, 64*(6), 884–892. doi:10.15288/jsa.2003.64.884

Brody, J. A. (1982). Aging and alcohol use. *Journal of American Geriatrics Society, 30*(2), 123–126. doi:10.1111/j.1532-5415.1982.tb01287.x

Carrol Chapman, S. & Wu, T., (2012). Substance abuse among individuals with intellectual disabilities. *Research in Developmental Disabilities, 33*, 1147–1156. doi:10.1016/j.ridd.2012.02.009

Center for Behavioral Health Statistics and Quality. (2016). *Key substance use and mental health indicators in the United States: Results from the 2015 National Survey on Drug Use and Health* (HHS Publication No. SMA 16-4984, NSDUH Series H-51). Retrieved from http://www.samhsa.gov/data

Centers for Disease Control and Prevention. (2006). *Trends in health and aging*. Washington, DC: Government Printing Office.

Centers for Disease Control and Prevention. (2011). Vital signs: Overdoses of prescription opioid pain relievers—United States, 1999-2008. *Morbidity and Mortality Weekly Report, 60*(43), 1487–1492.

Centers for Disease Control and Prevention. (2013). Vital signs: Overdoses of prescription opioid pain relievers and other drugs among women—United States, 1999-2010. *Morbidity and Mortality Weekly Report, 62*(26), 537–542.

Centers for Disease Control and Prevention (2017). Therapeutic drug use. Retrieved from https://www.cdc.gov/nchs/fastats/drug-use-therapeutic.htm

Cohen, G. D. (1995). Mental health promotion in later life: The case for social portfolio. *American Journal of Geriatric Psychiatry, 3*, 277–279. doi:10.1097/00019442-199503040-00001

Community Anti-Drug Coalitions of America. (2016). *Comprehensive Addiction and Recovery Act (CARA)*. Retrieved from http://www.cadca.org/comprehensive-addiction-and-recovery-act-cara

Comprehensive Addiction and Recovery Act of 2016. (n.d.). Retrieved from https://www.govtrack.us/congress/bills/114/s524/summary

Corasaniti, N. (2016, October 15). "We should take a drug test" before debate, Donald Trump says. *The New York Times*. Retrieved from https://www.nytimes.com/2016/10/16/us/politics/donald-trump-hillary-clinton-drug-test.html

Daniulaityte, R., Falck, R., & Carlson, R. G. (2012). "I'm not afraid of those ones just 'cause they've been prescribed": Perceptions of risk among illicit users of pharmaceutic opioids. *International Journal of Drug Policy, 23*(5), 374–384. doi:10.1016/j.drugpo.2012.01.012

Disabled World. (2018). *Addiction and substance use among people with disabilities*. Retrieved from https://www.disabled-world.com/medical/pharmaceutical/addiction/serious.php

Dorfman, R. A., Lubben, J. E., Mayer-Oakes, A., Atchison, K., Schweitzer, S. O., DeJong, F. J., … Matthias, R. E. (1995). Screening for depression among a well elderly population. *Social Work, 40*(3), 295–304. doi:10.1093/sw/40.3.295

Drake, R. E., Essock, S. M., Shanner, A., Carey, K. B., Minkoff, K., Kola, L., … Rickards, L. (2001). Implementing dual diagnosis services for clients with severe mental illness. *Psychiatric Services, 52*, 469–476. doi:10.1176/appi.ps.52.4.469

Emlet, C., Hawks, H., & Callahan, J. (2001). Alcohol use and abuse in a population of community dwelling, frail older adults. *Journal of Gerontological Social Work, 35*(4), 21–33. doi:10.1300/j083v35n04_03

Gask, L., Sibbald, B., & Creed, F. (1997). Evaluating models of working at the interface between mental health services and primary care. *British Journal of Psychiatry, 170*, 6–11. doi:10.1192/bjp.170.1.6

George, L. K. (1992). Community and home care for mentally ill older adults. In J. E. Birren, R. B. Sloane, G. D. Cohen, N. R. Hooyman, B. D. Lebowitz, & M. I. Wykle (Eds.), *Handbook of mental health and aging* (2nd ed., pp. 793–813). San Diego, CA: Academic Press.

Glazier, R., & Kling, D. (2013). Recent trends in substance use among people with and without disabilities. *Disability and Health Journal*, *6*(2), 107–115. doi:10.1016/j.dhjo.2013.01.007

Grant, B. F., Harford, T. C., Dawson, D. A., Chou, P. S., & Pickering, R. P. (1994). Prevalence of *DSM-IV* alcohol abuse and dependence: United States, 1992. *Alcohol Health and Research World*, *18*, 243.

Greenwald, B. S., Kramer-Ginsberg, E., Bogerts, B., Ashtari, M., Aupperle, P., Wu, H., ... Patel, M. (1997). Qualitative magnetic resonance imaging findings in geriatric depression. Possible link between later-onset depression and Alzheimer's disease? *Psychological Medicine*, *27*, 421–431. doi:10.1017/s0033291796004576

Haight, B. K., Michel, Y., & Hendrix, S. (1998). Life review: Preventing despair in newly relocated nursing home residents' short- and long-term effects. *International Journal of Aging and Human Development*, *47*, 119–142. doi:10.2190/a011-brxd-hafv-5nj6

Hanson, M., & Guthiel, L. A. (2004). Motivational strategies with alcohol involved older adults: Implications for social work practice. *Social Work*, *49*(3), 364–372. doi:10.1093/sw/49.3.364

Helzer, J. E., Burnam, A., & McEvoy, L. T. (1991). Alcohol abuse and dependence. In L. N. Robins, & D. A. Regier (Eds.), *Psychiatric disorders in America: The epidemiologic catchment area study* (pp. 81–115). New York, NY: Free Press.

Illinois Rural Health Association. (2006). *Mental health in rural Illinois: Recovery is the goal: An analysis of mental health care in rural Illinois*. Springfield, IL: Author.

Jeste, D. V., & Palmer, B. (1998). Secondary psychoses: An overview. *Seminars in Clinical Neuro Psychiatry*, *3*, 2–3.

Kaplan, M. S., Adamek, M. E., & Martin, J. L. (2001). Confidence of primary care physicians in assessing the suicidality of geriatric patients. *International Journal of Geriatric Psychiatry*, *16*(7), 728–734. doi:10.1002/gps.420

Katon, W., Robinson, P., Von Korff, M., Lin, E., Bush, T., Ludman, E., ... Walker, E. (1996). A multifaceted intervention to improve treatment of depression in primary care. *Archives of General Psychiatry*, *53*, 924–932. doi:10.1001/archpsyc.1996.01830100072009

Katon, W., Von Korff, M., Lin, E., Unutzer, J., Simon, G., Walker, E., ... Bush, T. (1997). Population based care of depression: Effective disease management strategies to decrease prevalence. *General Hospital Psychiatry*, *19*, 169–178. doi:10.1016/s0163-8343(97)00016-9

Katz, I. R., & Parmelee, P. A. (1997). Overview. In R. L. Rubinstein & M. Lawton (Eds.), *Depression in long term and residential care* (pp. 1–28). New York, NY: Springer.

Klein, W. C., & Jess, C. (2002). One last pleasure? Alcohol use among elderly people in nursing homes. *Health and Social Work*, *27*(3), 193–203. doi:10.1093/hsw/27.3.193

Kofoed, L. L. (1984). Abuse and misuse of over-the-counter drugs by the elderly. In R. M. Atkinson (Ed.), *Alcohol and drug abuse in old age* (pp. 49–59). Washington, DC: American Psychiatric Press.

LaGreca, A. J., Akers, R. L., & Dwyer, J. W. (1988). Life events and alcohol behavior among older adults. *The Gerontologist*, *28*(4), 552–558. doi:10.1093/geront/28.4.552

Lambert, D., & Agger, M. S. (1995). Access of rural AFDC Medicaid beneficiaries to mental health services. *Health Care Financing Review*, *17*, 133–145.

Levkoff, S. E., Chen, H., Fisher, J. E., & McIntyre, J. S. (2006). *Evidence-based behavioral health practices for older adults: A guide to implementation*. New York, NY: Springer Publishing.

Liberto, J. G., Oslin, D. W., & Ruskin, P. E. (1992). Alcoholism in older persons: A review of the literature. *Hospital and Community Psychiatry*, *43*, 975–984. doi:10.1176/ps.43.10.975

Mackenzie, C. S., Gekoski, W. L., & Knox, V. J. (1999). Do family physicians treat older patients with mental disorders differently from younger patients? *Canadian Family Physician*, *45*, 124–129.

Manchikanti, L., Fellows, B., Ailinani, H., & Pampati, V. (2010). Therapeutic use, abuse, and nonmedical use of opioids: A ten-year perspective. *Pain Physician*, 13(5), 401–435.

Meeks, S., Carstensen, L. L., Stafford, P. B., Brenner, L. L., Weathers, F., Welch, R., & Oltmanns, T. F. (1990). Mental health needs of the chronically mentally ill elderly. *Psychology and Aging*, *5*, 163–171.

Meeks, S., & Murrell, S. A. (1997). Mental illness in late life: Socioeconomic conditions, psychiatric symptoms, and adjustment of long-term sufferers. *Psychology and Aging*, *12*, 296–308. doi:10.1037/0882-7974.12.2.296

Mehta, K. M., Yaffe, K., & Covinsky, K. E. (2002). Cognitive impairment, depressive symptoms, and functional decline in older people. *Journal of the American Geriatrics Society*, *50*(6), 1045–1050. doi:10.1046/j.1532-5415.2002.50259.x

Memmet, J. L. (2003). Alcohol consumption by elderly Americans. *Journal of Studies on Alcohol*, *64*(6), 884–892.

Miech, R., Johnston, L., O'Malley, P. M., Keyes, K. M., & Heard, K. (2015). Prescription Opioids in Adolescence and Future Opioid Misuse. *Pediatrics, 136*(5), e1169–e1177. doi:10.1542/peds.2015-1364.

Mueller, K., Kashinath, P., & Ullrich, F. (1997). Lengthening spells of "uninsurance" and their consequences. *Journal of Rural Health, 13*(1), 29–37. doi:10.1111/j.1748-0361.1997.tb00831.x

Musnick, M. A., Blazer, D. G., & Hays, J. C. (2000). Religious activity, alcohol use, and depression in a sample of elderly Baptists. *Research on Aging, 22*(2), 91–116.

National Health Interview Survey. (2000). Retrieved from http://www.cdc.gov/nchs/about/major/nhis/quest_data_related_1997_forward.htm

National Household Survey on Drug Abuse. (2000). Retrieved from http://www.health.org/govstudy/bkd405/

National Institute on Aging. (2000). *Senior health facts*. Retrieved from www.seniorhealth.gov

National Institute on Drug Abuse. (2015). *Drugs of Abuse: Opioids*. Bethesda, MD: National Institute on Drug Abuse. Retrieved from http://www.drugabuse.gov/drugs-abuse/opioids

National Institute on Drug Abuse. (2018). Misuse of prescription drugs. Retrieved from https://www.drugabuse.gov/publications/research-reports/misuse-prescription-drugs/what-scope-prescription-drug-misuse

New Freedom Commission on Mental Health. (2004). *Subcommittee on rural issues: Background paper*. (DHHS Pub. No. SMA-04–3890). Rockville, MD. U. S. Department of Health and Human Services.

Proctor, E. K., Morrow-Howell, N., Doré, P., Wentz, J., Rubin, E., Thompson, S., & Li, H. (2003). Comorbid medical conditions among depressed elderly patients discharged home after acute psychiatric care. *The American Journal of Geriatric Psychiatry, 11*(3), 329–338. doi:10.1176/appi.ajgp.11.3.329

Proctor, E. K., Morrow-Howell, N., Rubin, E., & Ringenberg, M. (1999). Service use by elderly patients after psychiatric hospitalization. *Psychiatric Services, 50*(4), 553–555. doi:10.1176/ps.50.4.553

Qato, D. M., Alexander, G. C., Conti, R. M., Johnson, M., Schumm, P., & Lindau, S. T. (2008). Use of prescription\ and over-the-counter medications and dietary supplements among older adults in the United States. *Journal of the American Medical Association, 300*(24), 2867. doi:10.1001/jama.2008.892.

Regier, D. A., Boyd, J. H., Burke, J. D. Jr., Rae, D. S., Myers, J. K., Kramer, M., ... Locke, B. Z. (1988). One-month prevalence of mental disorders in the United States. Based on five epidemiologic catchment area sites. *Archives of General Psychiatry, 45*, 977–986.

Regier, D. A., Farmer, M. E., Rae, D. S., Locke, B. Z., Keith, S. J., Judd, L. L., & Goodwin, F. K. (1990). Comorbidity of mental disorders with alcohol and other drug abuse. *Journal of the American Medical Association, 264*, 2511–2518. doi:10.1001/jama.264.19.2511

Regier, D. A., Goldberg, I. D., & Taube, C. A. (1978). The defacto U.S. mental health service system: A public health perspective. *Archives of General Psychiatry, 35*(6), 85–93.

Robinson, G. K. (1990). The psychiatric component of long-term care models. In B. S. Fogel, G. L. Gottlieb, & A. Furino (Eds.), *Mental health policy for older Americans: Protecting minds at risk* (pp. 157–178). Washington, DC: American Psychiatric Press.

Rogers, A., & Barusch, A. (2000). Mental health service utilization among frail, low income elders: Perceptions of home service providers and elders in the community. *Gerontological Social Work, 34*(2), 23–38. doi:10.1300/j083v34n02_04

Rowe, J. W., & Kahn, R. L. (1997). Successful aging. *Gerontologist, 37*, 433–440.

Rudd, R. A., Seth, P., David, F., & Scholl, L. (2016) Increases in drug and opioid-involved overdose deaths—United States, 2010–2015. *Morbidity & Mortality Weekly Report, 65*, 1445–1452. doi:10.15585/mmwr.mm655051e1

Sarkisian, C. A., Hays, R. D., Berry, S. H., & Mangione, C. M. (2001). Expectations regarding aging among older adults and physicians who care for older adults. *Medical Care, 39*(9), 1025–1036. doi:10.1097/00005650-200109000-00012

Schonfeld, L. (1993). Behavioral treatment of addictions. *Addictive Behaviors, 18*(2), 105–106.

Schulberg, H. C., Madonia, M. J., Block, M. R., Coulehan, J. L., Scott, C. P., Rodriguez, E., Black, A. (1995). Major depression in primary care practice: Clinical characteristics and treatment implications. *Psychosomatics, 36*, 129–137. doi:10.1016/s0033-3182(95)71682-6

Scott-Lennox, J. A., & George, L. (1996). Epidemiology of psychiatric disorders and mental health services use among older Americans. In B. L. Levin & J. Petrila (Eds.), *Mental health services: A public health perspective* (pp. 253–289). New York, NY: Oxford University Press.

Special Committee on Aging. (1987). *Medicare prescription drug issues: Report to the Chairman, Special Committee on Aging*. Washington, DC: General Accounting Office.

Steinhagen, K. A., & Friedman, M. B. (2008). Substance use and misuse in older adults. *Aging Well, 3*, 20. Retrieved from http://www.todaysgeriatricmedicine.com/archive/071708p20.shtml

Stolee, P., Kessler, L., & Le Clair, J. K. (1996). A community development and outreach program in geriatric mental health: Four years' experience. *Journal of the American Geriatrics Society*, *44*, 314–320. doi:10.1111/j.1532-5415.1996.tb00922.x

Substance Abuse and Mental Health Services Administration. (2015). *Results from the 2014 National Survey on Drug Use and Health: Detailed tables. 2015.* Retrieved from http://www.samhsa.gov/data/sites/default/files/NSDUH-DetTabs2014/NSDUHDetTabs2014.pdf

Substance Abuse and Mental Health Services Administration. (2017). Comprehensive Addiction and Recovery Act: Building communities of recovery. Retrieved from https://www.samhsa.gov/grants/grant-announcements/ti-17-015

Taube, C. A., Morlock, L., Burns, B., & Santos, A., B. (1990). New directions in research on assertive community treatment. *Psychiatric Services*, *41*, 642–647. doi:10.1176/ps.41.6.642

Temple, M. T., & Leino, E. V. (1989). Long-term outcomes of drinking: A 20-year longitudinal study of men. *British Journal of Addiction*, *84*, 889–899. doi:10.1111/j.1360-0443.1989.tb00761.x

U.S. Department of Health and Human Services. (1999). *Mental health and older adults. Chapter five appearing in report of the surgeon general on mental health needs.* Bethesda, MD: U.S. Government Printing Office.

U.S. Department of Health and Human Services. (2000). *NIA's strategic plan to address health disparities in aging: Fiscal Years 2000–2005.* Bethesda, MD: U.S. Government Printing Office.

U.S. Department of Health and Human Services. (2005). Featured program: The gatekeeper model, *e-Communication*, *1*(2). Retrieved from http://www.samhsa.gov/OlderAdultsTAC

U.S. Department of Health and Human Services. (2006a). Featured program: The mental health and aging systems integration initiative, *e-Communication*, *2*(1). Retrieved from http://www.samhsa.gov/OlderAdultsTAC/

U.S. Department of Health and Human Services. (2006b). Featured program: The Recovery Center, *e-Communication*, *2*(1). Retrieved from http://www.samhsa.gov/OlderAdultsTAC

U.S. Department of Health and Human Services, Centers for Disease Control and Prevention, National Center for Health Statistics. (2004). *National Health Interview Survey*. Hyattsville, MD: Author.

U.S. Department of Health and Human Services, National Center for Health Statistics. (2001). *Behavioral risk factor surveillance system*. Bethesda, MD: Government Printing Office.

U.S. Department of Health and Human Services, National Center for Health Statistics. (2004). *Behavioral risk factor surveillance system (BFRSS)*. Bethesda, MD: Government Printing Office.

Waters, E. (1995). Let's not wait till it's broke: Interventions to maintain and enhance mental health in late life. In M. Gatz (Ed.), *Emerging issues in the mental health and aging* (pp. 183–209). Washington, DC: American Psychological Association.

Webster, P. C. (2012). Oxycodone class action lawsuit filed. *Canadian Medical Association Journal*, *184*(7), E345–E346. doi:10.1503/cmaj.109-4158

Weiss, T. (2017). Addiction and substance use among people with disabilities. *Disabled World*. Retrieved from https://www.disabled-world.com/medical/pharmaceutical/addiction/serious.php

West, N. A., & Dart, R. C. (2015). Prescription opioid exposures and adverse outcomes among older adults. *Pharmacoepidemiology and Drug Saftey*, *25*, 539–544. doi:10.1002/pds.3934

Part III

Tools for Policy and Program Development

Part III of this text provides some tools for the reader to use to be more adequately equipped to prepare program initiatives that flow from policy appropriations. The tools also are designed to prepare the practitioner or reader with some skills to more effectively advocate for policy change. This section helps bridge some of the skills and tools used within the disciplines of social work, public health, gerontology, and rehabilitation to begin to expand the boundaries of public policy development. Within this section of the book, Chapter 15 exposes the reader to health promotion frameworks, while Chapter 16 examines how media strategies impact public policy development. Chapter 17 relates to coalitions and coalition building, while Chapter 18 addresses needs assessments. Chapter 19 brings the tools together and attempts to facilitate using the tools to reach one's vision for policy change and program development.

15

Health Behavior Models and Health Promotion Frameworks

LEARNING OBJECTIVES

At the end of this chapter, readers will:

1. *Understand the relationship between health behavior models, health promotion frameworks, and success in program planning initiatives.*
2. *Understand specific components of health promotion models (Health Belief Model, Stages of Change Model, and Theory of Reasoned Action).*
3. *Understand how the integration of health promotion models can benefit programs and services for people growing older and/or people with disabilities.*

Erica and Theresa have now reviewed the demographics of communities, examined trends that impact aging and disability policies, reviewed databases to help understand the landscape of aging and disability statistics, and reviewed a range of policies that impact older adults. Throughout their investigation, they have tried to analyze why some people are more successful in changing their trajectory while others are not. They also have tried to analyze why some policies are effective while others are not effective in reaching the intended population. As they brainstormed, they realized that some policies do not take into consideration what motives and drives people to act or pursue action. Consequently, they decided that they need to have a stronger grasp of health behaviors and health promotion frameworks that impact the behaviors of people. This understanding will help build policies and programs that can truly meet individual needs. Through their discussions with consumers such as Betty, Angela, Joseph, and Ida, they were able to identify three specific theoretical frameworks that could be used to guide policies and programs for people growing older and people with disabilities.

***Betty**: Betty recently celebrated her 95th birthday, and lives in her own home in rural California in a small town known as Grimes, which boasts a population of 375 people. Betty still drives her own car although she does not pursue night driving anymore because of her macular degeneration. She has chickens on her property and barters eggs for other goods such*

(continued)

(continued)

as milk and yard chores. Betty is very careful about eating foods that are not processed and do not contain many preservatives. She believes that the secret to her long life has been that she cares for herself in the most holistic way possible. She believes that she is susceptible to many diseases because of the medical advice she has received through the years.

Angela and Joseph: *Angela (83) and Joseph (86) are currently living in Houston, Texas; however, they have worked in many corners of the world as a result of Joseph's distinguished career in the Air Force. Upon retirement from the Air Force, Joseph joined the National Aeronautics and Space Administration (NASA) and worked as an aeronautical engineer until his retirement at 69 years of age. Angela stayed at home while their three children were in school and then worked as a clerk at a local jewelry store. Angela credits their longevity and strong health outcomes to her approach toward planning, which includes thinking about the issue or problem at hand, helping her partner see this as a viable concern (even if he had never thought about it as being an issue in the past); planning, getting involved through some program or initiative, evaluating the strategies that she and Joseph have used, and revising or ending the strategies or techniques that they have used. Angela prides herself on having used these strategies for many years.*

Ida: *Ida, a resident of a Medicaid-funded long-term care facility in Denton, Texas, has lived with symptoms of multiple sclerosis since she was 52 years of age. Now 80 years of age, Ida is a widow, and her stepchildren look after her needs. Her stepchildren are spread throughout the Dallas area, and her daughter June and four grandchildren reside in Washington state. Despite her disability, she has been successful in remaining active until her 77th birthday. When asked what her secret to success was, she indicated that she always worried about being susceptible to her multiple sclerosis, understood the seriousness of the disability, and always tried to compensate for her inability to function with "cues to action" or focus on a specific strategy to help her with performance.*

WHAT ARE HEALTH PROMOTION FRAMEWORKS?

A vital tool in the development and design of programs and services for older adults should include health promotion frameworks or at least some features of these behavioral intervention models. The focus in this chapter is to explore health promotion frameworks, to showcase their role vis-à-vis health policy and programs, and to discuss three specific frameworks. Health promotion frameworks are theoretical conceptions of how health behavior can be addressed. These frameworks are conceived for the purpose of program and policy development. The health promotion frameworks discussed in this chapter are the Health Belief Model (HBM), the Theory of Reasoned Action, the Transtheoretical Model of Stages of Change.

HEALTH PROMOTION FRAMEWORKS AND HEALTH POLICY

The use of health promotions frameworks leads to three specific questions that play a role in the development of health policy: (a) what role do health promotion frameworks play in the development of health policy? (b) how are health promotion frameworks utilized in the health policy arena? and (c) what role does health promotion play in public policy and program development? This chapter addresses these three questions; however, prior to discussing these questions and answers, it is essential to understand some well-known health promotion frameworks. Although a number of health promotion frameworks exist in the literature (Glanz, Lewis, & Rimer, 1997), this chapter focuses on three that can be specifically applied to older adults.

The Health Belief Model

The HBM was originally conceptualized in the 1950s by social psychologists in an effort to understand why people did not use services for preventative or detection purposes. Although public health efforts in the 1950s evolved to provide for immunizations at no or little cost to the consumer, few people made use of these services. Thus, the question became apparent that there must be some reason why services were not being utilized, and understanding people's perception of their susceptibility to infectious diseases might be a key to improve utilization (Rosenstock, 1966). As the model evolved, it was used to help understand people's responses to symptoms (Kirscht, 1974) and compliance with medical regimens (Becker, 1974). See Figure 15.1.

The HBM was originally developed to provide a systematic approach or method to understand and predict one's behavior relative to preventative strategies. The initial model focused upon the relationships between health behaviors, health practices, and the use of healthcare services. As time progressed, the HBM was updated to include health motivation, which led to an understanding of the distinction between illness and sick-role behavior from health behavior. This theory has also been labeled as the genesis of systematic, theory-based research in health behavior. The HBM tries to predict health-related behavior through an understanding of specific "beliefs" one holds. The model is used in explaining and predicting preventive health behavior, as well as outlining responses to sick-role and illness behavior. People's motivation to act in specific ways when it comes to their health behavior can be categorized into three main arenas: individual perceptions, modifying behaviors, and likelihood of action. Individual perceptions are factors that affect the perception of illness or disease; they deal with the importance of health to the individual, perceived susceptibility, and perceived severity. Modifying factors include demographic variables, perceived threat, and cues to action. The likelihood of action discusses factors in the probability of appropriate health behavior; it is the likelihood of taking the recommended preventive health action. The HBM also suggests that the perception of one's personal health behavior and threats to one's behaviors is influenced by at least three specific factors: (a) one's general health values, which include one's interests

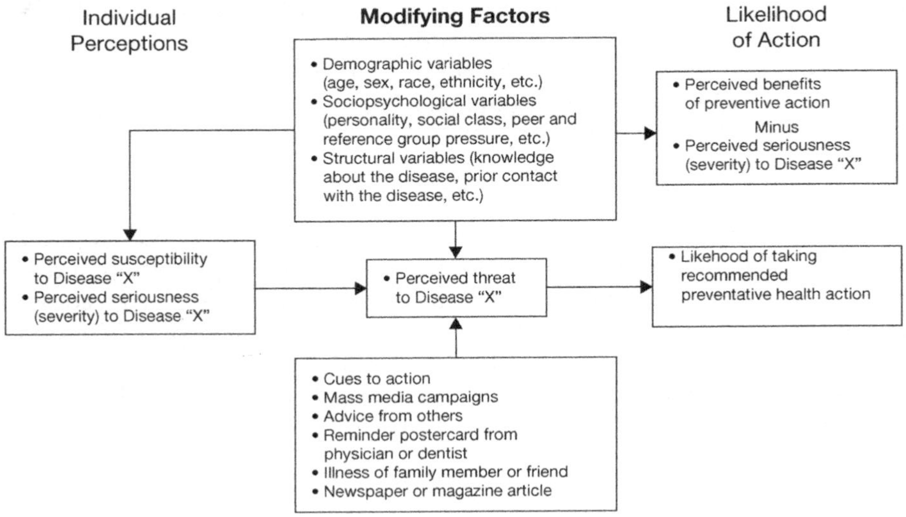

Figure 15.1 The Health Belief Model.

Source: Based on Rosenstock, I. M., Strecher, V. J., & Becker, M. H. (1988). Social learning theory and the Health Belief Model. *Health Education Quarterly*, *15*(2), 175–183. doi:10.1177/109019818801500203

and concern about one's own health; (b) specific health beliefs about vulnerability to a particular health threat; and (c) one's beliefs about the consequences of a specific health issue or diagnosis. Once an individual perceives a threat to his or her health and is simultaneously cued to action, and that person's perceived benefits outweigh his or her perceived barriers, then that individual is most likely to undertake the recommended preventive health action. Some variables (demographic, sociopsychological, and structural) can influence an individual's decision.

The components of the HBM include components identified by the authors as "perceived susceptibility," "perceived severity," "perceived benefits," "perceived barriers," "cues to action," and "self-efficacy." Understanding what these components mean, and how they interface with each other to explain one's behavior toward one's own health, can help program planners and practitioners to better plan and utilize healthcare resources.

Perceived Susceptibility

The authors of the HBM and its reiterations (Rosenstock, 1966; Rosenstock & Kirscht, 1984) define *perceived susceptibility* as one's perception of the likelihood of receiving the disease or the condition. In the application of this concept, it is important to consider the target population, define the population, and examine its at-risk levels. In addition, one may identify risk based upon the person's characteristics or behaviors. Each person has his or her own perception of the likelihood of experiencing a condition that would adversely affect his or her health and well-being. People's reaction to their perception of susceptibility to a disease or condition varies considerably. At one extreme are people who deny the possibility of contracting an adverse condition, while on the other end are people who are very obsessed with the possibility that they can be adversely affected by a given disease. People who are moderately susceptible seem to think that there is some chance of being affected by a specific disease or condition.

Perceived Severity

One's perceived severity refers to one's understanding of what the potential effects a given disease or condition would have on one's lifestyle and the consequences of the effects. These effects can be considered from the point of view of the difficulties that a disease would create. Examples are pain and discomfort, loss of work time, financial burdens, difficulties with family relationships, and susceptibility to future conditions. It is important to include these emotional and financial burdens when considering the seriousness of a disease or condition.

Perceived Benefits

Taking action toward the prevention of disease or toward dealing with an illness is the next step to expect after an individual has accepted the susceptibility of a disease and recognized it is serious. One's perception of the impact (or efficacy) that an advised action will have in an effort to reduce the risks or seriousness of the impact will dramatically affect one's perceived benefits. In an effort to identify perceived benefits, one should define the actions to be taken, how should they be taken, when should they be taken, and what positive effects can be expected.

Perceived Barriers

Action may not take place, even though an individual may believe that the benefits to taking action are effective. This behavior may be due to barriers. Barriers relate to the idea that a treatment or preventive measure may be inconvenient, expensive, unpleasant, painful, or upsetting. These ideas may lead a person away from taking the desired action.

Perceived barriers can also include one's opinion of the tangible and psychological costs associated with the actions or treatments advised. These barriers can be reduced through reassurance, correcting misconceptions or misinformation, developing incentives to action, and providing assistance to assure actions.

Cues to Action

Cues to action related to an individual's perception of the levels of susceptibility and seriousness provide the force to act. Benefits (minus barriers) provide the path of action. However, a cue to action may be required for the desired behavior to occur. These cues may be internal or external. These cues are strategies used to activate one's readiness. Cues can include providing information on how-to, creating awareness, and using reminder systems. A common example is refrigerator magnets with reminders to get a flu shot.

Self-Efficacy

Self-efficacy relates to confidence in one's ability to take action. In the self-efficacy phase, one accepts training and guidance in performing actions that lead to personal empowerment and control. In this stage, progressive goal setting is used. Coaching (verbal reinforcements), role modeling (demonstrating desired behaviors), and reducing anxiety are all components of this phase. This phase of the HBM was an addition, modeled from the work of Bandura, based on social learning theory (Bandura, 1977, 1982). Table 15.1 summarizes these components.

How Does This Model Apply to Health Policy, Program Planning, and Older Adults and People With Disabilities?

Essentially, the development of programs and resources, keeping in mind the mind-set of the specific target group of older adults one would like to reach can only enhance the benefit of any programs developed for older adults. A clear understanding of older adults' perceived benefits and barriers to action can make a striking difference in their compliance with specific regimes. For example, if an older adult perceives being susceptible to catching the flu, individual may be more likely to pursue seeking a vaccination against influenza. However, in other areas of health behavior that may be more taboo,

Table 15.1 Components of the Health Belief Model

Component	Definition
Perceived susceptibility	One's perception of how likely he or she is to contract a disease or condition
Perceived severity	The seriousness of a disease or event/condition to oneself
Perceived benefits	The benefits one sees in pursuing a specific intervention
Perceived barriers	Blocks that impede involvement for older adults (e.g., transportation or lack of insurance coverage) could be perceived barriers
Cues to action	Reminders that influence one's ability to comply
Self-efficacy	One's confidence in one's own ability to follow through

for example, sexual behaviors, an older adult may be less likely to feel susceptible or may have a wider range of barriers. HIV/AIDS awareness and protection is an illustrative example here. An older adult, recently widowed, new to the dating scene, may not feel at risk for sexually transmitted diseases (STDs) or consider protective measures against STDs because that individual may not perceive him- or herself to be of reproductive age. Consequently, these factors may play a role in one's overall willingness to exercise caution or take action against STDs.

Investing in Meaningful Health Interventions

Interventions are often embarked upon with great vigor, and often little foresight or planning from a theoretical perspective. Unfortunately, this approach leads to a diluted and limited impact when programs or interventions are developed. The HBM can be used as a guide to identify consumers' perspectives and enable the development of programs/resources to best utilize the resources invested in a program or intervention. A clear understanding, for example, of the specific benefits and barriers older adults may have to seeking help or engaging in a specific program can be very useful and helpful in the planning of the program and marketing of the program or intervention. Focus group approaches or community needs assessments can be very helpful in this process of identifying specific barriers and benefits.

The Theory of Reasoned Action

The Theory of Reasoned Action (TRA) and its companion Theory of Planned Behavior (TPB; Fishbein & Ajzen, 1975) have both come from studying human behavior and attempting to develop meaningful interventions to address such behaviors. The goal behind this theory is threefold: (a) to predict and understand motivational influences on behavior that is not under the individual's control; (b) to identify how and where to target strategies for changing behavior; and (c) to explain human behavior. This theory also assumes that human beings are rational, make systematic use of information given to them, and consider the implications of their decisions and actions before they decide to engage or not engage in certain activity.

The TRA framework is concerned with a person's motivation as a determinant of the likelihood for performing a specific behavior. The most important determinants of behaviors are behavioral intentions. Attitudes are determined by an individual's perception about outcomes of one's actions as a result of one's evaluation of this outcome or attribute. One's evaluation of the outcome or impact of taking action can seriously have some bearing on one's intentions toward taking some action. These intentions are also evaluated based upon the norms of one's culture and peer group and these two entities' influence on the person.

The components of TRA include behavioral beliefs, an evaluation of behavioral outcomes, attitude toward behavior, normative beliefs, subjective norms, the motivation to comply, behavioral intentions, and behavior. Behavioral intention refers to the perceived likelihood of performing the behavior.

One's attitude is influenced by both behavioral belief and one's subjective evaluation. The behavioral belief refers to the belief that one's actions or behaviors are associated with certain attributes or outcomes. One's subjective evaluation relates to the values one attaches to a behavioral outcome or attribute.

Subjective normative beliefs refer to the belief about whether there is approval or disapproval (acceptance level) for specific behaviors. The motivation to comply is the belief that one is motivated to do what a referent thinks.

Perceived behavioral control refers to the belief about one's sense of control that relates to the likelihood of the condition happening and its associated condition. One who does not perceive being impacted by a situation or condition may not pursue any action. Perceived power relates to how much power one has insofar as that individual can impact change or undergo behavior to pursue a specific action or task. Hence, the question one must consider is going to be, "What is the effect of each condition in making behavioral performance difficult or easy?"

The application of this TRA to health and help-seeking with older adults can be illustrated through two examples: mammography screening and Latino elders seeking mental healthcare (Godin & Kok, 1996). Although both sets of procedures may be necessary, they may not necessarily be used by older adults if the social support network does not perceive these as of value, does not see the benefits, and does not feel able to control the outcomes or results once results are presented.

Limitations to this model are several. This model does not take into consideration factors such as personality or basic demographic variables (Ajzen, 1998). Perceived behavioral control is also a variable that is difficult to measure and thus is difficult to ascertain or get a handle on. The theory is also based upon an assumption that human beings are rational, and they make systematic decisions based upon available information (Ajzen, 1980). Unconscious motives are not considered, and issues that may undermine rational behavior for older adults (such as dementia or early onset of Alzheimer's disease) may influence one's rational behavior.

Transtheoretical Model and Stages of Change Theory

This theory integrates stages of change into the processes and principles of change. It integrates the components from theories of psychotherapy and behavior changes. This model helps assess the readiness of individuals to follow through with interventions, which becomes critical when assessing where to invest health resources in order to maximize the impact of the investment. The stages of change actually run along a continuum from precontemplation to termination and follow-up, as illustrated in Figure 15.2.

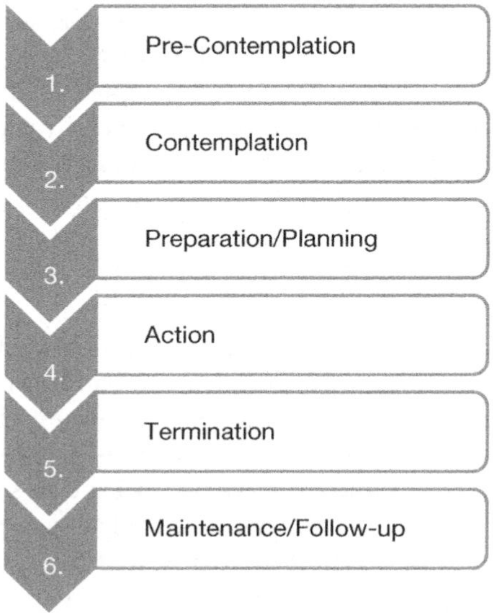

Figure 15.2 A model illustrating the stages of Change continuum.

Processes of Change

Each stage of change within this model provides for different stages along a continuum toward success and activation of new behaviors. The process of change may focus on one or several components of a model, and each stage will be utilized to facilitate change (Prochaska & Velicer, 1997). The individual stages are often components of health education or health interventions, shaped by specific health policies (Prochaska & DiClemente, 1983). This section provides an overview of the stages and the specific behavioral components and changes that can be expected at each stage. See Table 15.2.

Precontemplation and Contemplation Stages

These stages can be characterized as moving from unawareness to a consciousness-raising stage. At these stages, although an individual may have a specific problem or issue, whether it is recognized or acknowledged or not, the individual literally has no intention of changing behavior. The intervention strategies used during these stages focus on consciousness raising, dramatic relief, self-evaluation and self-reevaluation, and environmental reevaluation. In the process of consciousness raising, the goal is to provide information to target one's knowledge base. Advertisements and billboard campaigns often address the contemplation step. In the process of dramatic relief, role playing is often used as an intervention strategy, with the goal of creating awareness and insight into the problem. The process of environmental reevaluation examines how a problem affects one's physical environment. In the case of older adults, a falls prevention program may target not only creating an awareness for older adults, but the fact that one's frailty and need for additional support may be taxing on furniture in the absence of grab bars or aids for walking (cane or walker).

During the contemplation stage, an individual may recognize the problem and may actually be seriously thinking about changing relevant behavior. This stage is marked by an individual's self-evaluation and reflection. During this phase, some serious thought goes into changes that can be made, and there is recognition of a problem.

Preparation Stage

During the preparation stage, an individual recognizes the problem and has an intention to change behavior within the next month. Behavioral changes may occur but may not be consistent. This stage is also marked with some specific attempts to plan activities to put one's affairs in order, to be able to pursue a change effort plan consistently. An older adult may be contemplating attending a meal support program or nutrition site. Part of the planning process may include transportation or some assurance that handicapped accessible parking is available.

Action and Maintenance Stages

In the action and maintenance stages, an individual has demonstrated a consistent behavior change; however, the length of time for which this behavior change has been consistent will determine which stage the individual is actually engaged in. If the behavior change is consistent for 6 months or less, then the individual is considered to be in the action phase, as compared to the maintenance phase, in which one's behavior can be consistent for 6 months or more. Within this phase, an individual or group engages in specific action plans. The role of a program or facilitator during this phase is to assist with feedback, problem solving, social support, and reinforcement. During the maintenance phase of the plan, one may see assistance with coping strategies, reinforcements for prolonged behavior, seeking out alternatives, and strategies to avoid relapses. Helping relationships at this phase are focused on contingencies and reward, as well as stimulus and controls. Reminder messages or cues to action can be built into this phase, to help promote changes. Some examples may include reminder notices for checkups or check lists that summarize several of the healthy behaviors originally undertaken.

Termination Stage/Follow-Up

During the termination stage, social liberation is achieved, and the individual moves from an approach of being on the recipient end for services to becoming more of a peer helper, interested in sharing some of his or her own successes with others. In this stage, one can characterize an increase in social opportunities or alternatives, especially for those who are relatively deprived or oppressed. Empowerment approaches, policy development, and advocacy efforts can improve and increase opportunities for health promotion efforts for minority elders and those traditionally impoverished or ignored. Some of the same strategies can be implemented to help all people with change efforts, such as smoke-free zones, and healthy food choices.

Application of the Transtheoretical Model

The Transtheoretical Model offers promise for the development and implementation of specific interventions, particularly within the area of recruitment of subjects, retention of subjects, progress of individuals, the process of developing interventions, and outcomes.

Recruitment of a population using this model can yield high rates of participation. Since the model is structured so that people move through a process, based upon their

Table 15.2 Components of the Stages of Change Model

Concept	Definition	Application
Precontemplation	Unaware of the problem. Has not thought about change	Increase awareness. Identify need for change, tailor info to address risks and benefits
Contemplation	Thinking about change	Encourage specific plans
Preparation/ Planning	Develop a plan for change. Set gradual goals	Assist in the development of concrete action or plan for change
Action	Implementation of specific action plans	Provide feedback. Help with social support, reinforcement, and problem-solving skills
Maintenance	Continue desired actions. Repeat periodic recommended steps	Help with coping, give reminders, find alternatives, avoid relapses
Termination/ Follow-Up	Finalize intervention Or refer to other resources	Assist with strategies to maintain new behavior without direct intervention

readiness to change, the model can target participants at a range of stages, rather than simply those most prepared or ready for a commitment to action. Since this model makes no assumptions about people's readiness for change and assumes people will be at different levels, this model will engage many individuals with differing levels of participation.

Retention rates are another major positive consideration that can be seen with this model. Traditional programs quickly realize a mismatch between the program delivery or polices undergirding programs. If a program does not meet an individual's needs, or the individual is not ready to pursue change, he or she may quickly tire and drop out. In contrast, this model is designed to meet specific stages of change and needs of individuals; thus, people are less likely to drop out and more likely to remain within a specific stage until they are ready to move forward.

Another advantage of building programs or services around this framework is the notion of progress, which can be recognized much more readily and easily among individuals through the process of breaking down intervention strategies using the transtheoretical approach to program development (Prochaska, 1994). Unfortunately, most action-oriented programs identify a single outcome or set of outcomes that define success. Someone who fails to meet these criteria also fails to meet success. Conversely, when people, especially older adults, are grappling with the notion of making change, they may not easily or readily see success, when it is defined as an outcome maintained for 6 months or longer. The Transtheoretical Model offers the opportunity for measures to be collected, keeping in mind a full range of cognitive, emotional, and behavioral steps, which may take place through incremental stages, and much more slowly than moving directly to the ideal or desirable goal (Prochaska, Velicer, DiClemente, & Fava, 1988). Addiction or smoking-cessation programs have effectively integrated this model to help target where individuals or group interventions should begin (DiClemente, 1981, 1986; DiClemente et al., 1991). This approach works well with people growing older or people with disabilities, because one can experience success in the attainment of a new stage, rather than reaching a final goal.

Programs or interventions using these stages can be effective, especially if they take into consideration specific stages and develop materials or interventions accordingly (Prochaska, DiClemente, Velicer, Ginpil, & Norcross, 1985). For example, educational materials and psychoeducational programs can best be developed to target the various stages from precontemplation to action using this model. Incorporating this approach also reframes the notion of success; that is, rather than recognizing success based on the successful completion of new skills or mastering one's goals, one may recognize success if there has been movement from one stage to another, such as precontemplation to action (Prochaska & Velicer, 1997).

IMPLICATIONS OF THE HEALTH PROMOTION MODELS AND PROGRAM DEVELOPMENT FOR AGING AND DISABILITY-RELATED PROGRAMS AND SERVICES

The use of health promotion frameworks in the program planning process for older adults can have a number of positive outcomes, some of which are showcased in this chapter. Capturing health beliefs can enable program planners to tailor interventions and programs to meet the needs of different education levels or groups with ethnic variation. Another strength of using the models, especially a model such as Prochaska and DiClemente's (1983) Stages of Change Model, can relate to resources. If a program has a fixed amount of funding or resources, breaking down the stage and strategy to meet the needs of a specific change in a target group can have strong implications for success of a program and maximize the use of one's resources. Finally, in a climate with finite and limited resources, these models can be helpful in the process of defining and targeting effective strategies for service intervention and program delivery.

SUMMARY

The HBM, TRA, and Stages of Change are only three health promotion models used to help shape and understand health behavior. The models are vital to the development of aging policy, policy for people with disabilities, and programs and services for these target groups and interventions because models help practitioners stage interventions based upon the specific needs of a community or target group. They will become increasingly important and of value as we implement the legislative amendments to the Older Americans Act of 2006, which calls for health promotion and screening efforts within public health and mental health arenas.

ADDITIONAL RESOURCES

Websites

The National Commission for Health Education Credentialing: www.nchec.org

This is the official website for the National Commission for Health Education Credentialing and provides background on the responsibilities and competencies required of health educators. The competencies include assessing the individual and community needs for health education; planning effective health education programs; implementing health education programs; evaluating the effectiveness of health education programs; coordinating the provision of health education services; and acting as a resource person for health education and communicating health and health education needs, concerns, and resources. This site also provides information on how to become a certified health education specialist (CHES).

The American Journal of Health Behavior: www.ajhb.org

This site provides direct access to the *American Journal of Health Behavior*, which serves as the office publication of the American Academy of Health Behavior. The journal strives to improve the approach of health education, health promotion, and other multidisciplinary efforts through improving our understanding of systems approaches to health behaviors.

The Communication Initiative: www.comminit.com

This website provides a host of information that can assist the novice or inexperienced health educator to understand both health education and health education change strategies. The website also has links to various organizations worldwide that support health and education efforts both nationally and internationally. The site also deals with various change theories.

The American Public Health Association (APHA)/Health Education Special Interest Group: www.apha.org

This site provides access to APHA's special interest group, which addresses health education and health promotion concerns.

YouTube Videos

The HBM: www.youtube.com/watch?v=5uUhTgtsIsc

This YouTube Video reviews the HBM, its history, and its component parts. It is an excellent way for the viewer to easily understand the component parts of the model.

Changing Behaviors and Realizing Behavior Change: www.youtube.com/watch?v=AdKUJxjn-R8

This TED Talk helps the reader understand the concepts related to the Stages of Change Model. This easy-to-understand approach helps the reader put a theoretical framework into an easily understood framework.

DISCUSSION QUESTIONS

1. Consider the cases introduced at the beginning of this chapter. How would you utilize the Health Belief Model (HBM) to develop a health promotion framework and address the concerns presented in these cases?
2. Considering the cases presented at the outset of this chapter, how would you address building a health promotion message utilizing the Stages of Change framework?
3. What do you think the advantages and disadvantages of using a theoretical framework to build policies and programs would be?
4. How can you and your team utilize these frameworks to build healthy public policies for people growing older and older adults?

REFERENCES

Ajzen, I. (1980). *Understanding the attitudes and predicting social behavior*. Englewood Cliffs, NJ: Prentice Hall.

Ajzen, I. (1998). *Attitudes, personality and behavior*. Chicago, IL: The Dorsey Press.

Bandura, A. (1977). Self-efficacy: Toward a unifying theory of behavior change. *Psychological Review*, *84*, 191–215. doi:10.1037//0033-295x.84.2.191

Bandura, A. (1982). Self-efficacy mechanism in human agency. *American Psychologist*, *37*, 122–147. doi:10.1037//0003-066x.37.2.122

Becker, M. H. (1974). The Health Belief Model and personal health behavior. *Health Education Monographs*, *2*, 324–473.

DiClemente, C. C. (1981). Self-efficacy and smoking cessation maintenance: A preliminary report. *Cognitive Therapy and Research*, *5*, 175–187. doi:10.1007/bf01172525

DiClemente, C. C. (1986). Self-efficacy and the addictive behaviors. *Journal of Social and Clinical Psychology*, *4*, 302–315. doi:10.1521/jscp.1986.4.3.302

DiClemente, C. C., Prochaska, J. O., Fairhurst, S., Velicer, W. F., Rossi, J. S., & Velasquez, M. (1991). The process of smoking cessation: An analysis of precontemplation, contemplation and contemplation/action. *Journal of Consulting and Clinical Psychology*, *59*, 295–304.

Fishbein, M., & Ajzen, I. (1975). *Beliefs, attitudes, intention and behavior: An introduction to theory and research*. Reading, MA: Addison-Wesley.

Glanz, K., Lewis, F. M., & Rimer, B. K. (Eds.). (1997). *Health behavior and health education: Theory, research and practice*. San Francisco, CA: Jossey-Bass.

Godin, G., & Kok, G. (1996). The theory of planned behavior: A review of its applications to health-related behaviors. *American Journal of Health Promotion*, *11*(2), 87–98. doi:10.4278/0890-1171-11.2.87

Kirscht, J. P. (1974). The Health Belief Model and illness behavior. *Health Education Monographs, 2*, 387–408. doi:10.1177/109019817400200406

Prochaska, J. O. (1994). Strong and weak principles for progressing from precontemplation to action on the basis of twelve problem behaviors. *Health Psychology, 13*, 47–51. doi:10.1037//0278-6133.13.1.47

Prochaska, J. O., & DiClemente, C. C. (1983). Stages and processes of self-change of smoking: Toward an integrative model of change. *Journal of Consulting and Clinical Psychology, 51*, 390–395. doi:10.1037//0022-006x.51.3.390

Prochaska, J. O., DiClemente, C. C., Velicer, W. F., Ginpil, S., & Norcross, J. C. (1985). Predicting change in status for self-changers. *Addictive Behaviors, 10*, 395–406. doi:10.1016/0306-4603(85)90036-x

Prochaska, J. O., & Velicer, W. F. (1997). The Transtheoretical Model of health behavior change. *American Journal of Health Promotion, 12*, 38–48. doi:10.4278/0890-1171-12.1.38

Prochaska, J. O., Velicer, W. F., DiClemente, C. C., & Fava, J. L. (1988). Measuring the processes of change: Applications to the cessation of smoking. *Journal of Consulting and Clinical Psychology, 56*, 520–528. doi:10.1037//0022-006x.56.4.520

Rosenstock, I. M. (1966). Why people use health services. *Milbank Memorial Fund Quarterly, 44*, 94–124.

Rosenstock, I. M., & Kirscht, J. P. (1984). The Health Belief Model and personal health behavior. *Health Education Monographs, 2*, 470–473.

Rosenstock, I. M., Strecher, V. J., & Becker, M. H. (1988). Social learning theory and the Health Belief Model. *Health Education Quarterly, 15*(2), 175–183. doi:10.1177/109019818801500203

16

Media, Social Media, and Advocacy Strategies for Change

LEARNING OBJECTIVES

At the end of the chapter, readers will:

1. *Understand various strategies for policy advocacy through the use of the media.*
2. *Become familiar with social media strategies that can impact policy and program development within the aging and disability arenas.*
3. *Articulate strategies for advocacy through media artifacts.*

Erica and Theresa have found themselves buried deep into materials which will be helpful for their eventual blueprint for programs and services. After much deliberation, they decided that they would like to share their information with the public for a couple of reasons. First, information and promotion of the information would be helpful to people in efforts to education the general public on the status of policies, programs, and services. Second, reaching out to the target population can be helpful to rally support for public advocacy. As they pondered how to approach this issue, they realized that they needed to consider the demographic and target group (i.e., people advancing in age or people with disabilities) whom they wanted to reach and identify a range of media advocacy strategies. This chapter unfolds many of the strategies and approaches that Erica and Theresa decided to pursue.

ADVOCACY AND ITS ROLE IN PROGRAM AND POLICY DEVELOPMENT

Public advocacy has been at the heart and soul of policy development in aging services (Hudson, 2004). This advocacy effort has targeted social development and social change in efforts to develop and broaden the face of social policy over the past several decades. Initially, when policy development strategies were in the process of enactment, the advocacy forces driving policy development were elite groups working within governmental systems (e.g., policy advisors drafting the Social Security Act of 1935). Over time, an "interest group" era arose within the aging arena, and in the 1960s a proliferation of aging-oriented interest groups arose. These advocates were effective in shepherding legislation such as Medicare and the Older Americans Act of 1965. Groups such as the National Council of Senior Citizens, the National Association of Social Workers (NASW), and the National Association of Retired Federal Employees were all instrumental in developing policy and legislative changes. Further evolution of the policy advocacy arena included older adults and consumers themselves in this process. As advocacy organizations evolved, it also seemed to be prudent to include older adults as a component of the advocacy equation. Older adults, or consumers themselves, add credence to the importance of legislative efforts and the reasons for the development of new or revised policies or programs.

Within the efforts of advocacy for program and policy development, a number of initiatives are used to facilitate the advocacy process. Within Part III of this text, tools for advocacy development are discussed; this chapter deals with one subset of these strategies, namely using media as a part of the advocacy process.

Advocacy efforts count, and who better to consider developing and voicing these efforts than individuals who have expertise in the field of aging and have professional credentials (Coalition of National Health Education Organization Partners, n.d.). Advocacy efforts do not have to be time-intensive, for 1 minute can lead to a message to a legislator, 5 minutes can lead to photocopying and sharing an article with a colleague or legislator, and 10 minutes can generate enough time to send an email, fax, or letter to a legislator. Therefore, it may be helpful to gain some skills and expertise with the use of media strategies to develop advocacy efforts.

A number of successful efforts to improve health status or change health policy have been targeted using media advocacy strategies. Media advocacy and communications strategies have been effective in reducing health disparities through health communications or changing public perception on key health policy issues (Dorfman, 2005 Freimuth & Quinn, 2004). Effective media campaigns and the use of visual tools such as photography have been the key to success in public education and action on major issues such as the anthrax scare in 2001 or HIV/AIDS awareness (Bernhardt, 2004; Moore, 2004). Mueller, Page, and Kuerbis (2004) have analyzed how communication through media sources has influenced U.S. Congressional hearings and have concluded that communication of information strategies and media advocacy has been the single most influential force in the development of policy for social movement issues.

Health education campaigns have been found to be successful in the development of health policy or program development, and researchers have found that mass media campaigns have also influenced the changing of health behaviors (Cavill & Bauman, 2004; Randolph & Viswanth, 2004). Integrating a theoretical background into the development of health promotion messages and targeting the messages to a specific stage of behavioral change or mastery increases the chances of health promotion and media advocacy campaign efforts being effective. Changes in knowledge and attitudes have been possible in behavioral change campaigns through advocacy efforts.

One can draw from the field of health education, where health educators have developed a number of competencies revolving around the use of advocacy to advance health and health education efforts. Within their credentialing body, the National Commission for Health Education Credentialing, a framework for competencies have been developed. This "Competency-Based Framework for Graduate Level Health Educators," developed in 1999, lays out a number of competencies required for advocacy to advance the profession, and several can be borrowed by the aging profession. These include the use of a variety of methods and techniques to provide information through oral and written presentations and culturally sensitive methods and techniques, and exercise of organizational leadership through strategies to influence public policy. It is within this framework that we develop the use of media advocacy to educate on a specific topic of interest and attempt to advance policy and program development initiatives.

THE USE OF MEDIA ADVOCACY

What Is Media Advocacy?

Media advocacy is the strategic use of any form of media to help advance an organization's objectives or goals. In this context, media is a tool—not an end in itself, but a means to an end. Most health and human service professions, including social work and public health, have not taken advantage of media strategies for public education. Conversely, journalism and media specialists have not taken social welfare and health concerns under their wing for the promotion of health-related issues (American Public Health Association [APHA], 2008). Through media advocacy, one can frame issues and showcase their importance for the community.

Media advocacy explores a number of key issues and serves to present strategies that can be helpful in the development of innovative human service opportunities and educate the general public. Media advocacy can change both public perception and perception of key stakeholders, elite power, or key individuals within communities that impact policy or program-related issues for community development or community-based problems.

Media advocacy can be used to create a reliable, consistent stream of publicity or media focus for one's agency's issues and activities. It takes a focused approach to explain very specifically how targeted social problems or issues could and should be solved. Consequently, such a targeted approach will motivate community members and policy makers to step up to the plate and help with community change or endorse change efforts.

The National Council on Aging (2018) provides an Advocacy Toolkit outlining how the media can be used to inform, recast, encourage, and promote public policy that impacts older adults, When advocating through the media, problems or issues can be recast or reframed so that they affect all people, and not just a distinct group of individuals. Once problems are reframed, media strategies can be used to encourage community members, voluntary organizations, community leaders, and the faith-based community to find out more about problems or issues for older adults and establish some engagement from these stakeholders to get involved. Finally, media advocacy can be used to promote services within the community that address and meet the needs of a wide array of people that includes, but is not limited to, older adults.

When Using Media for Advocacy

Developing a media-based approach does not simply imply developing flyers or newspaper articles, but rather it attempts to develop a concerted approach to developing strategies for social change. These strategies include the message, the messengers, and devising strategies to meet the target audience.

The message should be carefully crafted to include a specific point one wants to convey, as well as the messengers or vehicles to convey the message. For example, in Chapter 15, health behavior models and various stages of the models are discussed. The Stages of Change Model would require different sound bites or messages, depending upon the stage that the information is targeted to address. Sound bites are also crucial in the process because they help frame what one hears and how one is called to action. Overburdening an audience with steps or activities may do more harm than good.

A second important step when considering using media for advocacy is to pick the right messengers. Questions to consider in this process are, "Do they have name recognition in the community?" or "Do they represent the class of individuals who are targeted?" and "Are they considered credible sources of information?" Examples of good messengers include elected officials, respected aging officials, and well-known volunteer advocates.

FORMS OF MEDIA ADVOCACY

Media strategies come in a variety of forms, including newspaper articles, news releases, letters to the editor, radio spots or television interviews, media events or press briefings, fact sheets, media artifacts, and social media. While these are effective strategies, they are only a fraction of strategies or approaches available. A number of creative approaches can also be used with media artifacts such as bumper stickers, refrigerator magnets, baseball caps, door knockers, T-shirts, posters, billboard advertisements, newsletters, postcards, and flyers.

Newspaper Articles

Newspaper articles can be used to effectively target people who are literate and subscribe to a local paper. Articles are generally written at a fifth-grade reading ability and can be effectively persuasive and educational on specific issues. Developing a strong relationship with a newspaper columnist can help enhance one's ability to advocate on specific issues, and this individual can also be a source of background on specific community-based issues.

News Releases

News releases are mechanisms to provide the "W-5s" of a story, meaning the who, what, when, where, and why of an upcoming news story. Usually this "W-5" approach provides a news reporter with the background to be able to decide whether an article will be newsworthy or not. According to the Media Advocacy manual from the APHA, the standard format for a news release is as follows

- Organization's name: Although the name of the organization should be across the top of the release, using letterhead will also help with the legitimacy of the release.
- Contact information: This information should follow the organization's name. Ideally one would want to put the contact name and telephone number/fax number/email address for one who can speak on behalf of the organization, such as a staff person who is knowledgeable and easy to contact. This information is usually presented on the top right-hand corner of the page.
- Release date: The release date alerts the reporter when a press release item should be either published or broadcast. If it is available for immediate release, then it should be labeled as "For Immediate Release," and this can appear on the left-hand corner of the page, immediately following the title. If it is preferable that the news release be held until a particular date, the release date should read "Embargoed until [release date/time]."
- Headline: This component of a news release is probably the most important and will be what sparks attention. It generally is a short phrase or "sound bite" that summarizes the point of the news release. It is generally found under the contact information and before the body of the release.
- Body: This is the portion of the document where the story is told. It contains the "who, where, what, when, and why" of the story. Generally speaking, one can

see the news release framed as what is known as the inverted pyramid style of disclosure. In such a format, the conclusion, or most important of the details, is found initially, followed by supporting information. This inverted pyramid style is attractive because readers are often overwhelmed with information and news release items; hence, they find the most important information summarized in the headline and initial paragraphs.

A few additional pointers that may be helpful to the writer when preparing a news release item include the following

- The first paragraph, which becomes the lead, should be the most powerful paragraph. It should captivate the interest of the reader.
- Sentences and paragraphs should be kept short and in layperson's language. Jargon and slang should be avoided. Ideally, the final product should be one or two pages, single spaced.
- Conclude the release with a "tag": This "tag usually consists of one paragraph and provides a background on the organization, its goals, and so forth. Generally, it is prewritten and consists of what is known as a "boiler plate," outlining the background, goals, and mission of the not-for-profit organization sponsoring the news release.
- End your release. In the news industry, news releases usually include some symbols to denote that the news release has been concluded. This can be symbolized in one of three ways, at the end of the release: "—30—," "END," or "####" and can be found centered on the end of the page. If a news release has two pages, always end the first page with: "—more—" to indicate that there is a second page.

Letters to the Editor

Letters to the editor are often considered simple ways to communicate one's opinion to the general public. One can increase the chances of having a letter published by targeting smaller newspapers or magazines. A general rule of thumb is that shorter pieces are better and have more likelihood of getting printed. In addition to checking for how letters to the editor appear in specific magazines, some rules to follow include the following:

- Be brief: Try to focus the perspective to include only one idea or concept. Limit the letter to 300 or fewer words.
- Refer to previous stories: Refer to stories that have been recently published in the news.
- Include contact information: Not only would one want to include daytime contact information (name, telephone, email addresses), but also one's organizational affiliation and any degrees attained or titles that are relevant. The use of titles will help legitimize one's expertise.

Radio Spots or Television Interviews

Interviews with the media can be an effective way to share a message. Radio stations often broadcast talk shows that are interested in newsworthy information that can educate the public. Talk show hosts also often look for guests, so these programs can also be effective ways to promote one's message.

One must exercise care not to share too much information and overwhelm the listeners but instead to use the technique of "sound bites" of information.

Some additional tips to help a spokesperson prepare for the interview include the following:

- *Arrange an appearance*: The first step is to communicate with the talk show host or the producer. Writing or calling directly is acceptable. In your introduction, explain why people would be interested in the material you have to share about programs or policy issues for the person advancing in age or people living with disabilities. Tying the information to a local event also adds to the appeal for the producer.
- *Do your homework prior to the program*: One cannot stress enough the importance of getting to know both the host and the program. It is also a good idea to be pragmatic and find out about the interview—that is, will it be live or taped, how long is the interview, and will there be call-in questions. It might also be helpful to listen to at least a couple of broadcasts beforehand in order to get an idea of what to expect from the program.
- *Plan ahead for the interview*: Preparing ahead of the interview can ensure that the most important points you want to make are covered. Prepare in written format, ahead of time, the most important points to be made, and include anecdotes or personal stories that will put a human touch to the face of the interview. Consider questions that you can anticipate and arguments and counterarguments that may come your way during the interview so that you can prepare ahead for them. Since the media likes to give air time to opposing points of view and both sides of a story, it is prudent to prepare for these. Role-playing ahead of time with a colleague can also be very helpful in the preparation process.

Once the planning for the interview has been established, the following tips to keep in mind during the actual interview process can help assure success

- Speak naturally and enunciate so you can be heard clearly. Maintaining a calm and poised self are key to a successful interview. Avoid being defensive or showing any signs of anger, especially if challenged during the interview. Exercise caution not to say anything that you would prefer not seen in a tabloid or on the evening news.
- Avoid initials, trade language or jargon, and acronyms. Since advocacy using the media may involve reaching an audience who is not familiar with aging issues or trade terms like Area Agencies on Aging (AAAs), use language that will be easily understood by other people.
- Use the opportunity to share your message first use an interview situation as an opportunity to bring out a clear and consistent message repeatedly. Clarify and restate your message at every opportunity; then utilize the interview time to make points that will support your message. Delivering one main message over and over will help to ensure that it is heard.
- Be concise. Prepare "sound bites" ahead of time that can be used during the interview. These will aid in keeping messages short and concise. It has been estimated that sound bites usually last 8 seconds; hence, it is important that these are quick and easily roll off your tongue. A media trick has been reported to be dead space between questions. Generally, people who are not prepared for this dead space jump in and say something that could be regretted later on, which can be picked up on by a reporter. Having prepared sound bites ahead of time enables you to avoid this pitfall.

Some people have been known to bring tape recorders in order to tape themselves during the interview. In this manner, they have the opportunity to see whether they have made any errors or omissions that they would like to have corrected prior to airing their interviews.

Following are a few additional pointers for being interviewed for television, where the public will see as well as hear you

- Attire: Clothing creates images whether on or off camera. On camera, however, does pose some challenges that one must be prepared for. Jewelry, if loud and flashy, can create a reflection off TV camera lights. Clothing colors that seem to work best on television are solid designs in gray, blue, and brown. Solid black or white on camera creates too much of a contrast with the lights and can sometimes blend in with the background.
- Focus on the host and not the camera: Make a point of focusing on the host, interviewer, or commentator. Maintaining eye contact with this individual, along with a comfortable style and smile, will go a long way.
- "Smile, you're on candid camera": Above all else, keep in mind that you are always on stage. With this knowledge, be guarded with your actions and comments. It is when one least expects it that their candid comments are caught.

At the conclusion, remember that this may be only the beginning of a long-standing working relationship with the reporter, so consider sending a personal thank-you note to the reporter. Generally speaking, they will also provide a tape of the interview, which can be used as a learning tool to evaluate your performance and things to consider for the next interview opportunity.

Media Events or Press Briefings

Media events or press briefings are the two most common venues used for disseminating information about programs, policies, services, or issues. The difference between the two strategies is that a press briefing is held to provide journalists with information or background on a particular topic as well as new developments or key findings and updates. These events can be informal and also be used as a venue to develop a relationship with the media. A news conference, on the other hand, usually is an opportunity to announce a major story such as a new initiative, research development, policy change, or program initiative.

Both media events and press briefings can actually be time-intensive, so they may not always be the best way to share information with a mass of people if resources are slim. This being said, if one chooses to move into the realm of media events or press briefings, it is usually preferable to host these in a large group setting. The following points should be kept in mind when planning media events

- *Consider the location*: Choosing a location that is easily accessible and well known assures that it is convenient for journalists to find and attend. When considering a location, keep in mind that journalists may need to bring their equipment; hence, it will be important to assure that there is adequate space at the back of a room, and plenty of electrical outlets. Popular sites to consider are usually hotels or press clubs, but a local aging or public health service provider, a local area agency on aging, or a public health department can all be adequate choices for a location.
- *Consider the time*: Timing of events is important to ensure that journalists will show up. Experts suggest that midweek events (Tuesdays, Wednesdays, or Thursdays) are best, and events scheduled in the morning (10 a.m. or 11 a.m.) meet the needs of journalists who are on the run.
- *Follow-up prior to the event*: Prior to the event, forward an advisory to remind journalists of the event. This may be faxed or emailed. Once initiated, a follow-up with

a telephone call can always be helpful since newsrooms are swamped with requests. This trail of contacts also helps to build rapport with the media.

- *Develop a press kit:* A press kit is generally a way of providing educational materials on a given topic that can be distributed the day of a media event. It can contain news releases, fact sheets, biographies of speakers or key individuals, case studies related to your event, and general information about an aging agency or services. The materials should provide a backdrop on issues for those receiving the information and can provide some background information for the journalists that they can draw from when producing articles or other related materials.
- *Prepare an agenda beforehand*: Since it is important to ensure that an event is well orchestrated, select a moderator for the event ahead of time, as well as an agenda and speakers, and determine who will make introductions, prepare remarks, and so on.
- *Presentations*: Formal statements should be prepared to be as brief as possible not to exceed 15 to 20 minutes. Experts suggest that a general rule to consider is to limit presentations to five speakers during a press conference, and limit speakers' time availability to 5 minutes. The setting for a media conference is not to provide dissertations to the audience, but to educate and provide plenty of opportunities for the media to ask questions.
- *Helping hands*: Press conferences can be time-sensitive; thus, having as many individuals as possible available who can help orchestrate an event and make it appear to move smoothly is helpful. Pairs of hands can assist with passing out press kits, attending to sign-in sheets, directing journalists to key presenters, or being available to manage any last-minute details or crises.
- *Interviews and photo opportunities*: Ensure some time at the end of the event for both interviews and photo opportunities.
- *Initiate some follow-up once the event is over*: Minding one's manners, such as following up with personal thank-you notes can go a long way toward building relationships with reporters. Forwarding a press kit to journalists who were unable to attend also fosters relationships. Finally, if your press conference reaps any news stories, respond to these in writing and provide some commentary that can be woven by journalists into future stories. Each attempt to communicate with a journalist provides the opportunity to build a relationship.

Fact Sheets

Fact sheets are resources that can be very helpful to educate on a topic quickly and provide a summary of important points. Fact sheets generally identify the main message and provide some empirical data (statistics, graphs, etc.), as well as some anecdotal stories to put a human touch on the materials. Fact sheets are excellent resources to use when educating local legislators about a problem or issue that requires their attention and are commonly used by local advocates. A key to keep in mind when developing fact sheets is to be brief, keeping them to one page.

Media Artifacts

In addition, there are also a variety of other methods and techniques that utilize media artifacts and present a message. The key to using media artifacts is to find something that can be useful and valued to your target population, and use either the distributor, a printer, or one's own ability to use the computer and office supplies to develop sound-bite messages. Many people are familiar with the use of artifacts by marketing companies to develop items for promoting goods or services. In this vein, the ideas are similar; however, this slogan may include a sound-bite that will help convey a message regarding a particular service or issue.

The author's bias is that these media artifacts can be very useful to convey a message that reaches the majority of people through some creative mechanism. These artifacts are also a creative way to encourage students to transform policy or program development term papers into mechanisms that can impact older adults and their caregivers.

The following list provides a range of artifacts that can be used to develop these materials

- Websites
- T-shirts
- Sun visors
- Door hangers
- Buttons
- Bumper stickers
- Refrigerator magnets
- CD cases
- Purse size makeup mirrors
- Purse size "emergency kits"
- Calculators
- Refrigerator magnets
- Posters
- Billboards
- Umbrellas
- Shoelaces
- Packaging for crackers and snack food items
- Photographs
- Loose change containers
- Blogs
- Social media
- Tweets (Twitter) and Facebook postings

Social Media

Over the past decade, social media strategies have boomed, and technology use taking advantage of social media strategies has been on the rise. Although these strategies are popularized by millennials and Generation X, one must be mindful of the demographic who are the end users (Picazo-Velalsis, Gutierrez-Martinez, & Luna-Reyes, 2012). Many people with disabilities who rely on technology for their day-to-day communication and connection to others may relate to the use of technology. These strategies can be very effective in reaching specific demographic segments of the population and can be exceptionally helpful when building policy awareness campaigns or promoting programs for the population advancing in age or living with disabilities. Social media approaches include Facebook, Twitter, Instagram, email, LinkedIn, and blogs, to name a few examples. These techniques are discussed in more detail in the following paragraphs.

Facebook

Facebook has cultivated a calling from numerous agencies and individuals across the life span into its membership. It is one of the most quickly growing ways to stay connected to people and also offers opportunities for organizations and individuals to keep in touch with one's support network. Increasingly, organizations are developing a Facebook page and integrating it along with other social media strategies into its network of marketing strategies. Older adults are increasingly becoming adept at computer applications and Facebook membership; however, we still see a digital divide along socioeconomic lines. Rural communities still struggle with access to the Internet and secure, high speed connections, while urban areas do not face these challenges. In contrast, people living with disabilities, especially those more likely to be homebound, are frequent users of Facebook and stay connected to both a social network and organizational network. Although this is an effective strategy to get a message out to the public, if used, it should not be the only strategy utilized for marketing policy or program-oriented messages to the target group. In addition, be mindful possible hacking of your account and safeguard against potential damage such hacking might cause.

Twitter and Instagram

Twitter and Instagram can be useful strategies to share consistent messages to a particular demographic. While not all older adults and people with disabilities may have the capacity to utilize Twitter or Instagram, both social media strategies can be utilized to reach a demographic who tend to relate to social media. This approach may be helpful to reach supporters quickly. For example, if one is trying to reach people who can contact their legislator expediently about a specific bill about to be voted on, tweeting on Twitter may be effective. Similarly, tweets may be useful to send out reminders about an event taking place in a specific location.

LinkedIn

LinkedIn accounts provide opportunities to promote one's agency, programs, and services to a professional arena. This approach may not necessary always reach consumers who are advancing in age or people with disabilities but it will likely reach stakeholders with a specific interest in issues that impact older adults and people with disabilities. Tapping into LinkedIn can be a very useful strategy to reach networks who may have influences with the elite power paradigm. Supporters through LinkedIn may also be very strong advocates for social justice and support policies that will influence people growing older adults and people with disabilities.

Email

Email strategies are being used increasingly to cut postage costs and provide a broader reach. One must be mindful of the potential for email messages finding their way to the clutter or spam boxes of the recipients. It is, however, a great strategy to reach people repeatedly. When utilizing email, keep messages brief, and add attachments as necessary.

Blogs

Blogs on specific topics can be useful strategies to reach a younger demographic and people with disabilities. Current research studying whether this is an effective strategy to reach older adults is limited. Blogs can also be an effective mechanism to field test ideas or secure feedback on policy or program initiatives that an agency is interested in getting up and running. It can also be a very effective strategy to discuss the pros and cons of particular policy or programmatic changes that one would like to see implemented and to secure feedback.

WHAT STRATEGIES ARE BEST TO USE?

Consider the Audience

When attempting to decide which strategies are best to use, one must consider numerous factors. The first consideration is the audience. Who are the target individuals whom one wants to reach? What demographic characteristics comprise this target audience? Demographics to consider include the average age to address, the ethnic makeup, marital status, income level, educational levels, and occupational makeup of the group. The age cohort is important because one would hope that messages may also consider some of the cohort-related issues that the individual may find of specific importance and have relevance over the course of their lifetime (see Chapter 2 for historical landmarks). One would not consider targeting messages using the Internet or blogs if the audience is not computer literate.

Consider the Message

A second consideration is the message to address using the strategy. Is the message intended to ensure that older adults are aware of the benefits of a flu vaccine, perceived susceptibility, perceived seriousness, or all of these issues? Should it address the subjective norms or beliefs as a part of the strategy? Health behaviors play a critical and vital role in the development of these messages as well.

Consider Time

A number of other considerations, which may be more pragmatic or logistical, are also relevant when developing media strategies. These include such concerns as time, financial resources, human resources, specific health promotion strategies, and a message to target. Time considerations include how much time is available to get the message out. Is the plan to meet a deadline for the next month, to meet some goals established for National Diabetes Awareness month, for example, or is there a longer-range plan to develop a health fair 6 months down the line? Conversely, is one's organization planning for media approaches for the next year and designing some educational tools to be used monthly for themes? Along with the consideration of time, one must also consider how much time is available to work on a specific issue, and how much time a specific anticipated strategy will take to pursue.

Consider Financial Resources

Financial resources are another consideration when devising media strategies. Working within a limited budget may also limit the specific type of strategies one could pursue. When limited resources are available, one may consider using public resources such as radio or the local newspapers. Soliciting corporate partners can also be a helpful venue for developing financial support for media efforts. For example, grocery stores often partner with regional or national associations and utilize their grocery bags to showcase specific events; these can be useful for promotion of a health message or media approach. Depending on one's financial situation, one may also be able to purchase the services of a social marketer to develop a marketing campaign that is more substantial.

Consider Human Resources

Human resources may include the personnel available to develop a marketing campaign, or to promote and market a message through chosen media. Individuals with expertise may not necessarily be available within a health or human services agency. This situation may make it worthwhile to utilize the expertise of a local academic setting such as a community college or a university and tap into a service learning project with the local institution. Human service workers or people with a liberal arts background may have the expertise to manage resources or conduct case management functions; however, these same individuals may lack a theoretical background to convey health promotion messages or use health behavior frameworks in the design of media strategies. Conversely, resources with expertise in marketing or the technical aspects of using various media may not be familiar with the specific nature of aging issues and the content, so partnerships bridging these human resources are very important. Figure 16.1 presents useful planning for building a blueprint for a media strategy.

Issue to Promote What is the issue that you or your constituency group wants to address?	**Target Group (Aging, Disability, or both)** Is your target group older adults (what age group; people with disabilities or a specific disability?	**Media Strategies to Be Used** What specific strategies will you use identified within this chapter?	**Messages/ Sound Bites to Be Executed** What are the sound bite messages that you want to get across?	**Pyramid Statement** What messages should be included in the pyramid statement?

Figure 16.1 A planning tool for a social media campaign.

Erica and Theresa sat down with the planning tool showcased in Figure 16.1 and decided to look at which strategy they would use to gain access to the public and identify what messages they wanted to impact others regarding their blueprint. Both women, although overwhelmed initially at the prospect of trying to develop a strategy for utilizing the media to showcase their blueprint, found that by looking at the pros and cons of each approach and resources needed, they could organize their ideas and approaches.

USING MEDIA ADVOCACY FOR POLICY DEVELOPMENT AND PROGRAM PLANNING

The use of media as an advocacy tool in the fields of public health and human services for aging adults and those with disabilities does not have a long-standing tradition (Tappe & Galer-Unti, 2001). In public health, the use of media has sometimes been coined as "social marketing." However, this approach has been used primarily for targeting health interventions and has addressed the individual at the initial stages of readiness for change (precontemplation and contemplation). A further discussion of how these stages fit into the health behavior repertoire is discussed in Chapter 15. In contrast to a social marketing approach, media advocacy can be effectively carried out using artifacts that send a simple take-home message. There are several benefits to incorporating media advocacy into a repertoire of skills for advocacy development. First, it is quick and can be inexpensive. Second, it helps assure that one's message is known, and by using a variety of strategies with the media, one may be able to amplify the impact. Last, other fields and occupations take advantage of media strategies to promote their message. There is no reason advocates within the fields of aging and disability need to be left behind (Baker, Leitner, & McAuley, 2001).

SUMMARY

This chapter reviews a number of specific media advocacy strategies and provides some innovative approaches to sending a message relevant to program or policy development. These strategies can be used as stand-alone methods or in combination with each other. Media artifacts can also be a creative way to get one's message out to the general public in a simple manner in areas that can be highly technical. These strategies build on understanding one's health and help-seeking behavior and enable advocates to influence a wide number and array of people with limited resources and energy.

ADDITIONAL RESOURCES

Websites

APHA, Advocacy For Public Health: www.apha.org/policies-and-advocacy/advocacy-for-public-health

This site provides tips, an advocacy priorities webinar, and a *Legislative Advocacy Handbook* that includes the 10 rules for advocacy efforts. The site also provides links for the reader to advocacy activities, policy statements, advocacy priorities, reports and fact sheets, and ideas for taking action. Links are also available to how-to sites related to advocacy efforts to influence policy makers, public meetings, and letter writing.

Centers for Disease Control and Prevention, Health Marketing Basics: www.cdc.gov/healthcommunication/index.html

This website provides helpful tips related to health marketing, beginning with an introduction to the concept, identifying a "market mix," and developing a marketing plan. It also provides some insight into market exchange and target markets.

The AGS Foundation for Health in Aging Advocacy Center: www.HealthinAging.org

This website, hosted by the American Geriatrics Society, offers tools for advocacy on issues that are important for the health and well-being of older adults. It provides links to sites with state-of-the-art information on the diseases and disorders of older adults, physician referral services, and aging stories.

A Journalist's Guide to the Internet: reporter.asu.edu/

This website, developed by a journalist (Dr. Christopher Callahan, Dean, Walter Cronkite School of Journalism and Mass Communication), provides a step-by-step guide and links to advocacy efforts from a journalist's perspective. Links include maps, sources, directors, Listservs, search tools, online newspapers, newsgroups, federal and state government links, and much more.

The Gerontological Society of America, Expert Referral Service: www.geron.org/press-room/expert-referral-service

This website provides links to experts in virtually any area in the field of aging. These can be helpful for the advocate seeking expert testimony on a specific topic within the field of aging.

Health Literacy Consulting: www.healthliteracy.com/tips

This website helps organizations communicate effectively to their target audience. Developed by a private consultant, it provides resources on health literacy, ideas for writing and editing effectively, and links to resources that can be used to promote health literacy through advocacy.

NASW Advocacy: www.socialworkers.org/advocacy

This website provides range of tips for effective advocacy from a social work perspective. It provides links for grassroots advocacy, a legislative advocacy network, legislative issues, congressional testimony, letters and comments, and a tool kit for effective lobbying action. The site also provides links to enable one to look up legislative bills and provides a link to useful publications that have been utilized in recent advocacy efforts.

YouTube Videos

How to create lead advertisements in Facebook: www.youtube.com/watch?v=9b9V9jMEVX4

This video provides a step-by-step approach to using and utilizing Facebook in a unique way—that is, to create advertising or secure contacts interested in your program or projects. It is useful for nonprofits and initiatives seeking to utilize Facebook to secure a following of supporters.

How to Create Your Own Blog: www.wix.com/html5bing/hiker-blog?experiment_id=developing%20blog%5Ebp%5E79371013446593%5Eyoutube%20videos%20on%20developing%20blogs&utm_campaign=ms_us_b_1_June_2016%5Ebl_blog&utm_medium=cpc&utm_source=bing

This site provides step-by-step instructions for the development of a blog. It also provides templates for the novice user to make one's life with blogging manageable.

Twitter for Beginners: www.youtube.com/watch?v=SBDYYGER5iM

This video provides a tutorial on the use of Twitter as a social media source. It provides the novice with basics from setting up an account to utilizing it for various purposes.

Podcast

Bryan Hewing on the use of social media. **Listen now:** https://bcove.video/2OULZRM

DISCUSSION QUESTIONS

1. What media strategies would work well in your community to showcase issues or programs and services that people growing older or living with a disability could benefit from? How would you implement these using the worksheet provided in Figure 16.1?
2. How would you design a pyramid statement for a press release that would address a policy or program-related issues within your community?
3. Compare and contrast how you would use similar or different media strategies across the lifespan, to appeal and reach different demographic groups.

REFERENCES

American Public Health Association. (2008). *APHA media advocacy manual*. Washington, DC: Author.

Baker, P., Leitner, J., & McAuley, W. J. (2001). Preparing future aging advocacy advocates: The Oklahoma Aging Advocacy Leadership Academy. *The Gerontologist*, *41*, 394–400. doi:10.1093/geront/41.3.394

Bernhardt, J. M. (2004). Communication at the core of effective public health. *American Journal of Public Health*, *94* (12), 2051–2053. doi:10.2105/ajph.94.12.2051

Cavill, N., & Bauman, A. (2004). Changing the way people think about health enhancing physical activity: Do mass media campaigns have a role? *Journal of Sports Sciences*, *22*(8), 771–790. doi:10.1080/026404104 10001712467

Coalition of National Health Education Organization Partners. (n.d.). *Making your advocacy efforts count*. Retrieved from http://www.healtheducationadvocate.org

Dorfman, L. (2005). More than a message: Framing public health advocacy to change corporate practices. *Health Education and Behavior*, *32*(3), 320–336. doi:10.1177/1090198105275046

Freimuth, V. S., & Quinn, S. C. (2004). The contribution of health communication to eliminating health disparities. *American Journal of Public Health*, *94*(12), 2053–2058. doi:10.2105/AJPH.94.12.2053

Hudson, R. B. (2004, Spring). Advocacy and policy success in aging. *Generations*, *28*(1), 17–24.

Moore, J. K. B. (2004, July). *Photography as a tool for advocacy and policy change: Successes from CARE and photosensitive's HIV positive campaign*. Paper presented at the XV International Conference on AIDS, Bangkok, Thailand. Retrieved from http://www.abstract-archive.org/

Mueller, M., Page, C., & Kuerbis, B. (2004). Civil society and the shaping of communication-information policy: Four decades of advocacy. *The Information Society*, *20*(3), 169–185. doi:10.1080/01972240490456845

National Council on Aging. (2018). Advocacy Toolkit. Available at https://www.ncoa.org/public-policy-action/advocacy-toolkit

Picazo-Velalsis, S., Gutierrez-Martinez, L., & Luna-Reyes, F. (2012). Understanding risks, benefits, and strategic alternatives of social media in the public sector. *Government Information Quarterly*, *29*(4), 504–511. doi:10.1016/j.giq.2012.07.002

Randolph, W., & Viswanth, K. (2004). Lessons learned from public health mass media campaigns: Marketing health in a crowded media world. *Annual Review of Public Health*, *25*, 419–437. doi:10.1146/annurev.publhealth.25.101802.123046

Tappe, M. K., & Galer-Unti, R. A. (2001). The health educators' role in promoting health literacy and advocacy for the 21st century. *Journal of School Health*, *71*(10), 477–482. doi:10.1111/j.1746-1561.2001.tb07284.x

17

Coalitions and Coalition Building for Advocacy and Policy Development

LEARNING OBJECTIVES

At the end of the chapter, the reader will:

1. *Be familiar with the role coalitions play in advocacy and policy development.*
2. *Understand the various types of coalitions that impact the policy landscape.*
3. *Be familiar with the various roles that exist within groups and coalitions that contribute to the success or nonsuccess of the group process.*

> *Theresa recently met Susan through a mutual connection and discovered that Susan was interested in participating in a local coalition that was targeting improved transportation services for the mobility impaired. Susan had voiced concerns about the local rural transportation provider who was assigned to pick up Susan's father, Gus, and take him to an adult day program. Susan was encouraged to join the local Coalition for Citizens with Disabilities because they were currently spearheading an effort to improve transportation services in Susan's rural region. Theresa had explained to Susan that consumer advocacy was important in efforts to improve service delivery and can be of great help to social workers who are also trying to pursue advocacy efforts in policy and program development.*

WHY ADVOCACY?

Many disciplines have advocacy embedded at the heart of the activities they aspire to carry out. In addition, several disciplines, such as social work, include advocacy within their own code of ethics and major activities for the profession. While advocacy takes on a host of different definitions, at the heart of all definitions is the act of speaking in favor of another's cause or speaking or writing in support of something. As many professions seek to challenge injustices within communities, increasingly, the act of advocacy is being built into the range of activities that professionals engage in. Advocacy is the bridge between what is seen as a social, health, or community need, and the outcome, such as policy development or program-or practice-related activities.

 DOI:10.1891/9780826128393.0017

In many profession, such as social work, one of the core values is to advocate for social justice. The National Association of Social Workers (NASW) *Code of Ethics* notes that through the value of social justice, social workers are called to challenge social injustice. According to the *NASW Code of Ethics* (2017)

> *Social workers pursue social change, particularly with and on behalf of vulnerable and oppressed individuals and groups of people. Social workers' social change efforts are focused primarily on issues of poverty, unemployment, discrimination, and other forms of social injustice. These activities seek to promote sensitivity to and knowledge about oppression and cultural and ethnic diversity. Social workers strive to ensure access to needed information, services, and resources; equality of opportunity; and meaningful participation in decision making for all people.*

Professions such as social work have a responsibility to a broader society through their commitment to social welfare. In essence, social workers strive to promote the general welfare of society, from local to global levels. They try to promote the development of human resources, communities, and environments. The *NASW Code of Ethics* also challenges social workers to advocate for some basic living conditions that respect human dignity and that promote human needs and foster human, economic, social, political, and cultural values of the core population. When translated to an aging population, social workers, as an example, strive to develop information and resources that will encourage and foster the dignity and worth of older adults and their families. This includes the process of advocacy for standards and living conditions that are consistent with the lifestyle and values that an older adult has been exposed to during his or her lifetime.

Within our service delivery systems there are a number of unresolved issues and areas for program development that will require advocacy. Gaps in service delivery are prime reasons why we would want to engage in advocacy efforts. Gaps in policy development are also major areas and reasons that require advocacy efforts on our part as health professionals and social workers. Examples include the need for services to be made available through Medicare, such as oral health screening and prevention services, and falls prevention education.

STRATEGIES FOR ADVOCACY: COALITION BUILDING

A number of strategies can be used to develop initiatives to impact one's advocacy efforts. These strategies can be used to promote the development of new programs and services and can include the use of and/or development of coalitions, the media and media advocacy, and consumer advocates. The following sections address each of these strategies in greater depth.

What Are Coalitions?

Coalitions can be defined as temporary alliances or factions that can be used for the benefit of a political strategy or goal. Essentially a coalition includes an organized group of people in a community who set out to work toward a common goal. The coalition can have individual, group, institutional, community, and public policy goals.

What Are Some Reasons for Developing Coalitions?

For a number of reasons, coalition building would be an effective strategy for the development of resources, policies, or programs. These include issues or concerns such as the following:

- Conducting needs assessments
- Addressing lack of resources
- Policy development
- Program planning
- Data collection strategies
- Action/evaluations
- Advocacy
- Road maps/blueprints/vision
- Evidence-based approaches

PARTNERS FOR COALITION ENTITIES

A number of community-based partners can serve to create effective partnerships in the coalition-building process. These partners, whether traditional or nontraditional in the sense of being vested in community efforts, can all contribute to the welfare of a community in an attempt to incorporate older adults and people with disabilities within the community and build on existing programs and services. Such partners include the following diverse interest groups listed in Table 17.1. These partners include academia, public health, human services, faith-based communities, law and safety enforcement, medical educators, consumers (older adults, caregivers, people with disabilities, and the general public), volunteer associations, and sport and recreational entities. This section will describe how each of these partners and relationships contribute as partner coalitions.

Table 17.1 Partnerships for Coalitions

Partner	Private or Public Entity
Academia	Public and private
Public health expertise	Public
Human service providers	Public and/or private
Consumer organizations	Private
Faith-based communities	Private
Law and safety enforcement	Public
Media/education	Public and/or private
Volunteer associations	Private
Sports and recreation entities	Public and/or private

Academia

Academia can prove to be an effective and helpful partner in the process of building coalitions for advocacy development in several ways. Educators' expertise lies in scholarship and training. Experts may provide information about the latest developments in the literature and ideas about the specific innovations within the field. They are usually also abreast of seminal documents such as task force reports and so on. In addition to their academic expertise, these experts can also provide student manpower and student input into the development of student projects, focus groups, or other mechanisms that can enhance the process for academic expertise.

Public Health Expertise

Public health expertise within a coalition can be an asset in several important ways (Minnix & Roadman, 2002). First, staff from public health departments can easily understand and interpret data such as vital statistics and epidemiological data, which can contribute to the rationale for program or policy changes. Second, public health has a strong advocacy arm and a tradition of building coalitions, which can also benefit the process.

Human Service Providers

Human service providers can provide some insight into three specific areas, which can be helpful in the coalition-building process. First, they can provide service statistics on the kinds of service needs seen within a specific geographic community and identify gaps in services. Second, they can provide staff who are knowledgeable about the needs and gaps in services within specific designated community areas. Last, they can provide some background into a consumer's perspective through the invitation and inclusion of consumers or their families as target groups and can involve these individuals on coalition forces.

Consumer Organizations

Consumer organizations play a critical role in the lifeblood of coalitions, especially when the coalition groups are designed to benefit the consumer of interest. Consumer groups within the realms of aging and disability are wide and varied, and despite the fact that they may represent individuals growing older or individuals with disabilities, they may not represent homogeneous ideas or values. Consumers from older adult constituency groups may be representative of caregivers, people from AARP, to support groups for conditions such as dementia, Alzheimer's, or cancer support. Consumers representing people with disabilities can run the gamut from autism to people with developmental disabilities, people with visual impairments, children and adults with severe and persistent mental illness, people who have hearing loss or deafness or are hard of hearing, and people with learning disabilities. Given the range of types of constituency groups, the different types of group affiliation may take the group into several different directions insofar as coalitions are concerned, based upon the mission and goals of the consumers.

Faith-Based Communities

Faith-based communities can also be key partners in coalitions since the leaders of faith-based communities have an active linkage with many people in their midst. Clergy and other religious leaders have the capacity to reach many people within their congregations, which can be helpful for community-based advocacy campaigns. Congregations may also be sought to provide expertise to community coalition efforts, and members can write to local, state, and federal legislators to promote the passage of specific legislation (such as seen in the process of passing Medicare Part D or the Americans with Disabilities Act [ADA]). Many faith-based communities also have social action committees, which can help promote the work of coalitions or provide perspectives that can contribute to the development of a coalition's work.

Law and Safety Enforcement

Law and safety enforcement entities can be helpful in the work of coalitions, especially in aging-related issues, since they are active in communities protecting and serving the needs of elders. They are often the first line of attack for needs and issues related to community safety; however, they can also offer a perspective on the needs and issues that older people will face related to public safety and victimization. They can also, in many cases, be called upon to share some degree of expertise related to the implementation of specific policies and programs.

Media/Education

The media can be an effective coalition partner because they can provide publicity and create public awareness about issues and concerns that the coalition is publicly involved in. The media can also be used to effectively persuade the public and community about specific initiatives that may impact people with disabilities and older adults and their family members and caregivers. Public radio and television stations can also be instrumental in developing and delivering messages that can further the work of a coalition's efforts. They can also be used to develop special educational segments that can showcase an issue or concern that the coalition is attempting to build awareness around and bridge resources for. An excellent example of the use of the media is Jackson County, Illinois, where a public television network (WSIU—affiliated with Southern Illinois University, Carbondale) created awareness of culture change within nursing homes known as the *Pioneering Movement*. Legislative efforts had been underway to develop a bill within the Illinois legislature to facilitate some efforts and expectations within nursing facilities to improve the culture within the nursing facilities of the state.

Volunteer Associations

Volunteer associations can also serve as effective partners on the coalition team. Volunteer associations often take on service projects, which can be community-oriented and provide partnership to coalitions with person power and members who offer their expertise pro bono. Lawyers or accountants who are members of voluntary associations are good examples of experts who can be called on to further a coalition's work on an issue. Once again, voluntary associations can also share their access to membership bases to help a coalition reach organizational membership. This is especially true now that the Internet and social media are powerful tools for information exchange. Voluntary groups such as local chapters of AARP can also be helpful in leveraging person-power to write letters or make telephone calls to one's local representatives and senators. They can also be helpful in bringing issues to the attention of their membership and securing community support.

Sports and Recreation Entities

Many retired people frequent facilities such as sports and recreation centers. These active seniors can also be a source of consumer group energy, which can be helpful to a coalition. Workers from these entities are often also in touch with a number of senior citizens, so they also can be an excellent source of contact or connection with older adults.

In summary, a number of partners can serve as effective members within a coalition, and resources that are often overlooked within communities can actually be available to provide intellectual, human, and promotional resources (Gallagher, Stanley, Shearer, & Klerman, 2006).

HOW DO WE BUILD COALITIONS?

Building coalitions can be an art form (built on some science), although some people may argue that one need only invite people to the table. Successful coalitions actually build some strategy and process into their design, which may in fact help the coalition to meet success (Butterfoss, 2013). Effective coalition leadership involves the use of strategic processes and mapping of resources to be sure that the necessary ingredients for success are in place (Sipe, 2005).

The first step in developing effective coalitions is to develop an issue-based approach to participation. Within this approach, an organizer or facilitator must consider what expertise is required and what the common goal is for all. This step requires communication skills, and once community partners are identified, it may be useful to develop one meeting dedicated to building a common vision or purpose. One tool that can be exceedingly helpful is known as the nominal group technique.

Theresa and Susan met following Susan's attendance at a couple of coalition meetings. Susan thought that the coalition could be helpful and a perfect avenue to work through issues and toward improving local programs and services. However, she was frustrated over the apparent infighting and wanted Theresa to help her strengthen her communication skills to enable her to be more effective with her local coalition. Theresa suggested that Susan consider some of the following ideas as part of better understanding the dynamics that were taking place within the coalition.

COMMUNICATION SKILLS FOR EFFECTIVE COMMUNITY NEGOTIATIONS

There are several communication skills that are essential in order to ensure effective community negotiations. These skills include active listening; conflict management; and an awareness of verbal and nonverbal messages, which are sent through specific roles stakeholder and community members play.

Active listening ensures that each participant or stakeholder is heard. This may include the use of techniques such as Nominal Group Techniques (NGT) or DELPHI. In the NGT process, each member is presented with 3- by 5-in. note cards and asked to present a written statement that reflects his or her contribution to the issue at hand. People are usually solicited for two or three statements in response to the facilitator's question. These are then collected and listed for all to view (using flip chart paper, computer projection, etc.). Items are ranked by the number of times they are identified by membership and then voted on in order of priority for the group. This process ensures that all stakeholders and members of the group, including the quieter and less vocal group members, are given the opportunity to present their perspective and opinions. The NGT process also enables the group to develop consensus on items of priority and moves toward the development of a community planning agenda.

The integration and use of consensus means that there is agreement on the general direction. However, ensuring that there is total agreement on every issue is not realistic when there is a range of divergent viewpoints and perspectives, but it is realistic to arrive at consensus where there is agreement on a range of issues at hand. One member may give on one item and then gain support in another area. In order to arrive at this point, it is important to understand sources of conflict.

Sources of Conflict

Several sources of conflict can be expected to arise when working with divergent personalities and differences in professional background, training, experiences, and personal agendas. Often conflict is perceived as negative and to be avoided. It can, however, provide the catalyst for effective and creative problem solving, since conflict resolution and relationship building are closely connected. Effective mastery of conflict in order to move toward creative problem solving begins with understanding sources of conflict. These can include differences in the interpretation of data, relationship conflict, structural conflicts, value conflicts, and interest conflicts.

Conflicts may arise from differences in perception and interpretation of data, for example, differences in the interpretation of balance sheets, financial information, or epidemiological data. Data related to incidence and prevalence may not hold the same meaning for a social worker as for a physician. Conversely, one's interpretation of issues related to psychiatry or psychiatric diagnosis may be interpreted in one way (based upon fear and stigma) for a community resident, and quite differently by a member of a treatment team. Thus, these issues may cause conflicts among various members of a coalition. However, an effective resolution is possible (Ospina & Saz-Carranza, 2005).

Conflicts may also arise because of age cohort differences in values (Huan & Yazdanifard, 2012; Karp & Osirias, 2001). It is possible to have at least five different cohorts working together within communities or coalitions (Pew Research Center, 2015). This age difference can result in differences across vision, values, pace, methodology and approach to policy development, program planning, and coalition building.

The Pew Research Center (2015) has characterized these different age cohorts, as shown in Table 17.2. For example, the oldest of these, born between 1901 and 1927, are described as having traditional values, being resilient and frugal, and placing importance on having a sense of purpose. This is in contrast to the cohort born between 1928 and 1945, who are identified as rule-oriented, hardworking, loyal, conformist, patriotic, and respectful of authority. Baby Boomers tend to be characterized as optimistic and striving for personal gratification, individuality, and independence and being youth-oriented with a focus on health and well-being. The next cohort, Generation Xers born between 1965 and 1980, tend to share characteristics of skepticism, and value having fun, seeking a work-life balance, being self-reliant, and having a global focus. Millennials, born between 1981 and 2000, are characterized as being proud of their accomplishments and societal contributions, optimistic, civically engaged, and interested in health and well-being. These differences in values and expectations can lead to sources of conflict when working toward coalitions and coalition building.

Table 17.2 Summary of Different Age Cohorts and Characteristics

Cohort	Age in 2015	% of Adult Population	Characteristics
The Greatest Generation (1901–1927)	88–114	2%	Traditional values, resilient, frugal, need for a sense of purpose. Relies upon face-to-face communication
The Silent Generation (1928–1945)	70–87	11%	Rule-oriented, hardworking, loyal, conformist, patriotic, respect for authority. Values open communication, relationships and person to person verbal communication
Baby Boomers (1946–1964)	51–69	30%	Optimistic, personal gratification, individuality, independent, youth-oriented, focus on health/wellbeing Values efficiency, but a balance between face-to-face, personal, and electronic media
Generation X (1965–1980)	35–50	27%	Skepticism, values having fun, seek a work-life balance, self-reliant, global focus Values team input
Millennials (1981–2000)	15–34	30%	Pride in accomplishments and contributions to society, realistic, civic engagement, optimistic, interested in health/well-being Prefers electronic communication and social media
Generation Z (2001–2020)	3–14	–	Technologically savvy, relationships based upon use of technological tools. Relies upon electronic communication and social media

Source: Pew Research Center. (2015). *The whys and hows of generations research*. Retrieved from http://www.people-press.org/2015/09/03/the-whys-and-hows-of-generations-research

Roles of Coalition Members

As a planner, one may want to be cognizant of the various roles that members play within the coalition-building process. If these have not naturally evolved, it may be helpful to ensure that there is representation from these various roles within the group so that there will be a skill set readily available to the group. These roles include, among others, initiator, negotiator, advocate, spokesperson, organizer, mediator, and consultant. These roles will be used in the coalition as several ways to foster the development of the coalition. Table 17.3 provides an overview of these roles.

Table 17.3 Roles of Group Members

Roles	Types of Roles
Initiator	Task oriented
Contributor	Task oriented
Information seeker	Task oriented
Opinion seeker	Task oriented
Information giver	Task oriented
Opinion giver	Task oriented
Evaluator-critic	Task oriented
Energizer	Task oriented
Procedural technician	Task oriented
Distractor	Individual oriented
Blocker	Individual oriented
Recognition seeker	Individual oriented
Self-confessor	Individual oriented
Playboy	Individual oriented
Encourager	Group/process oriented
Harmonizer	Group/process oriented
Compromiser	Group/process oriented
Gatekeeper	Group/process oriented
Expediter	Group/process oriented
Standard setter	Group/process oriented
Ego ideal	Group/process oriented
Group observer	Group/process oriented
Follower	Group/process oriented

Initiator

Initiators call attention to an issue such as a problem existing in the community, an unmet need, or a situation to be improved. They play a key role in getting the coalition going.

Negotiator

The negotiator represents an organization or group trying to gain something from another group. This individual seeks win-win situations and a middle ground that both sides can accept. Negotiators are vital when a range of factions exist at the coalition level.

Advocate

The advocate decides what clients is entitled to and what is keeping them from receiving what they need. Effective advocacy requires that the advocate have the capacity to assess various stakeholders' or coalition members' strengths and weakness.

Spokesperson

The spokesperson presents an organization's views to others without coloring them with his or her own opinions. This role is critical in showcasing the issues and strategies or promoting the outcomes found by the group.

Organizer

The organizer creates groups of people who share a similar concern. The organizer's tasks include developing the leadership potential of others, stimulating others to act, and identifying targets for change.

Mediator

The mediator role helps two sides work out a compromise. The individual who plays the role of the mediator is neutral, not siding with either party. One major task for the mediator is to ensure that both sides understand the other's positions and help these two side arrive at a consensus. The mediator is also responsible for helping to arrive at priorities and build consensus within the group.

Consultant

The consultant provides advice, suggestions, or ideas to another person, group, or organization. Two characteristics are important for the consultant: (a) knowing more than the group that is being initiated as a coalition and (b) being able to see his or her advice ignored without getting personally involved or hurt.

Individual Roles and Perspectives

In addition to the specific roles that are important to be represented within the group, it is also important for the coalition leadership to have a grasp of specific personality dynamics. Personality dynamics are such that membership will affiliate with either a task-oriented relationship, a process-oriented relationship, or the role of a distracter. Distracters tend to divert one away from the goal while the former two help move toward goals, either through accomplishing tasks or building relationships.

Understanding the Roles Participants Will Take On

Group members take on a variety of roles, which can either contribute to or hinder the development of a healthy group process. There are essentially three main types of roles group members fall into. These roles are helpful in understanding the group process and include group task roles, group building and maintenance roles, and individual roles. An understanding of each of these roles can lead to the development of understanding how each of them can either facilitate or impede the process of task development.

Group Task Roles

The roles of group tasks include the initiator, contributor, information seeker, opinion seeker, information giver, opinion giver, elaborator, coordinator, orientor, evaluator-critic, energizer, and procedural technician. The initiator/contributor tries to find new ways to meet a group goal. The information seeker seeks facts and clarification from facts and asks if these are adequate. The opinion seeker asks for facts and clarification from those making suggestions. The elaborator spells out suggestions and ideas to deduce how an activity will work if adopted by the group. The coordinator pulls ideas and suggestions together and coordinates activities. The orientor summarizes the past, points to where the group departs from goals, and charts future direction. The evaluator/critic subjects the group to standards, questions the group, and plays devil's advocate. The energizer pushers for higher quality activity. The procedural technician contributes to the logistics of the group and distributes materials. The recorder writes suggestions, records group decisions, and serves as the group memory.

Group Building and Maintenance Roles

Group building and maintenance roles have been identified as the encourager, harmonizer, compromiser, gatekeeper, expediter, standard setter or ego ideal, group observer/commentator, and follower. These roles are designed to strengthen the process of group building, develop a stronger bond among the group members, and serve as the glue that binds the process.

The encourager praises and shares warmth with the group. The harmonizer reconciles and mediates, relieving tension. The compromiser meets others halfway. The gatekeeper keeps communication channels open. The standard setter sets standards for the group. The group observer records group process and contributes the same. The follower goes along with the movements of the group.

Individual or Distractor Roles

There are several roles that lead to individual rather than group gain. These roles include the aggressor, the blocker, the recognition seeker, the self-confessor, and the playboy. The aggressor deflates the status and esteem of others, disapproves values of others, attacks efforts for change, and shows envy. The blocker is negative and stubbornly resistant, opposes without reason, and returns to settled or rejected issues. The recognition seeker calls attention to oneself and away from the project at hand through boasting about one's personal achievements. The self-confessor, on the other hand, is known for input about his or her shortfalls. The playboy can be cynical, nonchalant, or out of the field.

What Influences These Roles Within Coalitions?

A number of factors influence these roles among members of coalitions. These factors include individual members' needs and resources, the situation of the group, and the culture and environment of the group. In addition, human factors can lead to barriers to effective coalition building such as mutual trust, negotiation skills, communication skills, appropriate leaders, clear goals, and unified commitment will also affect the group as a whole and as individual members.

Thus far, this chapter has outlined a variety of issues related to coalitions, group development, and coalition building for aging policies and programs. The next segment provides examples of coalitions that have been effective in the aging arena.

> *Susan found that understanding the roles and agendas that various coalition members brought to the "table" enabled her to be more thoughtful and strategic in how she positioned her view of needs. She was now eager to get involved on subcommittees in order to specifically deal with the transportation needs of her rural community. She felt that a stronger grasp of what roles various coalition members played (task, maintenance, or distractor) greatly enhanced her ability to participate with the coalitions. Now she was eager to get involved with some other coalitions!*

MODEL COALITIONS AND THEIR OUTCOMES

The National Coalition on Mental Health and Aging

The National Coalition on Mental Health and Aging (NCMHA) has 47 partners to date in the United States and serves as a forum for information sharing among state and local coalitions. Information sharing can relate to a number of issues including best practices, grant opportunities, and national initiatives. It also serves as a vehicle for older adult consumers to share their perspectives at a national level on issues related to mental health and substance abuse. The coalition has also provided a voice in Washington, DC, and in 1995 provided representation and testimony to the White House Conference on Aging. The coalition has been in existence since 1991 and has grown to reach nearly all of the states in the United States over the past 25+ years.

The Ontario Healthy Communities Coalition

The Ontario Healthy Communities Coalition, established in 1992, works to promote the ability of communities to strengthen their social, environmental, and economic well-being. These communities are a direct result of the Healthy Communities Initiative but have spread throughout Ontario through the use of local and regional coalitions. One of the secrets to their success has been the collective vision of membership, despite the roles and agendas that may be brought to monthly meetings. The coalition has broadened its span and made training materials and its model available to other communities and countries, including in the United States.

Quad Counties Mental Health and Aging Coalition

The Quad Counties Coalition is a collection of service providers who joined forces from four counties in southern Illinois, as a result of a demonstration project implemented by the Office of Mental Health, State of Illinois. This demonstration project was in response to the Surgeon General's report on Mental Health (U.S. Department of Health and Human Services [DHHS], 1999), which called attention to an intervention to address system integration issues. The coalition has made use of partnerships with service providers, public health, aging, mental health, faith-based, and media communities to improve the point-of-service access for older adults, and to improve public awareness of aging and mental health issues. In 2006, the group was recognized for its innovation and success by the American Media Association.

The National Federation of the Blind

Founded in 1940, the National Federation of the Blind (NFB) is the nation's largest and most influential membership organization of persons who are blind. The purpose of the NFB is twofold: to help blind persons achieve self-confidence and self-respect and to act as a vehicle for collective self-expression by the blind.

The Coalition of Health and Disability Advocates

Health and Disability Advocates (HDA) seeks to assure that low-income older adults and children and adults with disabilities lead secure and dignified lives. HDA advocates for policies that promote economic security and provide health coverage. HDA's efforts are coordinated with and informed by individuals who rely on government programs, direct service providers, community-based organizations, the private sector, and state and federal agencies. HDA's advocacy efforts identify systemic barriers to self-sufficiency, employment, and access to healthcare and promote policy solutions to eliminate those barriers. HDA strives to protect and strengthen federal and state safety net programs. These include Supplemental Security Income (SSI), Social Security Disability Insurance (SSDI), Medicaid, and Medicare.

The Coalition of Citizens With Disabilities

This organization serves as an umbrella for organizations/coalitions that serve specific disability groups. Coalition of Citizens with Disabilities (CCD) was instrumental in working with regional and state-based chapters/groups in a massive letter writing/telephone blitz to elected representatives during the passage of the ADA of 1990. Through the concerted efforts of this coalition, the ADA became a focused effort spearheaded by the CCD to educate and promote the importance of the passage of this bill within the House of Representatives and Senate.

The Pioneer Network Coalition

The Pioneer Network Coalition's mission is to transform the culture of long-term care settings for older adults and people with disabilities into person-centered care opportunities. The national office facilitates state-wide efforts to promote state coalition activities. These activities often include educational programs and networking meetings for providers, communications including a newsletter and a website, and education of policy makers and regulators about culture change. Consumer involvement and education is also an important activity for state coalitions.

While these three examples merely provide a thumbnail sketch for coalitions, their success has embodied the principles outlined in this chapter.

SUMMARY

In summary, coalition building is not an easy venture, nor is it reasonable to expect the novice program or policy advocate to have the leadership skills necessary to successfully build coalitions. The art and science of effective coalition building lies both in understanding group dynamics and providing leadership to work toward a common agenda and goal. This chapter reviews some of the salient ingredients for effective coalition building.

ADDITIONAL RESOURCES

Websites

Coalition Building Tool Kit: https://ctb.ku.edu/en

This website links one to a section on coalition building, which is a part of a Community Toolbox series, developed through the University of Kansas. It provides examples, related topics, tools, and checklists for effective coalition building.

National Coalition Building Institute: www.ncbi.org

This website serves as the home page for the National Coalition Building Institute, an international nonprofit leadership training organization. It provides training on coalition building, as well as a manual for leaders and activists for building coalitions.

The Partnership Self-Assessment Tool: https://atrium.lib.uoguelph.ca/xmlui/bitstream/handle/10214/3129/Partnership_Self-Assessment_Tool-Questionnaire_complete.pdf?sequence=1&isAllowed=y

This assessment tool enables coalitions to assess how well their collaboration is doing in the areas of leadership, administration, and resources. It provides insight into how to improve the process and helps the group showcase its strengths to potential funders. This web-based resource from the Center for the Advancement of Collaborative Health originated from the New York Academy of Medicine.

Coalition Sustainability: Long-Term Successes and Lessons Learned: www.joe.org/joe/2002february/a2.php

This site provides an article that examines the impact of a coalition and its impact 10 years following the inception and development. It reviews lessons learned from the longevity of the project and provide guidance for other programs and coalitions.

Videos

SDN Interviews: The Coalition for Disability Access in Health Science and Medical Education: www.youtube.com/watch?v=-T4079LwZy4

This video focuses on the concept of building a coalition to improve access to information for people with disabilities and build upon resources for medical education.

Coalition for Disability: http://videos.myacpa.org/home

This video gallery showcases a coalition that has been active in spearheading services for people with disabilities.

How to Build a Coalition: www.youtube.com/watch?v=43E23A-UyIc

This video provides an overview of strategies to build a coalition for older people and prepare for care transitions.

DISCUSSION QUESTIONS

1. What coalitions currently exist in either your community or your state? Is it possible for you to participate either as a community representative or an observer?
2. What local agendas have led to the development of specific coalitions for either older adults or people with disabilities? What has been the impact of these efforts?
3. If people have been involved with local coalitions, what variables have helped the coalition to be successful? What variables have led to slow the progress of the coalition?

REFERENCES

Butterfoss, F. D. (2013). *Ignite! Getting your community coalition fired up for change*. Bloomington, IN: AuthorHouse.

Gallagher, K., Stanley, A., Shearer, D., & Klerman, L. (2006). Challenges in data collection, analysis, and distribution of information in community coalition projects. *Journal of Adolescent Health, 37*(3), S53–S60. doi:10.1016/j.jadohealth.2005.05.008

Huan, L. J., & Yazdanifard, R. (2012). The difference of conflict management styles and conflict resolution in the workplace. *Business and Entrepreneurship Journal, 1*(1), 141–155. Retrieved from http://www.scienpress.com/Upload/BEJ/Vol%201_1_9.pdf

Karp, H. B., & Osirias, D. (2001). Generational conflict: A new paradigm for teams of the 21st century. *Gestalt Review*, *5*(2), 71–87. doi:10.5325/gestaltreview.5.2.0071

Minnix, W. L., Jr, & Roadman, C. H, II. (2002). Health care coalition building. *Journal of the American Medical Directors Association*, 3(6), 397–399 doi:10.1016/S1525-8610(04)70536-8.

National Association of Social Workers. (2017). *NASW code of ethics*. Retrieved from https://www.socialworkers.org/About/Ethics/Code-of-Ethics/Code-of-Ethics-English

Ospina, S., & Saz-Carranza, A. (2005, August 5). *Paradox and collaboration in coalition work*. Paper presented at the 2005 Annual Meeting of the Academy of Management, Honolulu, HI.

Pew Research Center. (2015). *The whys and hows of generations research*. Retrieved from http://www.people-press.org/2015/09/03/the-whys-and-hows-of-generations-research

Sipe, C. (2005, September-October). Building an active aging coalition. *The Journal on Active Aging*, 60–67.

U.S. Department of Health and Human Services. (1999). *Mental health: A report of the surgeon general—executive summary*. Rockville, MD: U.S. Department of Health and Human Services, Substance Abuse and Mental Health Services Administration, Center for Mental Health Services, National Institutes of Health, National Institute of Mental Health.

18

Needs Assessment Tools

LEARNING OBJECTIVES

At the end of this chapter readers will:

1. *Understand what a needs assessment is and be acquainted with a framework within which to conduct a needs assessment.*
2. *Be familiar with the core concepts of a needs assessment.*
3. *Be familiar with strategies that encompass a needs assessment.*

> *Erica and Theresa have identified a number of areas of strength as they have pursued their community-wide scan. Now that they have done so, they want to identify a strategy for others to use within the realm of needs assessments. Consider how they unfold this process within this chapter.*

INTRODUCTION

Broadly defined, a needs assessment is a systematic process of activities that are conducted in order to help an individual or system set priorities and make decisions about a program, make decisions about ways to improve an organization, or identify ways to allocate resources. Priorities can be based on identified needs. Needs assessments can be used for a number of different purposes; however, the main role can be seen as estimating the extent of demand for a specific service or program (Kirst-Ashman & Hall, 2002). Many successful health education and promotion programs have been designed through the use of innovative and comprehensive needs assessment approaches (Bibbs, 2001; Calderon, Baker, & Wolf, 2000;Fouad et al., 2004; Fuller, Bentley, & Shotton, 2001; Jordan et al., 2002; Weist, Lowie, Flaherty, & Pruitt, 2001).

Needs are usually identified as the difference between what is or the present state of the way things are and what should be or a desired state of affairs. Hence, needs assessments try to identify what is, determine the discrepancies, look at the reason for these differences, and build resources to meet these gaps (Witkin & Altschuld, 1995). Needs assessments are very important for the process of developing new resources or determining whether there are new trends in needs at individual or community levels. The impact of bioterrorism on resources for communities caring for older adults is one such example (Shadel et al., 2002). A needs assessment can also help to identify a gap in resources within a community level that resulted from policy changes (Thompson,

 DOI:10.1891/9780826128393.0018

Howard, & Jin, 2001). Needs for new programs or needs for policy revisions can also be identified through needs assessments. Ideally, this is the first step when building a case to rationalize the need for a new program or service.

WHO IS RESPONSIBLE FOR CARRYING OUT NEEDS ASSESSMENTS?

Needs assessments can be carried out by a wide cast of people. Social workers and public health workers, as well as city planners, can carry out needs assessments, as can government organizations. Local citizens or groups of people can also be responsible for carrying out a needs assessment. These groups have been known to band together and work as a citizen's action group. Many groups can actually carry out needs assessments, such as city or governmental planning groups (to identify community needs or needs for resources), local Area Agencies on Aging (for the purpose of identifying programmatic needs), faith-based organizations, and local charity groups.

WHY WOULD INDIVIDUALS, GROUPS, OR ORGANIZATIONS BE INTERESTED IN CONDUCTING A NEEDS ASSESSMENT?

Regardless of the size, individuals, groups, communities, or organizations would be interested in carrying out a needs assessment as a strategy to make sure that resources are in place to help meet the needs of all members of a specific constituency group or community. We often think of the planning process in a casework situation as one mechanism that a caseworker may use to develop a profile of individual needs. Similarly, peer support groups for older adults would assess the needs prior to the onset of a group intervention to decide what to focus on within the group intervention. Communities or organizations will conduct needs assessments to help define to what extent a given population may be subject to a specific issue or phenomenon.

A prime example of a community needs assessment is the area plan, which is conducted on a regular basis by local Area Agencies on Aging to help develop a profile, statewide, of needs or areas to focus on as services or resources are built, revised, or developed. The use of a needs assessment is also vital in the development of new programs and services or revision or development of new policies or legislative efforts. Without an accurate picture of the current strengths and resources within a community, it becomes difficult to develop realistic and strategic resources in a rational and comprehensive manner.

CORE CONCEPTS OR BUILDING BLOCKS THAT SERVE AS A FOUNDATION FOR NEEDS ASSESSMENTS

A number of core concepts serve as building blocks or as the foundation for needs assessments. Some of these concepts include need, target groups, systems, outcome, plan of evidence, and evidence base. In this section, each of these concepts is examined and showcased.

Need

Need is defined as a gap in programs or services where some form of support or resources are required.

Target Groups

Target groups refer to the specific groups who will be the beneficiary of action or for whom an organization intends to lobby for change. Usually target groups are identified in the process in order to develop a blueprint for action. For example, specific age groups of older adults into (60+ preretirement, 65+ retired, young old, middle old, and frail elderly are examples of target groups) may be targeted.

Systems

Systems generally include three levels of systems, defined as micro-, meso-, and macrosystems. Micro refers to the most basic of systems and considers the individual or issues that impact the individual person. At the individual level, an advocate or organization is working to examine a person and that individual's specific needs.

Meso or the mesosystem refers to a group or two or more people within a system. A family may be considered a mesosystem, as well as a group work intervention.

Macro refers to a community or broader system, which takes in the bigger picture. Policy decisions or governmental legislation usually affect the macro level.

Stakeholders are people who have a specific interest in a policy, program, or interest group. They are generally people who may be affected by a new policy, practice, or lack of resources.

Outcomes

Outcomes are the end product of some specific action or intervention. Outcomes can occur at the micro, meso, or macro levels. Outcomes can also be thought of as one's expectations, or what one would like to accomplish as a result of a program, policy, or intervention.

Plan of Action

A plan of action can be thought of as a blueprint or road map to describe a series of activities, responsible parties, and due dates. A plan of action can relate to the implementation of a needs assessment, program, evaluation of a program, or policy initiative.

Evidence Base

Evidence base refers to the process of using empirical data to justify a program or service. It consists of factual objective data rather than opinion or interest group initiatives. It also provides an objective perspective of the issue at hand. A number of secondary data sources are often used in the process of objective assessment, as outlined in Chapter 4.

STRATEGIES FOR DEVELOPING A NEEDS ASSESSMENT

Several strategies can be used in the process of developing this inventory of community resources and gaps in the resources. Kirst-Ashman and Hall (2002) identify five specific strategies; social indicators, key informants, community forum, a survey, and agency-related data. Each is important and can make a significant contribution in part or in combination with other methods to a composite sketch of a community's needs.

Social Indicators

Social indicators include demographic indicators that provide a profile of the community or specific geographic area. Such indicators can be extracted from census data or vital statistics and provide an overview of the context of a community. These indicators can also provide some context for comparing a community with a state, regional, or national picture or comparative contexts among different countries. A number of websites can be used to gain access to this information, including the U.S. Census Bureau (www.census.gov), local area health departments (linked via the individual state departments of public health websites), local Area Agencies on Aging websites, state-based departments on aging, and the Centers for Disease Control and Prevention (www.cdc.gov).

A number of variables can be used as social indicators to provide profiles of a specific community. Some of the specific social indicators that could be useful in the planning process include the following variables:

- Population profile (number of people in 5-year increments, used to create a population pyramid, or the rate of people/percentage of people over 65 years of age)
- Population pyramid (male and female)
- Education level
- Housing
- Employment profiles
- Ethnicity
- Marital status
- Literacy rates
- Unemployment and poverty rates
- Number of people affected with mobility limitations
- Number of people affected with specific health conditions
- Morbidity rates
- Mortality rates

These items provide a sampling of potential variables that can be used to present a demographic profile of the community to be served. These variables can develop a composite sketch of a community and provide a profile to make the case for needed services, programs, or policies. Table 18.1 provides some useful sources of information that can provide social indicator data.

Key Informants

Key informants are people who can give you an idea about what is happening from their perspective within a specific community of interest. The key informant approach asks especially knowledgeable individuals about the needs of a given community who are sought out to share their opinions about needs in a particular area (Kirst-Ashman & Hall, 2002). Key informants can be individuals who are well connected with the communities for which they serve. Key informants can run the gamut from being the mayor, precinct captain, representatives from aging-related services, or local elders in the community who are well connected with people or resources within a given

Table 18.1 Data Sources for Needs Assessments

Source	Website/Homepage
U. S. Census Bureau	(www.census.gov) Local area health departments (vital statistics)
Local Area Agencies on Aging websites (Eldercare locator)	(eldercare.acl.gov/Public/Index.aspx) State-based departments on aging (contact information available in Table 18.3)
The CDC	(www.cdc.gov)
CDC: Healthy Aging Data	(www.cdc.gov/aging/agingdata/index.html)
Administration for Community Living: AGID	(agid.acl.gov/)

AGID, AGing Integrated Database; CDC, Centers for Disease Control and Prevention.

community or region. Key informants can provide much insight into community resources, strengths, activities, individuals, and groups.

Typically, we tend to think of key informants as individuals who are formal leaders in the community; however, Kretzmann and McKnight (1993) suggest that key informants can be drawn from all walks of life within the community and suggest that those individuals well connected through social ties can also provide much insight into the natural resources and assets within a community. Their workbook, *Building Communities From the Inside Out: A Path Toward Finding and Mobilizing a Community's Assets*, provides a step-by-step approach to utilizing and mobilizing disenfranchised groups to better understand the community and its available assets. They also make the argument that the most effective key informants are people who have had longstanding consumer roots within communities and can provide a perspective on some of the hidden talents and resources within community settings. Older adults, especially retirees, can often fit into this realm and provide skills, expertise, and consultation on a range of issues, often at low or no cost. Hence, this pool of key stakeholders should not be discounted or ignored.

Community Forum

A community forum is designed to hear a variety of voices from the community. Public notice is given, and people from the community attend to share their perspectives. This approach assumes that the general public has some awareness of a community's needs. Usually there are widely advertised meetings within communities, which are held in community settings in order to bring together a cross section of people. Community forums held within senior centers or senior nutrition sites are generally well accepted by older adults who make use of these settings and are an excellent way to seek input from seniors about their perceptions of community-based needs for older adults. This approach is commonly used by area agencies on aging when deciding on priorities for a community's area plan.

The steps to conducting an area plan are not complex and are generally relatively inexpensive to carry out. A facilitator identifies a specific date, time, and setting for a community forum to take place. Once these details are decided, local advertising can take place, which can be followed up with public service announcements, or announcements within a local meal site. During the actual "speak out" or community forum, people are given an opportunity to present ideas in front of a group using a microphone. The facilitators or assessment team should be available to transcribe these ideas and provide transcripts of the meeting. If resources permit, these can also be audio- or video-recorded and transcribed. Participants may also provide written testimony to the facilitation team, which can be incorporated into the assessment plan.

Field Study and Survey Data

In field studies and survey data, information is collected in order to identify issues and trends related to a specific topic area. Academic partners or university entities are often very helpful in this process. In this approach, the needs assessment is based on gathering data in the community through focus group sessions, and through a completed survey instrument, with preidentified questions. Methodologists would refer to the survey questionnaire as a quantitative approach to data collection, since the responses developed within the survey instrument are usually closed ended and have been predetermined.

Rates Under Treatment or Agency Service Data

The rates under treatment approach uses a specific count of people who are currently receiving services (e.g., home healthcare) to estimate the actual need for services within a given community. These service statistics relate to the numbers of clients who use a specific service. Once it is clear what issues or programs/services one would like to explore, a specific set of variables can be identified, and service statistics can be used to develop a profile of these variables of concern. Service statistics can include the number of home-delivered meals provided, case management and screening, transportation services provided, and in-home counseling of recipients to name a few. Table 18.2 provides an overview of some service statistics for services provided via a local area agency on aging.

Healthcare professionals and social workers may want to contact their state department on aging office for an overview of state, regional, and area-based service statistics. A contact listing is provided in Table 18.3.

Focus Groups

The focus group approach takes advantage of a specific, select group of individuals who can share their insights on a particular phenomenon or situation. This approach can be useful to identify gaps in services or potential and innovative solutions and help with the construction of new survey instruments that can be used in the quantitative approach to data collection. Methodologists would identify the focus group approach as a qualitative method of data collection.

Table 18.2 A Sample Overview of Service Statistics

Access Services	Persons Served	Units of Service	Areas Served
Case management[a]	3,250	6,100	13 Counties
Information and assistance[a]	9,000	14,000	13 Counties
Outreach[a]	5,500	5,500	13 Counties
Transportation[a]	650	19,066	10 Counties[b]
In-home services			
Home-delivered meals	2,000	320,000	13 Counties
Residential repair (home modifications[a])	40	40	13 Counties
Community services			
Congregate meals	2,400	230,000	13 Counties
Legal assistance[a]	650	9,000	13 Counties
Routine health screening	2,500	1,350	13 Counties
Health promotion	600	225	6 Counties
Physical fitness and group exercise	60	180	3 Counties
Medication management	60	200	13 Counties
Gerontological counseling (can be provided in-home)	25	285	13 Counties
Ombudsman	3,910	4,110	13 Counties

Family Caregivers Support Program (For Family Caregivers and Grandparents Raising Grandchildren)	Persons Served		Units of Service		Areas Served
	Caregivers	Grand parents	Caregivers	Grand parents	
Information	2400	10	4,000	10	13 Counties
Outreach	1,400	2	1,400	2	13 Counties

(continued)

Table 18.2 A Sample Overview of Service Statistics (*continued*)

Family Caregivers Support Program (For Family Caregivers and Grandparents Raising Grandchildren)	Persons Served		Units of Service		Areas Served
	Caregivers	Grand parents	Caregivers	Grand parents	
Case management	550	15	800	50	13 Counties
Counseling for family caregivers	35	3	225	60	13 Counties
Seminars, workshops, and education	115	20	90	4	13 Counties
Respite care (in-home and adult day service)	150	1	8,000	25	13 Counties
Supplemental "gap-filling" services	15	15	15	15	13 Counties
Legal assistance	40	4	300	50	13 Counties

Notes:
[a]These services are a priority for receiving Supportive Service funds.
[b]Every county has transportation services, but some counties rely on other funding sources to provide rides to senior adults.

Source: Egyptian Area Agency on Aging.

Table 18.3 Departments on Aging/Community Living Contact List in the United States

States/ Agency Name	Director	Address	Telephone	Email and/or Website Address
Alabama Department of Senior Services	Todd Cotton	PO Box 301851 201 Monroe St, Suite 350 Montgomery, AL 36130-1851	334-242-5743	www.alabamaageline.gov ageline@adss.alabama.gov
Alaska Department of Health and Social Services	Denise Daniello	150 Third Street, #103 PO Box 110693 Juneau, AK 99811-0693	907-465-3250	www.alaskaaging.org

(*continued*)

Table 18.3 Departments on Aging/Community Living Contact List in the United States (*continued*)

States/ Agency Name	Director	Address	Telephone	Email and/or Website Address
Arizona Division of Aging and Adult Services	Priscilla Kadi	Arizona State Unit on Aging Department of Economic Security 1789 West Jefferson Street, #950A Phoenix, AZ 85007	602-542-4446	https://des.az.gov/services/aging-and-adult/division-aging-and-adult-services
Arkansas Division of Aging and Adult Services	Craig Cloud	Department of Human Services PO Box 1437, slot S530 700 Main Street, 5th Floor, S530 Little Rock, AR 72203-1437	501-682-2441	www.daas.ar.gov aging.services@arkansas.gov
California Department of Aging	Lora Connolly	1300 National Drive, #200 Sacramento, CA 95834	916-419-7500	www.aging.ca.gov webmaster@aging.ca.gov
Colorado Commission on Aging	Todd Coffey	Department of Human Services 1575 Sherman St, 10th Floor Denver, CO 80203-1714	303-866-5288	www.colorado.gov/pacific/cdhs-boards-committees-collaboration/colorado-commission-aging tara.franck@state.co.us
Connecticut State Unit on Aging	Amy Porter	Department of Rehabilitation Services 55 Farmington Avenue, 12th Floor Hartford, CT 06106	860-424-5992	www.ct.gov/agingservices/site/default.asp aging.sda@ct.gov

(*continued*)

Table 18.3 Departments on Aging/Community Living Contact List in the United States (*continued*)

States/ Agency Name	Director	Address	Telephone	Email and/or Website Address
Delaware Division of Services for Aging and Adult with Disabilities	Kara Odom Walker	Department of Health and Social Services 1901 North DuPont Highway New Castle, DE 19720	800-223-9074	www.dhss.delaware.gov/dhss/dsaapd DelawareADRC@state.de.us
District of Columbia D.C. Office on Aging	Laura Newland	500 K Street, NE Washington, DC 20002	202-724-5626	dcoa.dc.gov dcoa@dc.gov
Florida Department of Elder Affairs	Jeffrey Bragg	4040 Esplanade Way, Suite 315 Tallahassee, FL 32399-7000	850-414-2000	elderaffairs.state.fl.us information@elderaffairs.org
Georgia Division of Aging Services	Abby Cox	Department of Human Services 2 Peachtree St. N.W. 33rd Floor Atlanta, GA 30303	404-657-5258	aging.georgia.gov
Hawaii Executive Office on Aging	Terri Byers	No. 1 Capitol District 250 South Hotel Street, Suite 406 Honolulu, HI 96813-2831	808-586-0100	health.hawaii.gov/eoa eoa@doh.hawaii.gov
Idaho Commission on Aging	Sam Haws	341 W. Washington Street, 3rd Floor PO Box 83720 Boise, ID 83702-0007	208-334-3833 x226	www.idahoaging.com deedra.hunt@aging.idaho.gov

(*continued*)

Table 18.3 Departments on Aging/Community Living Contact List in the United States (*continued*)

States/ Agency Name	Director	Address	Telephone	Email and/or Website Address
Illinois Department on Aging	Jean Bohnhoff	One Natural Resources Way, Suite 100 Springfield, IL 62702-1271	800-252-8966	www2.illinois.gov/aging/Pages/default.aspx aging.ilsenior@illinois.gov
Indiana Family and Social Services Administration, Division of Aging	Sarah Renner	402 W. Washington Street PO Box 7083, MS21 Room W-454 Indianapolis, IN 46204-7083	317-232-1731	www.state.in.us/fssa/2329.htm Patti.Bailey@fssa.IN.gov
Iowa Department on Aging	Linda Miller	Jessie Parker Building 510 East 12th St, Suite 2 Des Moines, IA 50319-9025	515-725-3333 800-532-3213	www.iowaaging.gov
Kansas Department for Aging and Disability Services	Tim Keck	New England Building 503 S. Kansas Avenue Topeka, KS 66603-3404	785-296-4986	www.kdads.ks.gov kdads.wwwmail@ks.gov
Kentucky Department for Aging and Independent Living	Lala Williams	275 East Main Street, 3E-E Frankfort, KY 40621	502-564-6930	chfs.ky.gov/agencies/dail/Pages/default.aspx DAIL.general@ky.gov
Louisiana Governor's Office of Elderly Affairs	Karen Ryder	525 Florida Street, 4th and 2nd Floors Baton Rouge, LA 70801-1732	225-342-7100	goea.louisiana.gov elderlyaffairs@goea.la.gov

(*continued*)

Table 18.3 Departments on Aging/Community Living Contact List in the United States (*continued*)

States/ Agency Name	Director	Address	Telephone	Email and/or Website Address
Maine Office of Aging and Disability Services	Amy MacMillan	11 State House Station 41 Anthony Avenue Augusta, Maine 04333	207-287-9200	www.maine.gov/dhhs/oads
Maryland Department on Aging	Rona Kramer	301 West Preston Street, Suite 1007 Baltimore, MD 21201	410-767-1100	www.mdoa.state.md.us webmail@ooa.state.md.us
Massachusetts Executive Office of Elder Affairs	Alice Bonner	One Ashburton Place, 5_{th} Floor Boston, MA 02108	617-222-7550	www.mass.gov/orgs/executive-office-of-elder-affairs elder.affairs@state.ma.us
Minnesota Board on Aging	Kari Benson	504 Cedar Street St. Paul, MN 55155	651-431-2500	www.mnaging.org mba.dhs@state.mn.us
Mississippi Division of Aging and Adult Services	John Davis	750 North State Street Jackson, MS 39202	601-359-4929 601-359-4915	www.mdhs.ms.gov/adults-seniors
Missouri Division of Senior and Disability Services	Jessica Bax	Department of Health and Senior Services PO Box 570 Jefferson City, MO 65102-0570	573-526-3626	health.mo.gov/seniors info@health.mo.gov
Montana Senior and Long-Term Care Division	Barb Smith	2030 11th Avenue Helena, MT 59601	406-444-4077	dphhs.mt.gov/sltc

(*continued*)

Table 18.3 Departments on Aging/Community Living Contact List in the United States (*continued*)

States/ Agency Name	Director	Address	Telephone	Email and/or Website Address
Nebraska Health and Human Services-State Unit on Aging	Cynthia Brammeier	PO Box 95026 301 Centennial Mall- South Lincoln, NE 68509	402-471-2307	dhhs.ne.gov/medicaid/Aging/Pages/AgingHome.aspx DHHS.Aging@Nebraska.gov
Nevada Aging and Disability Services Division	Dena Schmidt	3416 Goni Road, Building D-132 Carson City, NV 89706	775-687-4210	adsd.nv.gov adsd@adsd.nv.gov
New Hampshire Bureau of Elderly and Adult Services	Wendi Aultman	105 Pleasant Street Concord, NH 03301-3857	603-271-9203	www.dhhs.nh.gov/dcbcs/beas/index.htm
New Jersey Division of Aging Services	Louise Rush	PO Box 700 Trenton, NJ 08625-0707	877-222-3737	www.aging.nj.gov
New Mexico Aging and Long-Term Services Department	Lora M. Churh	2550 Cerrillos Road Santa Fe, NM 87505	505-476-4799	www.nmaging.state.nm.us
New York Office for the Aging	Greg Olsen	Two Empire State Plaza Albany, NY 12223-1251	844-697-6321	www.aging.ny.gov
North Carolina Division of Aging and Adult Services	Suzanne Merrill	2001 Mail Service Center 693 Palmer Drive Raleigh, NC 27699-2001	919-855-3400	www.ncdhhs.gov/aging Suzanne.Merrill@dhhs.nc.gov

(*continued*)

Table 18.3 Departments on Aging/Community Living Contact List in the United States (*continued*)

States/ Agency Name	Director	Address	Telephone	Email and/or Website Address
North Dakota Aging Services Division	Janet E. Engan	1237 West Divide Avenue, Suite 6 Bismarck, ND 58501	855-462-5465	www.carechoice.nd.gov carechoice@nd.gov
Ohio Department of Aging	Beverley L. Laubert	246 North High Street 1st Floor Columbus, OH 43215-2406	866-243-5678	aging.ohio.gov
Oklahoma Aging Services Division	Karen Poteet	50 NE 23rd Street City, OK 73105	405-521-2281	www.okdhs.org/services/aging/Pages/AgingServicesMain.aspx
Oregon Aging and People with Disabilities Program	Ashley Carson-Cottingham	Department of Human Services 500 Summer Street, NE, E12 Salem, OR 97301-1073	503-945-5858	www.oregon.gov/dhs/seniors-disabilities/Pages/index.aspx
Pennsylvania Department of Aging	Teresa Osborne	555 Walnut Street, 5th Floor Harrisburg, PA 17101-1919	717-783-1550	www.aging.pa.gov/Pages/default.aspx#.VL5ibC7bPwA aging@pa.gov
Puerto Rico Office for Elderly Affairs	Carmen Delia Sánchez Salgado	PO Box 191179 San Juan, PR 00919-1179	787-822-6559	www.agencias.pr.gov/agencias/oppea/Pages/default.aspx
South Carolina Lieutenant Governor's Office on Aging	Darryl Broome	1301 Gervais Street, Suite 200 Columbia, SC 29201	803-734-9900	www.aging.sc.gov askus@aging.sc.gov

(*continued*)

Table 18.3 Departments on Aging/Community Living Contact List in the United States (*continued*)

States/ Agency Name	Director	Address	Telephone	Email and/or Website Address
South Dakota Division of Long-Term Services and Supports	Yvette Thomas	3800 E. Hwy 34 c/o E. Capitol Ave. Pierre, SD 57507	605-773-4085	https:// dss.sd.gov/asa
Tennessee Commission on Aging and Disability	Jim Shulman	502 Deaderick Street, 9th Floor Nashville, TN 37243-0860	615-741-2056	www.tn.gov/aging laverdia.mccullough@tn.gov
Texas Department of Aging and Disability Services	Jon Weizenbaum	John H. Winters Human Services Complex 701 West 51st Street PO Box 149030 (W-619) Austin, TX 78714-9030	512-438-3030	www.dads.state.tx.us mail@dads.state.tx.us
Utah Division of Aging and Adult Services	Nels Holmgren	195 North 1950 West, 3rd Floor Salt Lake City, UT 84116	801-538-3921	daas.utah.gov nholmgren@utah.gov
Vermont Department of Disabilities, Aging, and Independent Living	Monica Caserta Hutt	HC2 South, 280 State Drive Waterbury, VT 05671-2020	802-871-3350 802-241-2401	www.dail.vermont.gov
Virginia Department for Aging and Rehabilitative Services	James Rothrock	8004 Franklin Farms Drive Henrico, VA 23229	804-662-7000	www.vadars.org

(*continued*)

Table 18.3 Departments on Aging/Community Living Contact List in the United States (*continued*)

States/ Agency Name	Director	Address	Telephone	Email and/or Website Address
Washington Aging and Long-Term Support Administration	Bill Moss	4450 10th Avenue SE Blake West Lacey, WA 98503	360-725-2300	www.dshs.wa.gov/altsa
West Virginia Bureau of Senior Services	Robert Roswall	1900 Kanawha Boulevard, East 3003 Town Center Mall Charleston, WV 25305-0160	304-558-3317	www.wvseniorservices.gov
Wisconsin Bureau on Aging and Disability Resources	Carrie Molke	Wisconsin Department of Health Services One West Wilson Street PO Box 7851 Madison, WI 53707-7851	608-267-5267	www.dhs.wisconsin.gov/dph/badr.htm carrie.molke@dhs.wisconsin.gov
Wyoming Aging Division	Lisa Osvold	2300 Capitol Avenue, 4th Floor Cheyenne, WY 82002	307-777-7995	health.wyo.gov/aging

Source: National Association of States United for Aging and Disabilities. (2016, June 17). *National Association of States United for Aging and Disabilities*. Retrieved from National Association of States United for Aging and Disabilities: About State Agencies List of Members: http://www.nasuad.org/about-nasuad/about-state-agencies/list-members

A focus group relies upon a small number of individuals who are well informed on a specific issue. Generally, it is best to select a manageable number—six to 12 participants works best. These people are invited to meet at a predesignated time and are selected because of the perspective that they can bring to the table on specific concerns and issues. Subjects are recruited by an invitational letter, asking them to attend a focus group on a specific date. Best results occur when the written invitation is followed up with an oral invitation. Prior to the meeting, a series of open-ended questions is drafted by the facilitators. Although not necessary, preparing these questions and placing each question on a color-coded sheet of paper, or 3- by 5-inch index card can be a real organizational asset during the focus group. A nominal group technique (NGT) process (Dunham, 1998) can also be used to discuss answers among the group members.

Since there are always people within a group who are more vocal and who will dominate a conversation, this approach assures that each member of a group will have the opportunity to contribute his or her thoughts and perspectives. Once all questions have been reviewed and the participants have had an opportunity to respond in writing, the facilitator generates a discussion to solicit feedback from the participants on their responses. This discussion can be handled by reviewing each question, one by one, and allowing participants to share responses and highlights from their index cards. This discussion can be tape-recorded and transcribed following the group discussion. Both the response cards and transcribed notes from the discussion can be used in the process of content analysis. The end results will be a set of transcriptions that then will be used to articulate main themes or issues from the focus group approach. Figure 18.1 provides an example of focus group questions, and an index card prepared in advance of coordinating a focus group.

Environmental Scans

An environment scan is an analysis and evaluation of internal conditions and external data and factors that affect the organization (Government of Saskatchewan, 2006). The process of an environmental scan identifies an understanding of the current environment in a particular field or subject area through the key components of the strengths, weaknesses, opportunities, and threats ("SWOT") analysis, using key informants and other resources. The major aim of an environmental scan is to identify trends, gaps, and issues as a basis for future planning.

A SWOT analysis provides an overview of a community area or organizational network. This SWOT process makes use of a small group discussion process among key stakeholders, who are divided into four specific groups. Each group examines the entity's SWOT. Once compiled, each of these aspects can be arranged into one complete picture to illustrate the culture or community.

Cario Senior Center's Focus Group Questions

1. Please list as many services that you are aware of for seniors (people 60 years of age and older) in Cairo and/ or other areas of Alexander County.
2. Happy Days is a Senior Center for Seniors in the community who are over the age of 60 and a resource center for caregivers of older adults. Can you list some reasons why people do and do not use the services?
   Do use   Do not use
3. How can the community be more involved with the Senior Center?
4. What resources or programs would you like to see for seniors in Cario and Alexander County
5. What could make this senior center a more vital resource for the community?
6. How do we get the word out to seniors about the Senior Centers and the services they offer?
7. Who are community people not here at this table whom we should be taking to about senior services?
8. Is there anything else that you think is important that we should be aware of to help us strengthen these resources for seniors?

Figure 18.1 Sample focus group questions.

The National Council on Aging, in collaboration with three other aging-related organizations, the Center for Healthy Aging, the Home Safety Council, and the Archstone Foundation, created an environmental scan to examine the issue of falls. Their document entitled *Falls Free: Promoting a National Falls Prevention Action Plan* examined the SWOT to demonstrate how these selected organizations and agencies were addressing falls prevention in older adults.

Once each of these areas is identified by the key constituents, some of the same basic strategies identified within this chapter can be used to identify the component parts of this needs assessment. Some examples of how these strategies have been incorporated can be found in areas such as chronic care and community-based resources (Branch, 2000); health visiting (Cowley & Houston, 2003; Cowley, Mitcheson, & Houston, 2004), and community health education (Cowley, Bergen, Young, & Kavanagh, 2000).

A MODEL FOR NEEDS ASSESSMENT

Key questions or issues to consider in the process of needs assessment can be placed in a model to help conceptualize and organize information. This model includes an examination of some of the questions raised in Figure 18.2.

Step 1: Identify the problem.

Step 2: Develop a definition of the problem so the assessment administrator and all stakeholders have a specific and clear understanding of what terms mean.

Step 3: Identify the extent of the problem through the use of existing and secondary data sources such as vital statistics and service statistics.

Step 4: Identify what key stakeholders tell about the problem and their perception of it.

Step 5: Identify what community members perceive about the problem through community forums.

Step 6: Analyze the various perspectives and look for agreement and areas of difference among perspectives.

Step 7: Develop an inventory of resources available within the community to deal with the problem and enable resolution.

Step 8: Identify what resources are still needed in order to bring the issue or problem/concern to resolution.

- **What is the problem?**
- **What is the extent of the problem?**
- **What do we know from the existing data, such as vital statistics, secondary data, and services statistics?**
- **How is the problem defined?**
- **What do key stakeholders tell us about the problem?**
- **What do community forums reveal about this problem?**
- **Who agrees and who disagrees—stakeholder perspectives?**
- **What resources are available within the community to deal with the problem or enable resolution?**
- **What resources are still needed to meet the gap in needs?**

Figure 18.2 Sample framework for needs assessment.

SUMMARY

A community needs assessment can be an ideal vehicle to enable the program planner or policy analyst the opportunity to identify the needs of the community, size up the strengths and weaknesses of the current program or policy, and identify strategies for moving forward and building resources. This chapter provides an overview of strategies to develop a needs assessment. When used in combination with a health behavior framework, a needs assessment can help one determine the needs of a community and attempt to build community support for this resource or policy change through media advocacy and coalition building.

ADDITIONAL RESOURCES

Websites

Community Tool Box: https://ctb.ku.edu/en/table-of-contents/assessment/assessing-community-needs-and-resources/conducting-needs-assessment-surveys/main

This website links to a section on conducting needs assessment surveys, which is a part of a Community Toolbox series, developed through the University of Kansas. It provides examples, related topics, tools, and checklists.

NOAA Coastal Services Center: www.coast.noaa.gov/needsassessment/#1

This website provides an overview of how to develop assessment instruments and questionnaires, facilitates an understanding of where needs assessments fit into the project development process and provides some basic steps to the novice on conducting needs assessments.

Handbook for needs assessment in Ohio's Aging Network: http://agefriendlycolumbus.org/wp-content/uploads/2016/08/2014_Central-Ohio-Older-Adult-Needs-Assessment.pdf

This link connects the reader to a handbook for needs assessments, which was developed by Ohio's Aging Network. It also provides some sample needs assessment surveys.

Conducting Environmental Scans: www.horizon.unc.edu/courses/papers/enviroscan/index.html

This link provides a primer for environmental scanning. The text was initially seen as a chapter in a primer for new researchers. It provides the novice with some basic skills in conducting environmental scans.

YouTube Videos

Community Needs Assessment in Action: www.youtube.com/watch?v=hi1pHf8LFb4

This YouTube video provides an overview of how one community developed its own community needs assessment to build healthcare resources.

Aha Moments in Needs Assessments: www.bing.com/videos/search?q=u+tube+videos+on+needs+assessments&&view=detail&mid=79B65BC40767A4C666F879B65BC40767A4C666F8&FORM=VRDGAR

This YouTube video provides the viewer with some hands-on examples of using needs assessments within communities for the purpose of building community health resources.

Podcast

Miriam Link-Mullison discusses needs assessments and public health. **Listen now:** https://bcove.video/2DwpDDU

DISCUSSION QUESTIONS

1. What steps would you take to begin to develop a community-based needs assessment within your community to address the needs of people growing older or people with disabilities using the framework provided in this chapter?
2. What data sources would you use in this process of needs assessment referred to in Question 1?
3. How can you use a series of Focus Groups to help identify needs for the community and community needs assessment?
4. How would you use the sample framework in Figure 18.2 to build a needs assessment?
5. How would you use a logic model to help build a community needs assessment?

REFERENCES

Bibb, S. C. (2001). Mary J. Nielubowicz essay award. Population-based needs assessment in the design of patient education programs. *Military Medicine, 166*(4), 297–300. doi:10.1093/milmed/166.4.297

Branch, L. G. (2000). Assessment of chronic care need and use. *Gerontologist, 40*(4), 390–396. doi:10.1093/geront/40.4.390

Calderon, J. L., Baker R. S., & Wolf, K. E. (2000). Focus groups: A qualitative method complementing quantitative research for studying culturally diverse groups. *Education Health, 13*(1), 91–105. doi:10.1080/135762800110628

Cowley, S., Bergen, A., Young, K., & Kavanagh, A. (2000). A taxonomy of needs assessment, elicited from a multiple case study of community nursing education and practice. *Journal of Advanced Nursing, 31*(1), 126–134. doi:10.1046/j.1365-2648.2000.01252.x

Cowley, S., & Houston, A. M. (2003). A structured health needs assessment tool: Acceptability and effectiveness for health visiting. *Journal of Advanced Nursing, 43*(1), 82–92. doi:10.1046/j.1365-2648.2003.02675.x

Cowley, S., Mitcheson, J., & Houston, A. M. (2004). Structuring health needs assessments: The medicalisation of health visiting. *Social Health Illness, 26*(5), 503–526. doi:10.1111/j.0141-9889.2004.00403.x

Dunham, D. (1998). *Nominal group technique: A user's guide*. Retrieved from https://sswm.info/sites/default/files/reference_attachments/DUNHAM%201998%20Nominal%20Group%20Technique%20-%20A%20Users%27%20Guide.pdf

Fouad, M. N., Nagy, M. C., Johnson, R. E., Wynn, T. A., Partridge, E. E., & Dignan, M. (2004). The development of a community action plan to reduce breast and cervical cancer disparities between African-American and White women. *Ethnicity and Disease, 14*(3), 53–60.

Fuller, J., Bentley, M., & Shotton, D. (2001). Use of community health needs assessment for regional planning in country South Australia. *Australian Journal of Rural Health, 9*(1), 12–27. doi:10.1046/j.1440-1584.2001.00353.x

Government of Saskatchewan. (2006). *Making life better*. Retrieved from http://www.gov.sk.ca/finance/accountability/2006/keyterms.htm

Jordan, J., Wright, J., Ayres, P., Hawkings, M., Thomson, R., Wilkinson, J., & Williams, R. (2002). Health needs assessment and needs-led health service change: A survey of projects involving public health doctors. *Journal of Health Services Research and Policy, 7*(2), 71–80. doi:10.1258/1355819021927719

Kirst-Ashman, K., & Hall, G. (2002). *Understanding generalist practice*. Pacific Grove, CA: Brooks/Cole.

Kretzmann, J. P., & McKnight, J. (1993). *Building communities from the inside out: A path toward finding and mobilizing a community's assets*. Evanston, IL: Center for Urban Affairs and Policy Research.

National Association of States United for Aging and Disabilities. (2016, June 17). *National Association of States United for Aging and Disabilities*. Retrieved from National Association of States United for Aging and Disabilities: About State Agencies List of Members: http://www.nasuad.org/about-nasuad/about-state-agencies/list-members

Shadel, B. N., Chen, J. J., Newkirk, R. W., Lawrence, S. J., Clements, B., & Evans, R. G. (2002). Bioterrorism risk perceptions and educational needs of public health professionals before and after September 11, 2001: A national needs assessment survey. *Journal of Public Health Management Practice, 10*(4), 282–289. doi:10.1097/00124784-200407000-00004

Thompson, A. H., Howard, A. W., & Jin, Y. (2001). A social problem index for Canada. *Canadian Journal of Psychiatry, 46*(1), 45–51. doi:10.1177/070674370104600107

Weist, M. D., Lowie, J. A., Flaherty, L. T., & Pruitt, D. (2001). Collaboration among the education, mental health, and public health systems to promote youth mental health. *Psychiatry Service, 52*(10), 1348–1351. doi:10.1176/appi.ps.52.10.1348

Witkin, B. R., & Altschuld, J. W. (1995). *Planning and conducting needs assessments: A practical guide*. Thousand Oaks, CA: Sage.

19

From Tools to Vision

LEARNING OBJECTIVES

At the end of this chapter readers will:

1. *Understand how to use tools such as health behavior models, the media, coalitions, and needs assessments to bring a vision to fruition.*
2. *Understand how to use advocacy tools for policy and program development.*
3. *Understand how to use advocacy tools to influence the practice arena for older adults and people with disabilities.*

> *Erica and Theresa have been investigating a number of angles and perspectives to identify how to develop a blueprint for their department on aging. Through their investigation, interviews with case subjects, and assessment of current policies and programs, they have decided that they need to put their tools utilized and findings together to develop a vision. This chapter outlines their current perspectives and discussion with each other, following their assessment and investigation.*

USING TOOLS AND STRATEGIES TO REACH YOUR VISION

At this point, we have introduced a number of tools and strategies. It seems prudent to consider how to use them to reach one's vision for policy development or program development. The purpose of this chapter is to review the various tools and strategies, along with policies that have been addressed thus far, and integrate these issues and skills with one's vision for either program planning or policy development.

Although some of the concepts presented may have been familiar to the reader, other issues, or concepts may be completely new. The key becomes how to use these skills and integrate them into one's repertoire of skills for policy development, policy analysis, or program planning/development. What mechanisms can one realistically develop, in an effort to showcase gaps within the current existing public policy, or existing programs and services? How would we use these measures to develop a policy brief, a white paper, a position paper, or media artifacts to showcase an issue? How do we use these strategies to bring our vision to fruition?

 DOI:10.1891/9780826128393.0019

First, when considering a white paper, or when considering writing testimony of any sort, it is very important to consider who the audience will be, and within this context, examine the philosophical paradigms of each of these individuals. It may be helpful to map out these considerations on paper as part of a strategy. Once the key players have been mapped out, identify what to expect each of these key players' philosophical paradigm may in fact be, and prepare to ask for support for one's own position. Once the researcher has a clear picture of the key players' perspectives, prepare data to address their concerns.

Second, build a case for the need for revision of an existing policy or program/service. Earlier in this book we discuss evidence-based policy development and present several sources of data. These sources can provide a useful backdrop to support renewed initiatives.

Third, know how existing legislation or program guidelines actually work and what has been signed into legislation. This knowledge is very helpful when one is attempting to showcase the need for changes.

Fourth, build a short presentation addressing the concerns that can be used when meeting with a legislator or program director. This presentation can be in the form of a brief or one-page fact sheet. It can be based on a white paper or legislative analysis that one has developed previously. Samples of media artifacts to fulfill this purpose are presented in Chapter 18.

Fifth, build a media campaign utilizing social media strategies to reach a specific demographic segment of the population. This approach will not reach all intended users, but can reach a specific segment.

Greenfield, Oberlink, Scharlach, Neal, & Stafford (2015) identified four major challenges that have impacted the development of resources and services for older adults, which may dampen one's enthusiasm despite the tools and resources provided in this textbook. These include:

- *Limited public policy supports, particularly at the national level*: Outside of Medicare and Social Security, there is relatively little federal funding for older adults specifically. This challenge opens the landscape for developing programs and services within a variety of dimensions for older adults. Although federal funding may be scarce, many municipalities are integrating some forms of taxation efforts to provide additional funding and resources to older adults and people with disabilities.
- *Engaging people outside of the field of aging and disabilities to take interest in aging and disabilities*: A key insight from Greenfield et al. (2015) is that adequately addressing challenges and opportunities for older residents and families extends beyond a local municipality's department on aging, disabilities, or public health offices. The portfolios of aging and disabilities transcend across the life span and touch the lives of stakeholders across a variety of sectors. As discussed in Chapter 17 on coalitions and coalition development, issues that matter for the elderly, people with disabilities, and their families and caregivers also resonate with many other groups within the public and private sectors, such as transportation, housing, community education, and physical design. Fragmentation endemic to professional practice, government philanthropy, health and social services, and academia makes it all the more challenging to create shared agendas and vision around the fields of aging and disabilities.
- *Fragmentation across service sector efforts*: Many interest groups working with people who growing older or have disabilities may have different or competing values and goals. Age cohort differences, as seen in Chapter 17 can also account for differences in values, vision, and goals. These differences impede the rapid development of joint policy agendas, pooling of resources, exchange of information, and messaging around collaborative and collective action and impact.

- *Evaluation challenges*: Policy makers and private funders are increasingly seeking evidence for programs' effectiveness, especially in terms of the anticipated benefits relative to the costs of running such programs. This reality needs to be taken into consideration as we move forward in building effective public policy for older adults and people with disabilities and as we attempt to cultivate programs that result from public policy.

FROM TOOLS TO POLICY DEVELOPMENT

Policy development is a competency that improves over time. When engaging in policy development, remember always to befriend your local legislator, regardless of party affiliation. If you are a known entity, you are more likely to reap success than if you are a one-time caller. Once you have established a relationship, you have some inroads, which will make the process much smoother when you actually have an issue of concern or policy revisions that you would like to see implemented.

When building support for a particular bill introduced into the legislature, use your skills and training from both needs assessment and coalition building to garner support. The needs assessment data will be helpful when arguing for a need or service. Building a coalition pursues the issue with a unified and stronger voice from a range of stakeholders.

FROM TOOLS TO PROGRAM DEVELOPMENT

When considering program development, all tools and strategies related to policy development apply equally. Some additional strategies or tools to use for program development include the health behavior models. Keeping in mind the stages of change, and which stage a person/community may be attuned to will provide a multitude of results. In addition, these tools will enable the program planner to target the intervention so that resources are maximized, and to enable minimal inputs.

SUMMARY

This chapter attempts to integrate the theories and concepts presented in Part III of this book and suggest how a program planner or policy advocate can apply them.

DISCUSSION QUESTIONS

1. Consider some of the cases presented throughout this textbook, specifically the cases of Margie, who lives in a rural community, beautifully wooded but with limited resources, or Joan, who has disabilities but wants to manage independently.
   a. How would you go about devising a plan to build resources for either of these individuals (or any of the cases introduced in this book).
   b. What skills discussed in Part III of the book would you utilize, and how would you go about putting the tools into action?
2. How would you combine health behavior models, the use of media, and coalitions to address either a policy revision or program development?
3. What tools do you feel are missing or you still need to develop missing to more adequately address policy gaps or build programs to address policy initiatives?

REFERENCES

Greenfield, E. A., Oberlink, M., Scharlach, A. E., Neal, M. B., & Stafford, P. B. (2015). Age-friendly community initiatives: Conceptual issues and key questions. *The Gerontologist, 55*(2), 191–198. doi:10.1093/geront/gnv005

Pew Research Center. (2015). *The whys and hows of generations research*. Retrieved from http://www.people-press.org/2015/09/03/the-whys-and-hows-of-generations-research

Part IV

Realities and Visions for the Future

This last part of the text outlines specific programmatic areas that do not necessarily flow from aging policies or from federally mandated policies but are realities and challenges for the future. Gaps and areas for development, model programs, challenges for the future, and visions for the future related to policy development for people advancing in age or people with disabilities are addressed. The tools and concepts presented earlier will be integrated and woven throughout. This part of the text challenges the reader to think about the top 10 issues that will be faced by policy analysts and program planners.

20

Challenges for Policy and Program Planning for the Future: Realities and Visions for the Future

LEARNING OBJECTIVES

At the end of this chapter, readers will:

1. *Be aware of the challenges that the aging- and disability-oriented service delivery systems are facing as part of the service delivery network.*
2. *Be able to identify realities that face our aging/disability service delivery system.*
3. *Identify how the aging/disability network can envision service delivery for the future.*

Erica and Theresa have poured over the notes that they have taken as they made their journey through the world of disability and aging, listened to case testimonies, and tried to make sense of the strengths and areas for development required for these groups. After much deliberation, they are prepared to consider developing a white paper for program planning and policy development. Within their deliberations, they have identified a number of challenges the system will face, which are articulated in this chapter.

INTRODUCTION

The preceding chapters address a number of areas that will affect the lives of people as they age or people who are older adults. Philosophical paradigms, statistics, evidence-based approaches, dealing with the media, making people aware of new technologies, and preparing for communities to best deal with issues of aging are all major issues of concern. A range of issues have been presented; however, this chapter provides an overview of the most significant ones to be addressed or to require intervention. Hence, the most challenging of issues for the future are framed in a "top 10 list."

© Springer Publishing Company DOI:10.1891/9780826128393.0020

THE TOP 10 LIST OF CHALLENGES FOR THE FUTURE IN THE AREAS OF DISABILITY AND AGING

The top 10 list of challenges for the future of service delivery within the aging and disability arena will include the following. Each will be described in detail to follow

1. Designing paradigms to meet the demographic and social needs of our graying and disabled populations through evidence-based approaches
2. Social Security—boom or bust?
3. Medicare: Will there be a pot of gold at the end of the rainbow for preventive services?
4. Understanding health behavior and planning with this understanding in mind
5. Using the media, advocacy, and coalitions for social change
6. Home- and community-based care
7. Mental health programs, services, and issues
8. Health programs, services, and issues
9. Long-term care
10. Diversity, health literacy, and special populations

Designing Paradigms to Meet the Demographic and Social Needs of Our Graying and Disabled Populations Through Evidence-Based Approaches

Reality

The evolving needs identified by our graying boomer population and population with disabilities will create an increased demand upon our public and private systems for resources and services. The financial resources available through public sources will see an increased demand for funding of services and resources at community, regional, and state levels. These demands will be experienced by both the public sector and private sources such as philanthropic or faith-based organizations. Consequently, an increased need to showcase how the donor investment has been utilized will be paramount. Evidence and best practices will guide program development for the future while needs assessments and data will transform both the development of programs and the mounting of program evaluations.

Vision

A vision for the future to meet the demand from this "top 10" list will include the increased need for accountability and evidence to support a specific program or service. Personnel in agency programs and services will become increasingly savvy with the use of statistics or data to provide a basis for program development and program design and to document the efficacy and impact of interventions. In addition, people involved in these programs and services will become more interested in using quantitative and qualitative outcomes to market programs to consumers, since there may be a feeling that consumers from the boomer era will be driven to decision making based upon empirical findings and evidence. The bottom line—considering that the boomer population has prided itself on decision making through consumer reports and the like, this perspective will also be an important dimension in the development of services and resources for both accountability and marketing. With an increased emphasis on evidence-based programs, agencies will also become more savvy with respect to delivering interventions that have been clinically defined as effective and have an evidence base to their framework.

Social Security

Reality

A major reality facing the Social Security program in the United States is whether to privatize the program or enable the program to remain as a public resource or program to benefit all. Debate will continue to ensue regarding the privatization of the Social Security retirement fund in order to maintain solvency into the Social Security trust fund. In reality, though, if such a measure were to occur, the system risks being thrust back into a situation of instability that led to the very development of the Social Security program—a stock market crash. While private interests may be eager to privatize, it may well be that the interests at heart for privatization are fueled by an innate desire to ensure that investors have funds available for investment. Hence, individuals with marginal resources, the working poor, and the vast majority of people living and working within the United States today could conceivably retire with limited funds available to them, both at the time of their retirement and long into their retirement years. This may result in cost shifting, since many of these same individuals, with limited funds available for retirement, will in effect require some assets for income. These assets could result in an increased flux of individuals funded through Medicaid or public aid resources and an increase in the elderly poor.

The changing demographics and increased numbers of people who have experienced multiple marriages, divorce agreements, and settlements resulting in pension splitting will skyrocket over the next few decades, resulting in more people than ever in situations where their current pension resources cannot adequately meet their needs. Consequently, the end result will be that some financial intervention will be required to meet the economic and social security needs of people into their retirement years.

Another reality worth considering is the reality that the Social Security Act does not merely cover retirement benefits for people who have retired, but also includes numerous other titles that fund a large number of need-based programs such as children's health insurance programs and maternal and child health programs. A reality for the future is that some of these programs may need to be revised in order to ensure costs and funds are available through the Social Security Trust Fund. Since many individual state revenues depend on these federal funds in order to remain solvent, it is unlikely that these programs will quickly receive support to dismantle.

Retirement ages currently have shifted, and people who previously could have retired without penalty at 64 years of age are now being forced to work longer and into their late 60s (up to 67 years of age for people born after 1954). While reality is that people will need to work longer in order for the fund to remain solvent, the reality is that many of the jobs will change, and technical skills required by specific jobs will also change. The challenge thus for the workforce will be to ensure that workers maintain their skills in order to help businesses remain competitive in the future and that small businesses also enable their workforce to upgrade skills in an effort to remain competitive.

A third challenge to the Social Security system will be the very retirement and pension systems paid by employers to employees. Increasingly, corporate entities have dismantled or dissolved company pension systems, with no ethical concern for how this may affect older workers. Thus, retiring employees will rely on the Social Security retirement system for support. This creates a challenge to the current Social Security fund, forcing many people to become dependent upon federal and public sources of funds for a financial safety net into their retirement.

A fourth challenge will be for people with disabilities to secure Social Security benefits. The increased financial pressure on the system to help people with disabilities in need of financial support will increase, and the eligibility criteria will become more stringent.

Finally, a challenge for the future will be to keep the Social Security fund solvent and available for financial resources to support older adults as they leave the workforce. Unlike other countries in the world, the United States opted to construct a "pay as you go" system, in which current revenues invested are used to finance current pension needs. Thus, a challenge may be to examine alternative forms of revenue investment in order to ensure that the fund retains the "pay as you go" features but also accommodates needs for the future. This is complicated by the fact that we currently have fewer people in the workforce than retirees, and there is more dependence upon the current workforce to fund the pensions of those collecting Social Security benefits. This of course was not the dynamic when the system was developed in the 1930s.

Vision

The vision for the Social Security fund for the future may include some options that are not popular views. The first unpopular view may include taxation for corporate entities to support individuals who provided backbone and essential labor services such as farmers and the working class. Since many of the same entities would be impacted in some way, and many may be active participants in the elite power structure, they may not be willing to be singled out to share their portion of corporate funding to a Social Security fund through additional corporate taxation and/or raising the maximum earnings cutoff limit for payroll taxes ($128,400 for 2018). Raising the cutoff (or eliminating it altogether, as has been proposed) would mean that more of the wealthy would be required to pay into Social Security.

A second vision for the future will be developing "Social Security passport accounts" for people entering into the workforce under the age of 30. These accounts will support individuals through investments for an individual cohort fund but will also address the needs of retirees of the present day. A portion of the funds will be invested into a "pay as you go" plan, and a second portion will go into a fund, designed to be invested and used at a later date (similar to the Social Security plan in Germany).

The third vision for Social Security will be that the plan provide an option for those beyond a specific income level to be able to privately invest their funds. Thus, a safety net will still prevail for the working class, but the option for those with incomes of $100,000 or more to invest a portion of their Social Security/retirement funds will also be a possibility.

Medicare

Reality

Medicare, a health insurance program for older adults who have worked at least 40 quarters during their vocational lifetime and contributed to the program will also face serious financial distress in the future. While the program currently funds a range of services through four component parts: Medicare Part A, Medicare Part B, Medicare Part C, and Medicare Part D, the reality is that these specific component parts may become increasingly stressed financially as time moves on.

A second reality is that currently there is much duplication of services per procedure by medical practitioners, who want to assure that they have taken the best care possible. Strategies to reduce the duplication of services will be necessary in efforts to reduce costs to the overall Medicare program. Consistent with the notion of reducing costs will also be the need to reduce long-term care costs through an increased emphasis on prevention services.

Vision

Consideration of the challenges that will be faced by the healthcare system and Medicare funding leads to several visions. An overall focus on holistic care for older adults to include prevention and screening services would greatly enhance the overall program, and address some of the costly long-term healthcare costs that are faced by individuals who do not have their healthcare problems detected early enough. In line with these prevention services the vision will include oral health screening services regardless of whether patients have their natural teeth or prosthodontics. In addition, services will also include care for the maintenance of one's natural teeth. A second area for prevention services will include physical activity, strength training, and falls prevention services/education.

Although Medicare is based on a micro-system program (services to individuals), another vision for the future will include opportunities for state departments on aging in collaboration with departments of public health to apply for Medicare funds to assure the funding of specific community health initiatives targeting prevention messages. This vision directly leads into the next on the "top 10" item.

Understanding Health Behavior and Planning With This Understanding in Mind

Reality

Currently few health promotion programs are utilized as a venue for modifying health behavior, but they are on the increase. The challenge will be to continue to ensure that these models are utilized. Planning for healthcare resources making use of such notions as the health beliefs of specific target groups, their perceived seriousness, perceived susceptibility, and perceived barriers can greatly improve the efficacy of specific resources. Using health behavior models to understand health behavior and plan for resources can be a tremendous asset for resource development, but also in preparation for meeting the needs of specific target groups. In addition, the use of health behavior models can greatly enhance the applicability of specific resources to specific target groups, regional variations, and age cohort groups and differences.

Vision

The vision is that all programs that target health behavior will utilize health behavior models to better describe and understand health behavior. Interventions will be developed with a theoretical framework to guide the actual intervention. Limited resources will encourage agencies and resources to move toward the development of resources and services that ensure the greatest impact for investment.

Using the Media, Advocacy, and Coalitions for Social Change

Reality

In Chapter 2, the lack of advances within the aging arena is compared to other areas of societal activity in the 20th and early 21st centuries; the contrast is stark and noteworthy. Limited energy can be devoted to the development of policies and programs to promote the field of aging. With this reality, it is paramount to produce and utilize strategies that will promote the development of programs and services for older adults. Since energies are finite, it becomes important to use the media, advocacy, and coalitions for social change efforts.

Policy development efforts can realize more progress when efforts are pooled together through coalitions. Change efforts often require an interface of various resources and services. Successful efforts to lobby and advocate for policy changes to congressional representatives and senators have been effectively enacted through joint efforts from multiple forces. The Americans with Disabilities Act (ADA) is a solid example of this type of coalition effort, in which resources were pooled together with the end result being the passage of the ADA. Coalitions also enable communication across lines and lead to improved program and service utilization.

Coalitions bring broad-based public support to an issue and can be used to leverage political support. Such advocacy efforts can facilitate broad-based social change at policy and programmatic levels.

The media can be an incredibly valuable asset in this process. They can showcase the issues and help facilitate awareness of the need and strategies for action through a number of venues. In addition, the media can showcase the need for health education and public education on issues that will impact older adults, now including the oldest members of the boomer generation.

Vision

Coalitions will help develop broad-based community support for initiatives and programs. The media will be used to help inform the public of issues and resources. Innovative approaches to the use of media such as media artifacts, fact sheets, and advertisement campaigns will also be used as strategies to improve broad-based community support for programs and initiatives.

Home- and Community-Based Care

Reality

Currently, most American people want to remain in their homes as long as possible. This growing phenomenon has led to the need for and importance of increased resources to deliver home- and community-based support and care. While this care may be possible within urban areas and larger centers, rural areas and communities with small population bases will be a challenge in the future.

The Older Americans Act (OAA) has focused on home-based supports to ensure one's activities of daily living (ADLs) can be carried out, but limited attention has been paid to resources that will allow for work or home-based support around one's home, and resources to carry out handyperson work and/or home repairs. This will be a growing issue as the community census of older adults increases and the numbers of natural social supports available to help the elders in the community decreases.

The concepts of autonomy, personal choice, and empowerment also play a critical role within community-based settings. Although older adults and people with disabilities would prefer to make decisions on who will provide in-home care, only a select number of states can provide this degree of autonomy. Community-based care and voucher systems are currently available only in specific states. These voucher systems enable family members to provide care or be considered a paid caregiver to an elder or disabled person requiring home care. The "cash and carry" systems need to be expanded to additional states and serve a broader range of potential users.

Rural communities may not have the same resources for older adults simply because the resources and service providers may not be available. Rural communities also face the dilemma that there are often more people per capita requiring resources, but fewer services or resources available. Transportation also poses a challenge for older adults and their need for services. Providers are often limited in the degree of service that they can provide because of the costs and increasing costs of travel to deliver services. In some ways, people who have been well connected to their peers and community will continue to have connections with people within their network to provide home-based supports. Unfortunately, those who have been perceived as deviant within communities will continue to be ostracized into old age and may be the most in need.

Home- and community-based care are not available to all people in the community, and the program is needs assessed. Thus, there is a wide pool of people who do not have access to services by virtue of the fact that their economic status is slightly above the eligibility requirements; however, these individuals are not financially well off and could not necessarily afford to pay for the home- and community-based services required to maximize their independence.

Another reality to consider is the number of older adults and people with disabilities who are in need of nutrition and food programs. An expansion of home-delivered meal programs is going to be necessary to meet the needs of people who are frail and would like to remain in their own homes and also be nutritionally sound.

Although a number of amendments to the OAA (2016) were passed that would impact home- and community-based services, this legislative mandate does not come with funding for improved services. Individual state authorities on aging (state departments on aging services) can take advantage of expansion of services if the funds are available. However, if funds are not available through state treasuries, expectations of such expansion will be unrealistic. The shrinking of budgets at the state and federal levels for human services will also impact community services.

Vision

Some ideal strategies to meet the needs of home- and community-based services will include an expansion of the voucher system available to an increased number of states.

Home-based supports can be expanded to include home maintenance and home repairs for people who would like to remain in their homes. In addition, improved training for home-health aides should occur in the future, because these individuals are often a vital link between family and the older adults. These home-health workers often serve as the eyes and ears for families to their beloved elders. However, home-health workers are often ill advised of behaviors and actions that can be symptomatic of issues that can foster greater concern or potential for life-threatening conditions, or signs of abuse and neglect. Enhanced training may also help bolster the workers' ability to recognize signs that can prevent further deterioration of health and provide some preventative approaches to care.

Cooperatives available as an alternative to home care system programs would enable people from a range of income levels to be cared for and will also become in vogue as the future unfolds. Given that there will be a growing population of people whose income will exceed the eligibility criteria for home-based services, this group will need some form of home-based supports. Cooperatives, which were fashionable especially in the 1960s, will be redeveloped by up-and-coming aging boomers to provide for the home-based services to meet the needs of this group in efforts to remain at home. In addition, the same constituents that creatively develop these cooperatives will also develop policies and lobby for legislation that will provide incentives for such initiatives both fiscally and socially.

Mental Health Programs, Services, and Issues

Reality

Mental health has been viewed as a stepchild to medicine, and in a stigmatizing manner for older adults. Although there is some provision for counseling in the OAA, it has not been sufficient to meet the needs of older adults. Services provide for a minimum of counseling or support services to people in need of acute services. The current mental health programs are based on policies for long-term chronic mentally ill and do not avail themselves to people who are afflicted with the normal issues of aging. Screening and assessment programs to reach older adults are not consistent across designated regions within state boundaries, let alone across states. The quality of these programs to meet the mental health needs of older adults is inadequate, and early detection programs are practically nonexistent. Peer support programs for older adults to discuss mental health issues are needed but are greatly lacking both in number and quality. Educational interventions to make people aware of services and supports to best understand the realities of aging are also needed.

Vision

Some visions for the future includes the Positive Aging Act, which attempts to enhance mental vitality among older adults, rather than let people remain under- or undiagnosed. The RAISE Family Caregivers Act will hopefully bring conversation and attention to the need for improved treatment, education, and intervention to individuals and families affected with Alzheimer's disease. The most recent amendments to the OAA (2016) impacting the mental health of older adults will enable the development of resources, including centers for mental health intervention and centers for excellence. Finally, programs that target the promotion of mental vitality will replace the intervention programs for mental health.

Health Programs, Services, and Issues

Reality

In the United States, healthcare is seen as a commodity, rather than a right. Attached to this commodity is a service or resource that is rising in cost, and those costs will continue to skyrocket over time. Hence, a challenge to deal with these rising costs will be to find solutions, one of which may be rationing of health services such as seen in Oregon.

A second challenge to the healthcare system is the need for an increased focus on prevention—prevention programs for chronic diseases and for diseases that may lead to more serious and costly healthcare issues.

A third challenge to the healthcare system is the focus on holistic care rather than disease-specific care. Oral healthcare is one such specific example, which can have a more extensive impact on one's overall health than merely the health of the oral cavity. The mouth is a mirror of the rest of the body (OAA, 2006), so the need is real for services and programs to examine oral healthcare within the continuum of healthcare services. The challenge will also include the expansion of current Medicare policy to include oral healthcare, since it is a myth that all older adults lose their natural teeth.

In Oregon, one option available to people, especially people diagnosed with a chronic health problem, is the option of assisted suicide. This controversial option poses challenges to state government and health authorities, because in the long run, individual choices to avoid the high cost of treatment for the inevitable may push lobbying for these options within the realm available to older adults. The assisted suicide option may be perceived as one solution to the high costs of healthcare; however, such an option is fraught with concern from religious groups and faith-based communities and will continue to be controversial as the option expands both domestically and internationally.

The costs of healthcare will continue to be a challenge in the future, especially costs associated with procedures that can be prevented in older adults. The costs of falls and hip fractures can often be avoided but will be an issue in attempting to curb healthcare costs.

Vision

Healthcare services for older adults in the future will include resources for preventive procedures to include dental care and falls prevention approaches. Models where supplemental insurance provides for these services may also be a wave of the future.

In an effort to deal with increasing costs of healthcare, some states within the United States will use the Oregon model of service delivery as a blueprint for state-based services. This approach may include some "rationing" of services and a legalized option for assisted suicide. In response to this option, individuals and interest groups will speak in support of the right to life.

Long-Term Care

Reality

Although only about 5% of older adults currently utilize long-term care facilities, a challenge still exists that limited resources are available for long-term care. These resources leave a lot to be desired. Older adults struggle with the multiple moves they may need to undergo as they proceed through the continuum of services from assisted living to congregate living, to nursing home, and finally to hospice care. The number of moves and changes one must endure during this time period is particularly challenging for older adults who have or are developing diminished cognitive capacity. In contrast, those with disabilities will be pushed toward moving from the institution back into the community.

Vision

A strategy to meet the challenge outlined for long-term care will include the development of campus settings with a range of housing options for older adults and people with disabilities. This continuum of services will move people from assisted living through hospice care all on the same campus. In addition, we will see more options available for people through institutional care that meets the varied preferences of people who will reside in these settings.

Diversity and Special Populations

Reality

Health disparities are rampant when we compare and contrast health outcomes among older adults who are in need of care or resources and who are people of color or members of a traditionally oppressed group. These health disparities only continue to grow as one ages and more health problems or issues evolve. Unfortunately, services and resources are not necessarily developed to meet the unique culture or health beliefs of specific culture groups, nor are programs and policies developed to be culturally sensitive. Health literacy is a venue for promoting health information, but once again, our system is not set up to deal best with educating individuals through the lens of culturally relevant resources. Health literacy will take on a more important function in the future as we move toward consumers assuming more responsibility for partnership in the healthcare delivery process.

Vision

The development of culturally relevant resources to narrow the gap between health services for the majority and those for disadvantaged populations could be an important strategy to cultivate. Programs and intervention efforts that target health literacy that are culturally relevant and developed at specific reading levels to accommodate educational attainment may also be some important strategies to bridge the gap resulting from health disparities.

SUMMARY

Aging and disabilities are realities in our society. Whatever we choose, whatever path we follow, we will still age, and policies, programs, and services will need to be in place to address the issues growing old brings to bear. Disability will also still exist within our communities, and programs/services will be needed to address these community needs. As we prepare to meet the challenges that our society presents, policies for aging and people with disabilities will require development and address. Although this chapter cites 10 major challenges that the future will bring, in reality, policy advocates will have to be prepared to address and deal with these challenges by using innovative strategies for policy development and policy change.

Policy development and program design to meet the needs of an aging and ability-challenged society are unique challenges that must be addressed. These issues require an understanding of the various players and philosophical paradigms that shape the values and visions within our society. Despite advances that may take place in science and technology, advances in aging policy have sadly lagged behind. Advances within disability policy have been much more forthcoming than those addressing the aging population. Part of this lag may be attributed to the lack of empirical evidence used to justify changes and the prevailing dearth of anecdotal evidence. Evidence-based policy development can be a strategy to help facilitate rationales for policy advocates to pursue. In effect, revised strategies will be necessary for policy advocates in their quest to meet the challenges that lie ahead.

Traditionally, we have focused on Social Security and Medicare as policies that most impact older adults in our nation. This text, however, has made the case that other policies also have an impact on the lives of older adults, including the Americans with Disabilities Act, the OAA, and the Community Mental Health Centers Act. Each of these pieces of legislation will continue to play a key role in the lives of older adults.

Policy and program development advocates in the future will also benefit from using a new set of skills in the pursuit of their goals. Competencies that will be invaluable in one's "tool kit" will include an understanding of health behavior models, coalition building strategies, needs assessment strategies, and skills for dealing with the media and preparing media artifacts. These abilities will be essential in building effective programs and policies for the future.

Finally, programs and services can only hope to benefit, and the challenges for the future can only be slowly addressed with a renewed set of strategies for program planning and policy development. This text has attempted to empower the policy advocate or program planner with some new skills and strategies that can impact programs and services in the future and overcome the challenges of today. The future of services to meet the needs of older adults is in our hands. Let us craft these wisely, skillfully, and with a renewed vision.

REFERENCE

Older Americans Act of 2016, Pub. L. No. 119-365, Cong. Rec., Vol. 152, U.S.C 3001 (2016).

Appendix A: Regional Support Centers

Regional Support Centers serve as the focal point for the development, coordination and administration of Administration for Community Living program and activities within designated Health and Human Services Secretariat (HHS) regions.

Region I: CT, MA, ME, NH, RI, VT

Kathleen Otte
Regional Administrator
John F. Kennedy Bldg, Rm 2075
Boston, MA 02203
Phone: 617-565-1158
Fax: 617-565-4511

Region II: NY, NJ, PR, VI

Kathleen Otte
Regional Administrator
26 Federal Plaza, Rm 38-102
New York, NY 10278
Phone: 212-264-2976
Fax: 212-264-0114

Region III and IV: AL, DC, DE, FL, GA, KY, MD, MS, NC, PA, SC, TN, VA, WV

Costas Miskis
Regional Administrator
Atlanta Federal Center
61 Forsyth Street, SW, Suite 5M69
Atlanta, GA 30303-8909
Phone: 404-562-7600
Fax: 404-562-7598

Region V and VII: IA, IL, IN, KS, MI, MN, MO, NE, OH, WI

Amy Wiatr-Rodriquez
Regional Administrator
233 N Michigan Ave, Suite 790
Chicago, IL 60601-5527
Phone: 312-938-9858
Fax: 312-886-8533

Region VI: AR, LA, OK, NM, TX

Percy Devine
Regional Administrator
1301 Young St, Rm 736
Dallas, TX 75201
Phone: 214-767-2971
Fax: 214-767-2951

Region VIII: CO, MT, UT, WY, ND, SD

Percy Devine
Regional Administrator
1961 Stout Street
Denver, CO 80294-3638
Phone: 303-844-2951
Fax: 303-844-2943

Region IX: CA, NV, AZ, HI, GU, CNMI, AS

David Ishida
Regional Administrator
90 7th Street, T-8100
San Francisco, CA 94103
Phone: 415-437-8780
Fax: 415-437-8782

Region X: AK, ID, OR, WA

David Ishida
Regional Administrator
701 Fifth Avenue, M/S/RX-33
Suite 1600
Seattle, Washington 98104
Phone: 206-615-2298
Fax: 206-615-2299

Appendix B: *Healthy People 2020* Objectives for Older Adults*

GOAL

Improve the health, function, and quality of life of older adults.

OVERVIEW

Older adults are among the fastest growing age groups, and the first "baby boomers" (adults born between 1946 and 1964) turned 65 in 2011. More than 37 million people in this group (60%) will manage more than one chronic condition by 2030 (American Hospital Association, 2007).

Older adults are at high risk for developing chronic illnesses and related disabilities. These chronic conditions include:

- Diabetes mellitus
- Arthritis
- Congestive heart failure
- Dementia

Many experience hospitalizations, nursing home admissions, and low-quality care. They also may lose the ability to live independently at home. Chronic conditions are the leading cause of death among older adults (Kramarow, Lubitz, Lentzner, & Gorina, 2007).

WHY IS THE HEALTH OF OLDER ADULTS IMPORTANT?

Health Services

Preventive health services are valuable for maintaining the quality of life and wellness of older adults. In fact, the Patient Protection and Affordable Care Act of 2010 includes provisions related to relevant Medicare services. However, preventive services are underused, especially among certain racial and ethnic groups (Kramarow et al., 2007; U.S. Department of Health and Human Services [USDHHS, 2010]).

Ensuring quality healthcare for older adults is difficult, but the Centers for Medicare & Medicaid Services (CMS) has programs designed to improve physician, hospital, and nursing home care, among others. Older adults use many healthcare services, have complex conditions, and require professional expertise that meets their needs. Most providers receive some type of training on aging, but the percentage of those who actually specialize in this area is small. More certified specialists are needed to meet the needs of this group (Institute of Medicine, 2008).

**Source*: Healthy People 2020 website: http://www.healthypeople.gov/2020/topics-objectives/topic/older-adults

Quality of Life

Through programs that address chronic illnesses, Federal Government agencies are improving the quality of life for older adults. To combat existing health disparities, many of these programs target minorities and underserved populations. The ability to complete basic daily activities may decrease if illness, chronic disease, or injury limit physical or mental abilities of older adults. These limitations make it hard for older adults to remain at home. Early prevention and physical activity can help prevent such declines. Unfortunately, less than 20% of older adults engage in enough physical activity, and fewer do strength training (Centers for Disease Control and Prevention, 2004; Christmas & Andersen, 2000; Sollitto, 2018). Minority populations often have lower rates of physical activity.

Most older adults want to remain in their communities as long as possible. Unfortunately, when they acquire disabilities, there is often not enough support available to help them. States that invest in such services show lower rates of growth in long-term care expenditures.

Injury Prevention

Each year, one out of three older adults falls (Hausdorff, Rios, & Edelberg, 2001; Hornbrook et al., 1994; Moyer & U.S. Preventive Services Task Force, 2012). Falls often cause severe disability among survivors (Centers for Disease Control and Prevention, 2010). Injuries from falls lead to:

- Fear of falling
- Sedentary behavior
- Impaired function
- Lower quality of life

Falls are the leading cause of death due to unintentional injury among older adults; deaths and injuries can be prevented by addressing risk factors.

Caregivers

Caregivers for older adults living at home are typically unpaid family members. Caregiver stress often results in unnecessary nursing home placement. One to 2 million older adults in the United States are injured or mistreated by a loved one or a caregiver (Bonnie & Wallace, 2003). A measure of elder abuse has been added to encourage data collection on this issue.

Understanding the Health of Older Adults

The *Healthy People 2020* objectives on older adults are designed to promote healthy outcomes for this population. Many factors affect the health, function, and quality of life of older adults.

INDIVIDUAL BEHAVIORAL DETERMINANTS OF HEALTH IN OLDER ADULTS

Behaviors such as participation in physical activity, self-management of chronic diseases, or use of preventive health services can improve health outcomes.

Social Environment Determinants of Health in Older Adults

Housing and transportation services affect the ability of older adults to access care. People from minority populations tend to be in poorer health and use healthcare less often than people from nonminority populations (Institute of Medicine, 2008).

Health Services-Related Determinants of Health in Older Adults

The quality of the health and social services available to older adults and their caregivers affects their ability to manage chronic conditions and long-term care needs effectively.

EMERGING ISSUES IN THE HEALTH OF OLDER ADULTS

Emerging issues for improving the health of older adults include efforts to:

- Coordinate care.
- Help older adults manage their own care.
- Establish quality measures.
- Identify minimum levels of training for people who care for older adults.
- Research and analyze appropriate training to equip providers with the tools they need to meet the needs of older adults.

There is growing recognition that data sources are limited for certain subpopulations of older adults, including the aging lesbian, gay, bisexual, and transgender populations. Research for these groups will inform future health and policy initiatives.

The specific Program Objectives for Older Adults are as follows:

Prevention

OA-1. Increase the proportion of older adults who use the Welcome to Medicare benefit.

OA-2. Increase the proportion of older adults who are up-to-date on a core set of clinical preventive services.

- **OA-2.1.** Increase the proportion of males aged 65 years and older who are up-to-date on a core set of clinical preventive services.
- **OA-2.2.** Increase the proportion of females aged 65 years and older who are up-to-date on a core set of clinical preventive services.

OA-3. (Developmental) Increase the proportion of older adults with one or more chronic health conditions who report confidence in managing their conditions.

OA-4. Increase the proportion of older adults who receive Diabetes Self-Management Benefits.

OA-5. Reduce the proportion of older adults who have moderate to severe functional limitations.

OA-6. Increase the proportion of older adults with reduced physical or cognitive function who engage in light, moderate, or vigorous leisure-time physical activities.

OA-7. Increase the proportion of the health care workforce with geriatric certification.

- **OA-7.1.** Increase the proportion of physicians with geriatric certification.
- **OA-7.2.** Increase the proportion of psychiatrists with geriatric certification.
- **OA-7.3.** Increase the proportion of RNs with geriatric certification.
- **OA-7.4.** Increase the proportion of dentists with geriatric certification.
- **OA-7.5.** Increase the proportion of physical therapists with geriatric certification.
- **OA-7.6.** Increase the proportion of registered dieticians with geriatric certification.

LONG-TERM SERVICES AND SUPPORTS

OA-8. (Developmental) Reduce the proportion of noninstitutionalized older adults with disabilities who have an unmet need for long-term services and supports.

OA-9. (Developmental) Reduce the proportion of unpaid caregivers of older adults who report an unmet need for caregiver support services.

OA-10. Reduce the rate of pressure ulcer-related hospitalizations among older adults.

OA-11. Reduce the rate of ED visits due to falls among older adults.

OA-12. Increase the number of States, the District of Columbia, and tribes that collect and make publicly available information on the characteristics of victims, perpetrators, and cases of elder abuse, neglect, and exploitation.

OA-12.1. Increase the number of States and the District of Columbia that collect and make publicly available information on the characteristics of victims, perpetrators, and cases of elder abuse, neglect, and exploitation.

OA-12.2. (Developmental) Increase the number of tribes that collect and make publicly available information on the characteristics of victims, perpetrators, and cases of elder abuse, neglect, and exploitation.

REFERENCES

American Hospital Association. (2007). *When I'm 64: How boomers will change health care*. Chicago, IL: American Hospital Association.

Bonnie, R. J., & Wallace, R. B. (Eds.). U.S. National Research Council, Panel to Review Risk and Prevalence of Elder Abuse and Neglect. (2003). *Elder mistreatment: Abuse, neglect and exploitation in an aging America*. Washington, DC: National Academies Press.

Centers for Disease Control and Prevention. (2004). Strength training among adults aged ≥65 years—United States, 2001. *Morbidity Mortality Weekly Review, 53*(2), 25–28. Retrieved from https://www.cdc.gov/mmwr/preview/mmwrhtml/mm5302a1.htm

Centers for Disease Control and Prevention. (2018). Injury prevention & control: Data and statistics (WISQARS). Atlanta, GA: Author. Retrieved from http://www.cdc.gov/injury/wisqars/index.html

Christmas, C., & Andersen, R. A. (2000). Exercise and older patients: Guidelines for the clinician. *Journal of the American Geriatrics Society, 48*(3), 318–324. doi:10.1111/j.1532-5415.2000.tb02654.x

Hausdorff, J. M., Rios, D. A., & Edelberg, H. K. (2001). Gait variability and fall risk in community living older adults: A one-year prospective study. *Archives of Physical Medical Rehabilitation, 82*(8), 1050–1056. doi:10.1053/apmr.2001.24893

Hornbrook, M. C., Stevens, V. J., Wingfield, D. J., Hollis, J. F., Greenlick, M. R., & Ory, M. G. (1994). Preventing falls among community-dwelling older persons: Results from a randomized trial. *The Gerontologist, 34*(1), 16–23. doi:10.1093/geront/34.1.16

Institute of Medicine, Committee on the Future Health Care Workforce for Older Americans. (2008). *Retooling for an aging America*. Washington, DC: National Academies Press.

Kramarow, E., Lubitz, J., Lentzner, H., & Gorina, Y. (2007). Trends in the health of older Americans, 1970–2005. *Health Affairs (Millwood), 26*(5), 1417–1425. doi:10.1377/hlthaff.26.5.1417

Mover, V. & U.S. Preventive Services Task Force (2012). Prevention of falls in community-dwelling older adults: U.S. Preventive Services Task Force recommendation statement. *Annals of Internal Medicine, 157*(3), 197–204. doi:10.7326/0003-4819-157-3-201208070-00462

Sollitto, M. (2018, March 21). How seniors can benefit from adopting an exercise regimen. Retrieved from https://www.agingcare.com/articles/exercise-benefits-for-the-elderly-95383.htm

U.S. Department of Health and Human Services, Centers for Medicare & Medicaid Services. (2010). *Medicare claims data*. Baltimore, MD: Centers for Medicare & Medicaid Services.

Appendix C: *Healthy People 2020* Objectives for Disability and Health*

BACKGROUND TO THE DISABILITY AND HEALTH OBJECTIVES

Goal

To promote the health and well-being of people with disabilities.

Overview

This section of *Healthy People 2020* focuses on promoting the health and well-being of people with disabilities. The U.S. Census 2000 counted 49.7 million people with some type of long-lasting condition or disability (Waldrop & Stern, 2003). An individual can get a disabling impairment or chronic condition at any point in life. Disability is part of human life, and an impairment or condition does not define individuals, their health, or their talents and abilities.

People with disabilities play an important and valued role in every community. All people, including people with disabilities, must have the opportunity to take part in important daily activities that add to a person's growth, development, fulfillment, and community contribution. This principle is central to all objectives outlined in this topic.

The Disability and Health objectives highlight areas for improvement and opportunities for people with disabilities to

- Be included in public health activities.
- Receive well-timed interventions and services.
- Interact with their environment without barriers.
- Participate in everyday life activities.

Without these opportunities, people with disabilities will continue to experience health disparities, compared to the general population. The 2020 objectives were developed with extensive input from disability communities, and this partnership between the public health and disability communities must continue over the decade in order to meet the Healthy People 2020 objectives.

WHY IS DISABILITY AND HEALTH IMPORTANT?

The largest set of U.S. health data for people with disabilities, the Disability and Health Data System (DHDS), measures health at the population level (Centers for Disease Control and Prevention, 2010). These data highlight improvements in health over the previous decade and clearly reveal specific health disparities for people with disabilities. Compared with people without disabilities, people with disabilities are more likely to

**Source*: Healthy People 2020 website at http://www.healthypeople.gov/2020/topics-objectives/topic/disability

- Experience difficulties or delays in getting the healthcare they need.
- Not have had an annual dental visit.
- Not have had a mammogram in past 2 years.
- Not have had a Pap test within the past 3 years.
- Not engage in fitness activities.
- Use tobacco.
- Be overweight or obese.
- Have high blood pressure.
- Experience symptoms of psychological distress.
- Receive less social–emotional support.
- Have lower employment rates.

Understanding Disability and Health

Public health efforts, from the individual to the national level, can affect the health and well-being of people with disabilities. These efforts must respond to known determinants of disability and health. There are many social and physical factors that influence the health of people with disabilities. The following three areas for public health action have been identified, using the International Classification of Functioning, Disability, and Health (ICF; World Health Organization [WHO], 2001) and the three WHO principles of action for addressing health determinants (WHO, 2008).

1. Improve the conditions of daily life by
   - Encouraging communities to be accessible so all can live in, move through, and interact with their environment.
   - Encouraging community living.
   - Removing barriers in the environment using both physical universal design concepts and operational policy shifts.
2. Address the inequitable distribution of resources among people with disabilities and those without disabilities by increasing
   - Appropriate healthcare for people with disabilities.
   - Education and work opportunities.
   - Social participation.
   - Access to needed technologies and assistive supports.
3. Expand the knowledge base and raise awareness about determinants of health for people with disabilities by increasing
   - The inclusion of people with disabilities in public health data collection efforts across the life span.
   - The inclusion of people with disabilities in health promotion activities.
   - The expansion of disability and health training opportunities for public health and healthcare professionals.

EMERGING ISSUES IN DISABILITY AND HEALTH

There are several emerging issues related to disability and health, including the need to

- Include disability and health courses.
- Assess drug and alcohol abuse and their treatment among people with disabilities.
- Include and improve strategies for emergency preparedness and response for people with disabilities.
- Include people with disabilities in all health promotion efforts.

REMOVING BARRIERS TO PARTICIPATION (ORGANIZATIONS)

- **Center for Universal Design**, North Carolina
- **National Center on Accessibility**, Indiana
- **Center for Inclusive Design and Environmental Access**, New York
- **Access Board**, Washington, DC
- **U.S. Department of Justice**, Washington, DC

Learn More

National Center for Health Statistics (NCHS) Identifying People with Disabilities in Public Health Surveillance.

Including People With Disabilities in Community and Health Promotion Activities (Publications).

- Fair Housing Act Design Manual. (1998). Retrieved from http://www.huduser.gov/publications/pdf/fairhousing/fairfull.pdf
- Removing Barriers to Health Clubs and Fitness Facilities. (1999). Retrieved from http://fpg.unc.edu/sites/fpg.unc.edu/files/resources/other-resources/NCODH_RemovingBarriersToHealthClubs.pdf
- Access Board ADA Guidelines for Recreation Facilities. (2010). Retrieved from http://www.access-board.gov/guidelines-and-standards/buildings-and-sites/about-the-ada-standards/background/ada-accessibility-guidelines-for-recreation-facilities
- Access Board Guidelines on Play Areas. (2005). Retrieved from http://www.access-board.gov/guidelines-and-standards/recreation-facilities/guides/play-areas
- ADA Hospitality: Accessible Meetings Events & Conferences Guide. (2018). Retrieved from http://www.adahospitality.org/accessible-meetings-events-conferences-guide/book
- Involving People with Disabilities as Members of Advisory Groups: Rural Practice Guidelines. (2007). Retrieved from http://mtdh.ruralinstitute.umt.edu/blog/?page_id=1031

EQUIPPING SERVICE SETTINGS/PROVIDING APPROPRIATE SERVICES

- North Carolina Office on Disability and Health. (1998). *Removing barriers to health care: A guide for health professionals*. Retrieved from http://fpg.unc.edu/sites/fpg.unc.edu/files/resources/other-resources/NCODH_RemovingBarriersToHealthCare.pdf
- The Lewin Group (on behalf of HHS). (2004). Dental services for children with special health care needs: Treatment guidelines and Medicaid reimbursement options. Retrieved from http://www.mchoralhealth.org/pdfs/dentalservicescshcn.pdf
- Oklahoma Dental Foundation. (2008). *Oral health care for children with special health care needs: A guide for family members/caregivers and dental providers*. Retrieved from http://www.okacaa.org/8.5 x 11 Oral Health Care for Children with Special Health Care Needs.pdf
- Association of State and Territorial Health Officials (ASTHO). (2013). *Access to preventive healthcare services for women with disabilities, fact sheet*. Retrieved from http://www.astho.org/Access-to-Preventive-Healthcare-Services-for-Women-with-Disabilities-Fact-Sheet/
- North Carolina Office on Disability and Health/Villanova University College of Nursing. (1999). *A provider's guide for the care of women with physical disabilities and*

chronic health conditions. Retrieved from http://fpg.unc.edu/sites/fpg.unc.edu/files/resources/other-resources/NCODH_ProvidersGuide.pdf
- Administration for Community Living. (2017). *Assistive technology fact sheet*. Retrieved from http://eldercare.acl.gov/Public/Resources/Factsheets/Assistive_Technology.aspx

REFERENCES

Centers for Disease Control and Prevention. (2010). *National Center for Health Statistics, DATA 2010*. Hyattsville, MD: Author. Retrieved from http://wonder.cdc.gov/data2010/focus.htm

Waldrop, J., & Stern, S. M. (2003). *Disability status: 2000 [Census 2000 Brief C2KBR-17]*. Washington, DC: U.S. Department of Commerce, Census Bureau. Retrieved from https://www.census.gov/prod/2003pubs/c2kbr-17.pdf

World Health Organization. (2001). *International classification of functioning, disability and health (ICF)*. Geneva, Switzerland: Author.

World Health Organization, Commission on Determinants of Health. (2008). *Closing the gap in a generation: Health equity through action on the determinants of health*. Geneva, Switzerland: World Health Organization.

THE *HEALTHY PEOPLE 2020* OBJECTIVES WITHIN THE AREA OF DISABILITY AND HEALTH ARE AS FOLLOWS

Systems and Policies

DH-1. Increase the number of population-based data systems used to monitor Healthy People 2020 objectives that include in their core a standardized set of questions that identify people with disabilities.

DH-2. Increase the number of tribes, States, and the District of Columbia that have public health surveillance and health promotion programs for people with disabilities and caregivers.

DH-2.1. Increase the number of State and the District of Columbia health departments that have at least one health promotion program aimed at improving the health and well-being of people with disabilities.

DH-2.2. Increase the number of State and the District of Columbia health departments that conduct health surveillance of caregivers for people with disabilities.

DH-2.3. Increase the number of State and the District of Columbia health departments that have at least one health promotion program aimed at improving the health and well-being of caregivers of people with disabilities.

DH-2.4. (Developmental) Increase the number of tribes that conduct health surveillance for people with disabilities.

DH-2.5. (Developmental) Increase the number of tribes that have at least one health promotion program aimed at improving the health and well-being of people with disabilities.

DH-2.6. (Developmental) Increase the number of tribes that conduct health surveillance of caregivers for people with disabilities.

DH-2.7. (Developmental) Increase the number of tribes that have at least one health promotion program aimed at improving the health and well-being of caregivers of people with disabilities.

DH-3. (Developmental) Increase the proportion of U.S. Master of Public Health (MPH) programs that offer graduate-level courses in disability and health.

Barriers to Healthcare

DH-4. (Developmental) Reduce the proportion of people with disabilities who report delays in receiving primary and periodic preventive care due to specific barriers.

DH-5. Increase the proportion of youth with special healthcare needs whose healthcare provider has discussed transition planning from pediatric to adult healthcare.

DH-6. Increase the proportion of people with epilepsy and uncontrolled seizures who receive appropriate medical care.

DH-7. Reduce the proportion of older adults with disabilities who use inappropriate medications.

Environment

DH-8. (Developmental) Reduce the proportion of people with disabilities who report physical or program barriers to local health and wellness programs.

DH-9. (Developmental) Reduce the proportion of people with disabilities who encounter barriers to participating in home, school, work, or community activities.

DH-10. (Developmental) Reduce the proportion of people with disabilities who report barriers to obtaining the assistive devices, service animals, technology services, and accessible technologies that they need.

DH-11. Increase the proportion of newly constructed and retrofitted U.S. homes and residential buildings that have visitable features.

DH-12. Reduce the number of people with disabilities living in congregate care residences.

- **DH-12.1.** Reduce the number of adults with disabilities aged 22 years and older living in congregate care residences that serve 16 or more persons.
- **DH-12.2.** Reduce the number of children and youth with disabilities aged 21 years and under living in congregate care residences.

Activities and Participation

DH-13. (Developmental) Increase the proportion of people with disabilities who participate in social, spiritual, recreational, community, and civic activities to the degree that they wish.

DH-14. Increase the proportion of children and youth with disabilities who spend at least 80% of their time in regular education programs.

DH-15. Reduce unemployment among people with disabilities.

DH-16. Increase employment among people with disabilities.

DH-17. Increase the proportion of adults with disabilities who report sufficient social and emotional support.

DH-18. (Developmental) Reduce the proportion of people with disabilities who report serious psychological distress.

DH-19. (Developmental) Reduce the proportion of people with disabilities who experience nonfatal unintentional injuries that require medical care.

DH-20. Increase the proportion of children with disabilities, birth through age 2 years, who receive early intervention services in home or community-based settings.

Appendix D: Overview of Relevant Legislation That Impacts Older Adults and People With Disabilities

Domain	Relevant Public Laws
Income	Social Security Act of 1935 (Pub. L. No. 271).
Health	Medicare (through the Social Security Amendments of 1965). Public Law 89–97, The Medicare Improvements for Patients and Providers Act of 2008 (Pub. L. No. 110–275). Death with Dignity Act, 3 Ore. Rev. Stat. SS, 127-800-995 (1994–1999). Patient Self Determination Act, 42 USC SS 1395 ET SEQ (1990). Patient Protection and Affordable Care Act (2010) (Pub. L. No. 111–148). The Health Maintenance Act of 1973 (outlines patient protection obligations)
Aging	The Older Americans Act of 1965, Public Law. Older Americans Act Amendments of 2006 (Pub. L. No. 109–365, 120 Stat. 2522. Omnibus Budget Reconciliation Act of 1987 (Pub. L. No. 100–203, 42 USC SS 1395i-3). RAISE Family Caregivers Act of 2018 (Pub. L. No. 115–119). IMPACT Act of 2014 (Pub. L. No. 113–185).
Mental Health	Mental Health Parity and Addiction Equity Act (Pub. L. No. 100–204) The National Mental Health Act of 1946 (Pub. L. No. 79–487). The Mental Health Study Act of 1955 (Pub. L. No. 84–182). The Mental Health Systems Act of 1980, provided improved services to people with mental illness. The Omnibus Budget Reconciliation Act of 1981 (Pub. L. No. 97–35), repealed the Mental Health Services Act and withdrew the federal government's involvement in service provision by the Alcohol, Drug Abuse, and Mental Health Administrator's consolidation of funding into single block grants to each state. The State Comprehensive Mental Health Services Plan Act of 1986 (Pub. L. No. 100–203). Paul Wellstone and Pete Domenici Mental Health Parity and Addiction Equity Act of 2008 (Pub. L. No. 110–343).

Domain	Relevant Public Laws
Disability	The Mental Retardation Facilities and Community Mental Health Centers Construction Act of 1963 (Pub. L. No. 88–164), authorized funding for professional training for community mental health centers for outpatient, inpatient and partial hospitalization, emergency care, and education for community caretakers. The Education for All Handicapped Children Act of 1975 (Pub. L. No. 94–142). Americans with Disabilities Act of 1990 (Pub. L. No. 101–336, 104 Stat. 327). Architectural Barriers Act of 1968 (Pub. L. No. 90–480, 82 Stat. 718), codified at 42 U.S.C. SS4151 et seq. Civil Rights Act of 1968 (Pub. L. No. 90–284, 82 Stat. 73). Developmentally Disabled Assistance and Bill of Rights Act (Pub. L. No. 94–103, 89 Stat 486 to 506). Developmentally Disabled Assistance and Bill of Rights Act of 2000 (Pub. L. No. 106–402, 104 Stat. 1191). Autism CARES Act of 2014 (Pub. L. No. 113–157). Fair Housing Amendment Act of 1988 (Pub. L. No. 42 U.S.C. 3601). Rehabilitation Act of 1973 (Pub. L. No. 93–112, 87 Stat. 355). (September 26, 1974). Rehabilitation Act Amendments of 1992 (Pub. L. No. 94–1442).

Appendix E: Aging and Disability Resource Centers

Alabama

ATRC	ADRC/AAA	107 Broad Street Wilcox County 36726	888-617-0500 334-682-5206	www.atrcregion6.com
Central Alabama Aging Consortium	ADRC serving the Central Alabama region	818 South Perry Street Montgomery County 36104	800-264-4680 334-240-4666	www.alabamaconnect.gov
East Alabama Area Aging and Disability Resource Center	ADRC serving the East Alabama region	PO Box 2186 1130 Quintard Ave Ste 300 Calhoun County 36202	256-237-6741 800-239-6741	www.alabamaageline.gov or www.earpdc.org
LRCOG	ADRC serving the Lee-Russell region	2207 Gateway Drive Opelika Lee County	334-749-5264	www.lrcog.com
LRCOG	ADRC serving the Lee-Russell region	2207 Gateway Drive Opelika Lee County	334-749-5264	www.lrcog.com
M4A	ADRC serving the Middle Alabama region	Post Office Drawer 618 Saginaw Shelby County 35137	205-670-5770	www.m4a-alabama.org
NARCOG	ADRC serving the North Central Alabama region	P.O. Box C Decatur Cullman County 35602	256-355-4515 ext. 261 800-AGELINE (243-5463)	www.alabamaageline.gov

(continued)

Alabama (*continued*)

Northwest Alabama Council of Local Governments	AAA	103 Student Drive POB 2603 Muscle Shoals Colbert County 35662	256-389-0530 800-838-5845	www.nacolg.com
OSCS	ADRC serving the greater Birmingham and Jefferson County region	1515 6th Avenue, South Suite 6 Birmingham Jefferson County 35233	205-325-1416 800-AGELINE (243-5463)	www.alabamaconnect.gov
Southern Alabama Regional AAA/ SARCOA	South Alabama Aging and Disability Resource Center	1075 South Brannon Stand Road Dothan Houston County 36305	334-793-6843 1-800-239-3507	www.sarcoa.org
SARPC	South Alabama ADRC/AAA	110 Beauregard St., Suite 207 P.O. Box 1665 Mobile AL Mobile County 36633	251-433-6541 1-800-AGELINE (243-5463)	http://aging southalabama.org
South Central Alabama Development Commission Area Agency on Aging	ADRC serving the South Central Alabama region	5900 Carmichael Place Montgomery County 36117	334-244-6903 800-AGELINE (243-5463)	www.alabamaageline.gov or www.scadc.net
Southern Alabama Regional AAA/ SARCOA	South Alabama Aging and Disability Resource Center	1075 South Brannon Stand Road Dothan Houston County 36305	334-793-6843 1-800-239-3507	www.sarcoa.org
Top of Alabama Regional Council of Governments	ADRC)serving the top of Alabama region	5075 Research Drive NW Huntsville Marshall County 35805	256-830-0818 800-AGELINE (243-5463)	www.alabamaconnect.gov

(*continued*)

Alabama *(continued)*

West Alabama Regional Commission	ADRC serving the West Alabama region	P.O. Box 509 Northport Tuscaloosa County 35476	205-333-2990 800-432-5030	www.3awa. org or www. alabamaageline. gov

AAAs, Area Agencies on Aging; ADRC, Aging and Disability Resource Center; ATRC, Alabama-Tombigbee Regional Commission; LRCOG, Lee-Russell Council of Governments; M4A, Middle Alabama Area Agency on Aging; NARCOG, North Central Alabama Regional Councils of Governments; OSCS, Office of Senior Citizen's Services; SARPC, South Alabama Regional Planning Commission.

Alaska

Bristol Bay Native Association	Bristol Bay and Kodiak	PO Box 310 1500 Kanakanak Rd. Dillingham 99576	907-842-6248 1-877-625-2372	tgardiner@ bbna.com
Kenai Peninsula Independent Living Center	Kenai Peninsula, Valdez-Cordova, Mat-Su	47255 Princeton Ave. Soldotna 99669	907-262-6333 1-877-625-2372	www. peninsulailc. org
Mat-Su Links ADRC	Matanuska-Susitna Borough	3161 E. Palmer-Wasilla Highway #2 Wasilla 99654	907-373-3632	www.linksprc. org
Municipality of Anchorage, DHHS, Senior Services Section	Anchorage	PO Box 196650 825 L Street, Ste 203 Anchorage 99501	907-343-7770 1-877-625-2372	www.muni. org/adrc
Southeast Alaska Independent Living Center	Southeast	225 Hospital Drive Juneau 99801	907-586-4920 1-877-625-2372	www.sailinc. org

ADRC, Aging and Disability Resource Center; DHHS, Department of Health and Human Services.

Arizona

Maricopa Arizona Links	Maricopa County	1366 E. Thomas Road, Suite 108 950 A Phoenix Maricopa County 85014	602-264-2255 888-783-7500 800-432-4040	www.aaaphx.org
Northern Arizona Links	Apache, Coconino, Navajo and Yavapai Counties (Non-Navajo Nation Residents)	43 South San Francisco Street Flagstaff, AZ Coconino County 86001	877-521-3500	www.nacog.org/aging/senior_services.asp
Pima Arizona Links	Pima County	8467 E. Broadway Tucson Pima County 85710	520-790-0504 520-790-7262	www.pcoa.org
Pinal-Gila Arizona Links	Pinal and Gila Counties	8969 W. McCartney Road Casa Grande Pinal County 85194-7432	520-836-2758	www.pgcsc.org
SouthEastern Arizona Council of Governments, Area Agency on Aging	Cochise, Graham, Greenlee, and Santa Cruz Counties	118 Arizona St. Bisbee Cochise County 85603	520-432-5301 ext. 220 520-432-5301 ext. 220	www.seago.org
Western Arizona Council of Governments, Area Agency on Aging, Region Four	La Paz, Mojave, and Yuma Counties	24 South 3rd Avenue Yuma Yuma County 85364	928-782-1886 928-753-6247	https://des.az.gov/services/aging-and-adult/aging-and-disability-services-ads

Arkansas

Choices in Living Resource Center	Statewide	P.O. Box 1437, Slot S-530 700 Main Street Little Rock Pulaski County 72203-1437	1-866-801-3435	www.choicesinliving.ar.gov

California

ADRC—Riverside	Riverside County	6296 River Crest Drive # K Riverside Riverside County 92507	951-867-3800	www.riverside.networkofcare.org or www.rcaging.org
Access to Independence	San Diego Area	8885 Rio San Diego Dr San Diego San Diego County 92108	(619) 293-3500	http://accesstoindependence.org
CalOptima	Orange County, CA	1120 W La Veta Ave Orange Orange County 92868	(800) 510-2020	www.adrcoc.org or www.caloptima.org
Dayle McIntosh Center	Orange County, CA	13272 Garden Grove Blvd Garden Grove Orange County 92843	714/621-3300 800-972-8285	www.adrcoc.org or www.daylemc.org
Del Norte Area Aging and Disability Resource Center	ADRC—Del Norte and Humboldt County	3300 Glenwood Eureka Del Norte County 95501	707- 442-3763	www.A1AA.org
FREED Center for Independent Living	ADRC—Nevada County, Sierra, Sutter, Yuba	117 New Mohawk Road, Suite A Nevada City Nevada County 95959	530-477-3333 800-655-7732 for Voice 530-477-8194 for TTY	https://freed.org

(*continued*)

California *(continued)*

Office on Aging	Orange County, CA	1300 S. Grand Ave Santa Ana Orange County 92705	800-510-2020	www.adrcoc.org
PASSAGES	ADRC—Butte, Colusa, Glen, Plumas, and Tehama Counties	491 Carmichael Drive, Suite 400 Chico 95928	530 898-5923	www.passagescenter.org
San Francisco DAAS, ILRCSF	ADRC—City and County of San Francisco	DAAS: 1650 Mission Street, 5/F ILRCSF: 649 Mission Street, 3/F San Francisco San Francisco County 94103	DAAS: 415-355-6700 415-543-6222	www.sfdaas.org or www.ilrcsf.org
San Diego AIS and a2i	ADRC—San Diego County	5560 Overland Ave. Suite 310 San Diego, CA 92123 (for AIS) 8885 Rio San Diego Drive, San Diego, CA 92108 (for a2i) San Diego San Diego County 92123	800-510-2020 in San Diego 800-339-4661	https://www.sandiegocounty.gov/content/sdc/hhsa/programs/ais/about_ais.html

a2i, Access to Independence; ADRC, Aging and Disability Resource Center; AIS, Aging and Independent Services; DAAS, Department of Aging and Adult Services; ILRCSF, Independent Living Resource Center San Francisco.

Colorado

Alamosa ARCH	Alamosa, Conejos, Costilla, Mineral, Rio Grande, and Saguache Counties	116 3rd Street Alamosa 81101	(719) 589-4511	https://resources.caregiver.com/listing/alamosa-arch-54c2c0cc9d6ff.html
Boulder ADRC	Boulder County	3482 North Broadway Boulder Boulder County 80306	303-441-3986	http://boulder.co.networkofcare.org/aging/services/agency.aspx?pid=BoulderCountyAgingDisabilityResourcesforColoradoADRC_894_1_0
DRCOG ADRC	Adams, Arapahoe, Broomfield, Clear Creek, Denver, Douglas, Gilpin, and Jefferson Counties	1290 Broadway, Suite 700 Denver Denver County 80203	303-480-6700	https://drcog.org/programs/area-agency-aging/aging-and-disability-resource-center
El Paso ADRC	El Paso and Teller Counties	15 South 7th Street Colorado Springs El Paso County 80905	719-955-0742	http://lrgv.tx.networkofcare.org/aging/services/index.aspx
Huerfano and Las Animas ADRC		615 Russell Avenue Walsenburg 81089	719-738-2378	www.srda.org/index.aspx?NID=88
Kit Carson ADRC	Cheyenne, Elbert, and Kit Carson Counties		719-346-7158 ext 139	

(*continued*)

Colorado (*continued*)

Larimer County (Fort Collins)	Larimer County ADRC—Aging and Disability Resources for Colorado	2601 Midpoint Drive Suite 112 Fort Collins Larimer County 80525	970-498-7750	http://larimer.co.networkofcare.org/aging
Lower Arkansas Valley Area Agency on Aging	LaJunta ARCH	13 West Third St, Room 110 La Junta Otero County 81050	719-383-3166	
Mesa County ARCH	Mesa, Garfield, Moffat, Rio Blanco, and Routt Counties	510 29 1/2 Road Grand Junction Mesa County 81502	970-241-8480	www.humanservices.mesacounty.us
Montrose ARCH	Counties of Montrose, Delta, Gunnison, San Miguel, Hinsdale, and Ouray	Montrose County	970-249-2436	
Northeastern ARCH	Logan, Morgan, Phillips, Sedgwick, Washington, and Yuma Counties	231 Main Street, Suite 211 Fort Morgan Morgan County 80701	970-867-9409	
Pueblo County ARCH	Pueblo County	2631 E. 4th Street Pueblo Pueblo County 81001	719-583-6317 719-583-6120	http://www.co.pueblo.co.us/hhs/paaa
Region 12 ADRC	Eagle, Grand, Jackson, Pitkin, and Summit Counties	249 Warren Ave. Silverthorne Summit County 80498		

(*continued*)

Colorado (*continued*)

San Juan Basin AAA	Archuleta, Dolores, La Plata, Montezuma, and San Juan Counties	450 Lewis Street Pagosa Springs Archuleta County 81147	970-264-0501	http://sjbaaa.org
Upper Arkansas ADRC	Chaffee, Custer, Fremont, and Lake Counties	139 East 3rd Street Salida Chaffee County 81201	719-539-3341	
Weld ARCH	Weld County	315 C. N. 11th Avenue P.O. Box 1805 Greeley 80631	970-346-6952	

AAAs, Area Agencies on Aging; ADRC, Aging and Disability Resource Center.

Connecticut

North Central Connecticut	North Central Region Community Choices: North Central Region	55 Farmington Avenue, 12th Floor Hartford, CT 06105-3730	1-866-218-6631	http://www.ct.gov/agingservices/cwp/view.asp?Q=486430
North Central Connecticut	Connecticut Community Care, Inc.	100 Great Meadow Rd. Wethersfield Hartford County 06109	860-257-1503	http://www.ct.gov/agingservices/cwp/view.asp?Q=486430
North Central Connecticut	Independence Unlimited	151 New Park Ave. Hartford Hartford County 06106	860-523-5021	

(*continued*)

Connecticut (*continued*)

North Central Connecticut	North Central Area Agency on Aging	151 New Park Ave. Hartford Hartford County 06106	860-724-6443	
South Central Connecticut	Agency on Aging of South Central CT	One Long Wharf Drive New Haven New Haven County 06511	203-785-8533	
South Central	Community Choices: South Central Region			www.ct.gov/agingservices/cwp/view.asp?a=2510&q=385896
South Central Connecticut	Center for Disability Rights	764 Campbell Ave, Suite A West Haven New Haven County06516	203-934-7077 1-800-994-9422	
Southwestern Connecticut	Disability Resource Center of Fairfield County	80 Ferry Blvd. #200 Stratford Fairfield County 06615	203-378-6977 1-800-994-9422	
Southwestern Connecticut	Southwestern CT Area Agency on Aging	10 Middle Street Bridgeport Fairfield County 06604	203-333-9288	www.swcaa.org
Tolland County, Windham County, Middlesex County, New London County	Senior Resources	19 Ohio Ave. Norwich New London County 06360	860-887-3561	

(*continued*)

Connecticut *(continued)*

Tolland County, Windham County, New London County	Disabilities Network of Eastern CT	19 Ohio Ave. Norwich New London County 06360	860-823-1898	
Tolland County, Windham County, New London County	Connecticut Community Care, Inc.	108 New Park Ave. Franklin New London County 06254	860-885-2960	
Western Connecticut	Independence Northwest	1183 New Haven Rd. Suite 200 Naugatuck New Haven County 06770	203-729-3299	www.independencenorthwest.org/index.php/contact-us
Western Region	Community Choices: Western Region	84 Progress Lane, Waterbury, CT 06705	203-757-5449 800-994-9422 203-757-4081	Margaret.geruno-murkette@ct.gov

District of Columbia

Washington DC	District of Columbia Office on Aging/DC ADRC	500 K St. NE Washington District of Columbia 20002	202-724-5626	https://dcoa.dc.gov/page/aging-and-disability-resource-center-adrc

ADRC, Aging and Disability Resource Center.

Florida

Alachua County, Bradford County, Citrus County, Columbia County, Dixie County, Gilchrist County, Hamilton County, Hernando County, Lafayette County, Lake County, Levy County, Marion County, Putnam County, Sumter County, Suwannee County, Union County	Elder Options, The Mid Florida Area Agency on Aging	100 SW 75th Street, Suite 301 Gainesville Alachua County 32607	352-378-6649 1-800-262-2243	www.aging resources.org
Baker, Clay, Duval, Flagler, Nassau, St. Johns, and Volusia counties	ElderSource, Area Agency on Aging for Northeast Florida	10688 Old St. Augustine Road Jacksonville Duval County 32257	904-391-6600 1-888-242-4464	http:// myeldersource.org
Based in Fort Myers, serving Charlotte, Collier, DeSoto, Glades, Hendry, Lee, and Sarasota counties	Area Agency on Aging for Southwest Florida, Inc.	15201 N. Cleveland Avenue Suite 1100 North Fort Myers Lee County 33903	239-652-6900 (admin) 239-652-6901	www.aaaswfl.org
Based in Orlando and serving Orange, Osceola, Seminole, and Brevard counties	Senior Resource Alliance	988 Woodcock Road 6Suite 200 Orlando Orange County 32803	407-514-1800 (admin) 407-514-0019	www.senior resourcealliance. org

(*continued*)

Florida (*continued*)

Based in St. Petersburg and serving Pasco and Pinellas counties	Area Agency on Aging of Pasco-Pinellas, a designated ADRC	9549 Koger Boulevard, Gadsden Building, Suite 100 St. Petersburg Pinellas County 33702	(727) 570-9696 (admin) for Pasco 1-800-861-8111 for Pinellas 727-217-8111	www.agingcarefl.org
Hardee, Highlands, Hillsborough, Manatee, and Polk counties	West Central Florida ADRC	5905 Breckenridge Park Drive Tampa Hillsborough County 33601	813-740-3888 (admin) 1-800-336-2226	www.agingflorida.com
Indian River, Martin, Okeechobee, Palm Beach, and St. Lucie Counties	Area Agency on Aging of Palm Beach/ Treasure Coast, Inc.	4400 North Congress Avenue West Palm Beach Palm Beach County 33407	561-685-5885 (admin) 561-214-8600	www.youraging resourcecenter.org
Miami-Dade county and Monroe County	Alliance for Aging	760 NW 107 Avenue, Suite 214 Miami Miami-Dade County 33172	305-670-6500 (admin) 305-670-4357	
Northwest Florida	Northwest Florida Area Agency on Aging	5090 Commerce Park Circle Pensacola Escambia County 32505	904- 494-7100 (admin) 1-866-531-8011 850-494-7101	www.nwflaaa.org

(*continued*)

Florida (*continued*)

Serving Broward County	ADRC of Broward County	5300 Hiatus Road Sunrise Broward County 33351	(954) 745-9567 (954) 745-9779 (Elder Helpline)	http://www.adrcbroward.org

ADRC, Aging and Disability Resource Center.

Georgia

Central Savannah River Area	Central Savannah ADRC	3023 Riverwatch Pkwy. Suite A, Bldg 200 Augusta Richmond County 30907-2016	706-210-2018 706-650-5645 888-922-4464	www.georgiaadrc.com or www.csrardc.org/csra/aging/aaa.htm
Coastal Georgia	Coastal Georgia ADRC	1181 Coastal Drive SW Darien Glynn County 31305	912-437-0852	www.georgiaadrc.com or http://www.coastalgeorgiardc.org/aaa.html
Georgia Mountains	Georgia Mountains ADRC	P.O Box 2534 Gainesville Hall County 30503-2660	770-538-2650 1-800-845-5465	www.georgiaadrc.com or www.legacylink.org
Heart of Georgia	Heart of Georgia ADRC	331 West Parker Street Baxley Appling County 31513-0674	912-367-3648 1-888-367-9913	www.georgiaadrc.com or www.hogarc.org
Metro Atlanta Region	Atlanta ADRC	Atlanta Regional Commission 40 Courtland St. NE Atlanta Fulton County 30303	800-676-2433 404-463-3333	www.georgiaadrc.com or www.agewiseconnection.com

(*continued*)

Middle Georgia	Middle Georgia ADRC	175 Emery Hwy Suite C Macon Bibb County 31217-3679	478-751-6466 1-866-552-4464	www.georgiaadrc.com or www.mg-rc.org
Northeast Georgia	Northeast Georgia ADRC	305 Research Drive Athens Clarke County 30605	706-369-5650 706-425-2954	www.georgiaadrc.com or http://www.negrc.org/aging/php
Northwest Georgia	Northwest Georgia ADRC	PO Box 1798 Rome Floyd County 30162	800-759-2963 or 706-295-6485 for Seniors 800-646-7721 or 706-802-5272 for Adults with Developmental Disabilities	www.georgiaadrc.com or www.northwestga-aaa.org/adrc.htm
River Valley	River Valley ADRC	1428 Second Avenue Columbus Muscogee County 31902-1908	706-256-2910 1-800-615-4379	www.georgiaadrc.com or www.rivervalleyrcaaa.org
Southern Crescent ADRC	Southern Crescent AAA and Department of Behavioral Health and Developmental Disabilities Region 1	P.O. Box 1600 Franklin Upson County 30217-1600	678-552-2842 706-407-0018 866-854-5652 678-552-2842 for Seniors 800-646-7721 706-802-5272 for Adults with Developmental Disabilities	www.georgiaadrc.com or www.scaaa.net/ADRC.htm

(*continued*)

Georgia (*continued*)

Southern Georgia	Southern Georgia ADRC	1725 South Georgia Parkway, West Waycross Ware County 31503-8958	912-287-5888 912-303-1705 for Adults with Developmental Disabilities	www.georgiaadrc.com or https://aging.georgia.gov/aging-and-disability-resource-connection-adrc
Southwest Georgia	Southwest ADRC	1105 Palmyra Road Albany Dougherty County 31701-1933	229-423-1124 1-800-282-6612	www.georgiaadrc.com or www.sowegacoa.org

ADRC, Aging and Disability Resource Connection; AAAs Area Agencies on Aging.

Guam

Entire Island of Guam (all 19 municipalities/all 26 villages)	Guam Aging and Disability Resource Center (Guam GetCare)	238 AFC Flores St., DNA Bldg., Ste 702 Hagatna Guam 96910	671-475-4646	https://resources.caregiver.com/listing/guide/aging-disability-resource-center-adrc

Hawaii

County of Hawaii (Island of Hawaii)	ADRC Hawaii—Kahi Malama	1055 Kinoole Street Suite 101 Kahi Malama Hilo Hawaii County 96720-3872	808-961-8600 808-961-8626	http://hawaiiadrc.org
City and County of Honolulu	ADRC Hawaii: a program of the Honolulu Elderly Affairs Division	715 South King Street Suite 200 Honolulu Honolulu County 96813-3021	808-768-7705 808-768-7700	http://hawaiiadrc.org

(*continued*)

Hawaii (*continued*)

County of Kauai (Island of Kauai)	Kauai ADRC	4444 Rice Street Suite 330 Lihue Kauai County 96766	808-241-4470	http://hawaiiadrc.org
County of Maui (Islands of Maui, Molokai and Lanai)	Maui County Office on Aging	2200 Main Street Room 547 Wailuku Maui County 96793	808-270-7755	http://hawaiiadrc.org

ADRC, Aging and Disability Resource Center.

Idaho

Area I	North Idaho AAA			
Area II	North Central Idaho AAA	124 New 6th Street Lewiston Nez Perce County 83501	208-746-3351	www.cap4action.org
Area III	AAA Serving	125 E 50th St Garden City Ada County 83714	208-908-4990	https://aging.idaho.gov/adr
Area IV	CSI Office on Aging	315 Falls Avenue PO Box 1238 Twin Falls Twin Falls County 83303	208-736-2122	officeonaging.csi.edu
Area V	Southeast Idaho AAA	214 E. Center P.O. Box 6079 Pocatello Bannock County 83201	208-233-4032	www.sicog.org

(*continued*)

Idaho (*continued*)

Area VI	Eastern Idaho AAA	935 Lincoln Road Idaho Falls Bonneville County 83401	208-522-5391	www.eicap.org

AAA, Area Agencies on Aging.

Illinois

Nine counties in Northwestern Illinois (Rockford)	ADRC of Rockford (Northwestern Illinois AAA)	1111 S. Alpine Road Rockford Winnebago County 61108	815-226-4901	www.nwilaaa.org
Bond, Clinton, Madison, Monroe, Randolph, St. Clair, Washington	AAA of Southwestern Illinois	2365 Country Road Belleville St. Clair County 62221	800-326-3221	www.answersonaging.com
Bureau, Henderson, Henry, McDonough, Knox, LaSalle, Mercer, Putnam, Rock Island, and Warren Counties	Western Illinois Area Agency on Aging and Disability Resource Center	729 34th Avenue Rock Island Rock Island County 61201	309-793-6800	www.wiaaa.org
Cook County	Progress Center for Independent Living	7521 Madison Street Forest Park 60130	708.209.1500	www.progresscil.org
Decatur	ADRC (Macon County Health Department)	1221 Condit Street Decatur Macon County 62521	217-423-6550	www.adrc-tae.acl.gov/tiki-login_scr.php

(*continued*)

Illinois (*continued*)

DuPage, Grundy, Kane, Kankakee, Kendall, Lake, McHenry and Will	AAA of Northeastern Illinois	245 W. Roosevelt Road Bldg. 6 West Chicago DuPage County 60185	630-293-5990	www.ageguide.org
East Central Illinois	East Central Illinois AAA in Bloomington, PSA 5 (Starting Point ADRC-Decatur)			
Suburban Cook County	AgeOptions AAA in Oak Park	1048 Lake Street, Suite 300 Oak Park Cook County 60301	703-383-0258	www.ageoptions.org

AAA, Area Agency on Aging; ADRC, Aging and Disability Resource Connection.

Indiana

Adams, Allen, DeKalb, Huntington, LaGrange, Noble, Steuben, Wells, and Whitley Counties	Aging and In-Home Services Northeast Indiana, Inc.	2927 Lake Ave Fort Wayne, IN 46805	260-745-1200 1-800-552-3662	www.agingihs.org
Bartholomew, Brown, Decatur, Jennings, and Jackson counties	Aging & Com. Serv. South Central Indiana	1531 13th Street Suite G-900 Columbus Adams County 47201	812-372-6918 866-644-6407	www.agingandcommunityservices.org

(*continued*)

Indiana (*continued*)

Benton, Carroll, Clinton, Fountain, Tippecanoe, Montgomery, Warren, and White counties	Area IV Agency on Aging and Community Action Programs, Inc.	660 North 36th St P.O. Box 4727 Lafayette, IN 47903	765-447-7683 1-800-382-7556	www.areaivagency.org
Blackford, Delaware, Grant, Henry, Jay, Madison, and Randolph counties in East Central Indiana	LifeStream Services, Inc.	1701 South Pilgrim Blvd. P O Box 308 Yorktown Delaware County 47396	765-759-1121 800-589-1121	www.lifestreaminc.org
Boone, Hamilton, Hancock, Hendricks, Johnson, Marion, Morgan, Shelby	CICOA Aging & In-Home Solutions (Area 8)	4755 Kingsway Dr. Ste. 200 Indianapolis Marion County 46205	317-254-5465 317-254-3660 800-432-2422	www.cicoa.org
Cass, Fulton, Howard, Miami, Wabash, Tipton	Area Five Agency on Aging & Community Services, Inc.	1801 Smith Street Suite 300 Logansport 46947	574-722-4451 800-654-9421	www.areafive.com
Clark, Floyd, Harrison, Scott	LifeSpan Resources, Inc.	33 State Street, Suite 308 PO Box 995 New Albany 47151	812-948-8330 888-948-8330	www.lsr14.org
Clay, Parke, Putnam, Sullivan, Vigo, Vermillion	Area 7 Agency on Aging and Disabled West Central Indiana Economic Development District, Inc.	1718 Wabash Avenue P.O. Box 359 Terre Haute 47807	812-238-1561 800-489-1561	www.westcentralin.com

(*continued*)

Indiana (*continued*)

Daviess, Dubois, Greene, Knox, Martin, and Pike Counties (Office in Vincennes)	Generations Aging and Disability Resource Center (Link-Age)	1019 N. 4th St PO Box 314 Vincennes Knox County 47591	812-888-5880 800-742-9002	www.generationsnetwork.org
Dearborn, Jefferson, Ohio, Ripley, Switzerland	Lifetime Resources, Inc.	13091 Benedict Dr. Dillsboro Dearborn County 47018	812-432-5215 812-432-6200	www.lifetime-resources.org
Elkhart, LaPorte, Marshall, Kosciusko, and St. Joseph counties (South Bend)	REAL Services, Inc., Aging and Disability Resource Center	1151 South Michigan Street P.O. Box 1835 South Bend St. Joseph County 46634	574-284-2644	www.realservicesinc.com/
Fayette, Franklin, Rush, Union, Wayne	Area 9 In-Home and Community Services Agency	520 South 9th Street Richmond 47374	765-966-1795 800-458-9345	www.iue.indiana.edu/departments/Area9
Lake, Porter, Jasper, Newton, Pulaski, and Starke counties	Northwest Indiana Community Action Corp.	5240 Fountain Drive Crown Point, IN 46307	219-794-1829	www.nwi-ca.com
Lawrence County, Orange County, Washington County, Crawford County	Hoosier Uplands/Area 15 Agency on Aging and Disability Services	521 West Main Street Mitchell Adams County 47446	812-849-4457 800-333-2451	www.hoosieruplands.org

(*continued*)

Indiana (*continued*)

Monroe, Owen	Area 10 Agency on Aging	631 West Edgewood Drive Ellettsville 47429	812-876-3383 800-844-1010	www.area10agency.org
Vanderburgh, Warrick, Spencer, Gibson, Perry, and Posey Co.	SWIRCA ADRC	P.O. Box 3938 16 W. Virginia St Evansville Vanderburgh County 47737-3938	812-464-7800 1-800-253-2188	www.swirca.org

ADRC, Aging and Disability Resource Center.

Iowa

Benton Cedar Iowa Johnson Jones Linn Washington	LifeLong Links ADRC Heritage AAA	6301 Kirkwood Blvd., SW PO Box 2068 Cedar Rapids 52406	319-398-5559	http://heritageaaa.org/lifelong-links---aging-disability-resource-center
Black Hawk, Butler, Bremer, Chickasaw, Buchanan, Grundy, Hardin, Marshall, Poweshiek, Tama	Northeast Iowa AAA	2101 Kimball Ave., Ste 320 PO Box 388 Waterloo Black Hawk County 50702-5057	866-468-7887	cjohnson@nei3a.org
Services available through website and toll-free number statewide	Iowa Department on Aging	510 E. 12th St., Suite #2 Des Moines	515-725-3335 800-532-3213	www.lifelonglinks.org

ADRC, Aging and Disability Resource Center; AAA, Area Agency on Aging.

Kansas

Allen, Bourbon, Cherokee, Crawford, Labette, Montgomery, Neosho, Wilson, Woodson	Southeast Kansas ADRC	1 West Ash Chanute Neosho County 66720	620-431-2980 1-800-794-2440	www.sekaaa.com
Barber, Barton, Clark, Comanche, Edwards, Finney, Ford, Grant, Gray, Greeley, Hamilton, Haskell, Hodgeman, Kearny, Kiowa, Lane, Meade, Morton, Ness, Pawnee, Pratt, Rush, Scott, Seward, Stafford, Stanton, Stevens, Wichita	Southwest Kansas ADRC	236 San Jose Avenue PO Box 1636 Dodge City Ford County 67801	620-225-8230 1-800-742-9531	www.swkaaa.org
Central Plains/ Wichita	Central Plains ADRC	2622 W. Central, Ste 500 Wichita Sedgwick County 67203	316-660-5210 800-367-7298	www.cpaaa.org
Chase, Clay, Cloud, Dickinson, Ellsworth, Geary, Jewell, Lincoln, Lyon, Marion, Mitchell, Morris, Ottawa, Pottawatomie, Republic, Riley, Saline, Wabaunsee	North Central Flint Hills ADRC	401 Houston Manhattan Riley County 66502	785-776-9294 1-800-432-2703	www.ncfhaaa.com

(*continued*)

Kansas (*continued*)

Chautauqua; Cowley; Elk; Greenwood; Kingman; Harper; McPherson; Reno; Rice; Sumner	South Central Kansas ADRC	304 South Summit Arkansas City Cowley County 67005	620-442-0268 1-800-362-0264	http://sckaaa.org
Johnson	Johnson County ADRC	11811 South Sunset Drive Suite #1300 Olathe Johnson County 66061	913-715-8800 1-888-214-4404	www.jocogov.org/dept/human-services/area-agency-aging/aging-disability-resource-center
Northwest Counties / Hays Area	Northwest Kansas ADRC	510 W 29th Street, Suite B Hays Ellis County 67601	785-628-8204 800-432-7422	www.nwkaaa.com
Osage, Franklin, Miami, Coffey, Anderson, Linn	East Central Kansas ADRC	117 South Main Ottawa Franklin County 66067	785-242-7200 1-800-633-5621	http://www.eckaaa.org
Shawnee, Jefferson, Douglas	Jayhawk ADRC	2910 SW Topeka Blvd Topeka Shawnee County 66611	785-235-1367 1-800-798-1366	www.jhawkaaa.org
Washington, Marshall, Nemaha, Brown, Jackson, Doniphan, Atchison	Northeast Kansas ADRC	526 Oregon Hiawatha Brown County 66434	785-742-7152 1-800-883-2549	www.nekaaa.org

(*continued*)

Kansas (*continued*)

Wyandotte, Leavenworth	Wyandotte-Leavenworth ADRC	1300 North 78th Street Suite #100 Kansas City Wyandotte County 66112	913-573-8531 1-888-661-1444	www.wycokck.org/aging

ADRC, Aging and Disability Resource Center

Kentucky

Barren River Area	Barren River AAA	177 Graham Avenue Bowling Green Warren County 42102	800-395-7654 877-293-7447	http://resourcemarket.ky.gov
Big Sandy Area	Big Sandy AAA	100 Resource Drive Prestonsburg Floyd County 41653	606-886-2374 800-737-2723 877-293-7447	www.bigsandy.org/index.php?option=com_content&view=section&id=13&Itemid=2
Bluegrass Area	Bluegrass AAA and Independent Living	699 Perimeter Drive Lexington Fayette County 40517	859-269-8021 866-665-7921	http://resourcemarket.ky.gov
Buffalo Trace Area	Buffalo Trace AAA	201 Government Street Suite 300 Maysville 41056	606-564-6894 800-998-4347 or 877-293-7447	http://resourcemarket.ky.gov
Cumberland Valley Area	Cumberland Valley AAA	P.O. Box 1740 342 Old Whitley Road London Laurel County 40743	606-864-7391 877-293-7447	http://resourcemarket.ky.gov

(*continued*)

Kentucky (*continued*)

FIVCO Area	FIVCO AAA	P.O. Box 636 3000 Louisa Street Catlettsburg Boyd County 41129	606-929-1366 877-293-7447 800-499-5191	http://resourcemarket.ky.gov
Kentucky River Area	Kentucky River AAA	917 Perry Park Road Hazard Perry County 41701	606-436-3158 877-293-7447	http://resourcemarket.ky.gov
KIPDA Area	KIPDA AAA and Independent Living	11520 Commonwealth Drive Louisville Jefferson County 40299	502-266-5571 888-737-3363	http://resourcemarket.ky.gov
Gateway Area	Gateway AAA	110 Lake Park Drive Morehead Rowan County 40351	606-780-0090 1-855-882-5307	http://resourcemarket.ky.gov
Green River Area	Green River AAA	3860 U.S. Highway 60 West Owensboro Daviess County 42302	270-926-4433 800-928-9093 877-293-7447	http://resourcemarket.ky.gov
Lake Cumberland Area	Lake Cumberland AAA	P.O. BOX 1570 374 Lakeway Drive Russell Springs Russell County 42642	270-866-4200 800-264-7093 877-293-7447	http://resourcemarket.ky.gov
Lincoln Trail Area	Lincoln Trail AAA	P.O. Box 604 613 College Street Road Elizabethtown Hardin County 42702	270-769-2393 800-264-0393 877-293-7447	http://resourcemarket.ky.gov

(*continued*)

Kentucky (*continued*)

Northern Kentucky Area Development District	Northern Kentucky AAA and Independent Living	22 Spiral Drive Florence Pendleton County 41042	859-283-1885	http://resourcemarket.ky.gov
Pennyrile Area	Pennyrile AAA	300 Hammond Drive Hopkinsville 42040	270-886-9484 800-928-7233 877-293-7447	http://resourcemarket.ky.gov
Purchase Area	Purchase AAA	1002 Medical Drive PO Box 588 Mayfield Graves County 42066	270-247-7171 877-352-5183 877-293-7447	http://resourcemarket.ky.gov

AAA, Area Agency on Aging; KY Independence for People with Disabilities and Aging, Kentuckiana Regional Planning and Development Agency.

Louisiana

Based in Baton Rouge, serving 13 surrounding parishes Assumption, Ascension, East Baton Rouge, East Feliciana, Iberville, Livingston, Pointe Coupee, St. Helena, St. Tammany, Tangipahoa, Washington, West Baton Rouge, West Feliciana	Capital ADRC	6554 Florida Blvd Suite 221 Baton Rouge East Baton Rouge Parish 70806	800-833-9883 800-833-9883	www.louisianaanswers.com

(*continued*)

Louisiana (*continued*)

Based in Lafayette, serving surrounding parishes Acadia, Evangeline, Iberia, Lafayette, St. Landry, St. Martin, St. Mary, Vermilion Parishes	Cajun ADRC	110 Toledo Drive Lafayette Vermilion Parish 70506	800-738-2256	www. louisianaanswers. com
Based in Metairie, serving four surrounding parishes Jefferson, St. Charles, St. James, and St. John the Baptist	Jefferson Council on Aging	6620 Riverside Dr./Suite 107 Metairie Jefferson Parish 70003	504-207-4690 800-635-1437	www. louisianaanswers. com
North Delta ADRC	North Delta AAA	1913 Stubbs Avenue Monroe, LA Ouachita Parish 71201	318-387-2572	www. louisianaanswers. com
Serving Avoyelles, Catahoula, Concordia, Grant, LaSalle, Rapides and Winn Parishes	Cenla ADRC	1423 Peterman Drive Alexandria Rapides Parish 71301	318-484-2260 800 454-9573	www. louisianaanswers. com
Serving Bienville, Bossier, Caddo, Claiborne, DeSoto, Natchitoches, Red River, Sabine and Webster Parishes	Caddo ADRC	1700 Buckner St./Ste 240 Shreveport Caddo Parish 71101	316-676-7900 800-793-1198	www. louisianaanswers. com

(*continued*)

Louisiana (*continued*)

Serving Lafourche and Terrebonne Parishes	Terrebonne ADRC	995 West Tunnel Boulevard Houma Terrebonne Parish 70360	985-868-8411 800-353-3265	www.LouisianaAnswers.com
Serving Orleans, Plaquemines and St. Bernard Parishes	Orleans ADRC	2475 Canal Street Suite 211 New Orleans 70119	888-922-8522	www.LouisianaAnswers.com

AAA, Area Agency on Aging; ADRC, Aging and Disability Resource Center.

Maine

4 county area: Penobscot, Piscataquis, Hancock, Washington	Eastern AAA ADRC	450 Essex Bangor Penobscot County 04401	207-941-2865 800-432-7812	www.eaaa.org
6 counties: Kennebec, Knox, Lincoln, Sagadahoc, Somerset, Waldo	Spectrum Generations Agency on Aging ADRC	One Weston Court Suite 203 Augusta Kennebec County 04330	207-623-0764 800-639-1553	http://www.spectrumgenerations.org
Aroostook	Aroostook Agency on Aging ADRC	1 Edgemont Drive Suite 2 Presque Isle Aroostook County 04769	207-764-3396 1-800-439-1789	www.aroostookaging.org
York and Cumberland Counties	Southern Maine Agency on Aging ADRC	136 U.S. Route One Scarborough Cumberland County 04074	207-396-6500 1-877-353-3771	www.smaaa.org

AAA, Area Agency on Aging; ADRC, Aging and Disability Resource Center.

Maryland

Allegany County	Maryland Access Point of Allegany County (Allegany County Human Resources Development Commission)	125 Virginia Avenue Cumberland Allegany County 21502	301-783-1752	www.alleganyhrdc.org/map.html
Anne Arundel County	Maryland Access Point of Anne Arundel County (Anne Arundel County Department of Aging and Disabilities)	Heritage Complex 2666 Riva Road, Suite 400 Annapolis Anne Arundel County 21401	410-222-4257, ext. 221	www.aacounty.org/Aging/agingServices/IA.cfm
Baltimore City	Maryland Access Point of Baltimore City (Office of Aging & Care Services)	417 East Fayette Street, 6th Floor Baltimore Baltimore County 21202	410-545-1555	www.baltimorehealth.org/index.html
Baltimore county	Maryland Access Point of Baltimore County (Baltimore County Department of Aging and Commission on Disabilities)	611 Central Avenue Towson Baltimore County 21204	410-887-2594	www.baltimorecountymd.gov/Agencies/aging/helpfulnumbers/mapbaltco.html or www.baltimorecountymd.gov/Agencies/neighborhoodimprovement/disabilities/index.html

(*continued*)

Maryland (*continued*)

Caroline County	Maryland Access Point of the Upper Shore (Upper Shore Aging, Inc./ Caroline County Senior Center)	403 South 7th Street, Suite 127 Denton Caroline County 21629	410-479-2535	www.uppershoreaging.org
Carroll County	Maryland Access Point of Carroll County (Carroll County Bureau of Aging & Disabilities)	125 Stoner Avenue Westminster Carroll County 21157	410-386-3800	http://ccgovernment.carr.org/ccg/aging
Cecil County	Maryland Access Point of Cecil County (Cecil County Department of Senior Services and Community Transit)	200 Chesapeake Blvd. Suite 2550 Elkton Cecil County 21921	410-996-8172 410-996-8169	http://www.ccgov.org/dept_aging
Charles County	Maryland Access Point of Charles County (Charles County Area Agency on Aging, Aging and Senior Programs Division)	8190 Port Tobacco Charles County 20677	301-934-0111 855-843-9725	www.charlescountymd.gov/cs/aging/aging-and-senior-programs
Dorchester, Somerset, and Wicomico Counties	Maryland Access Point of Wicomico County (MAC, Inc.)	909 Progress Circle Salisbury Wicomico County 21804	410-742-0505	www.macinc.org/md-access-point.html

(*continued*)

Maryland (*continued*)

Frederick County	Maryland Access Point of Frederick County (Frederick Department of Aging)	1440 Taney Avenue Frederick Frederick County 21702	301-600-1605	www.frederickcountymd.gov/Aging
Harford County	Maryland Access Point of Harford County (Harford County Office on Aging & Disability Resource Center)	145 North Hickory Avenue Bel Air Harford County 21014	410-638-3025	http://www.harfordcountymd.gov/services/aging/index.cfm
Howard County	Maryland Access Point of Howard County (Howard County Office on Aging)	6751 Columbia Gateway Drive Suite 200 Columbia Howard County 21046	410-313-5980	www.howardcountyaging.org
Kent County	Maryland Access Point of Upper Shore (Upper Shore Aging, Inc./Amy Lynn Ferris Adult Activity Center)	200 Schauber Road Chestertown Kent County 21620	410-778-2564	www.uppershoreaging.org
Montgomery County	Maryland Access Point of Montgomery County (Montgomery County Division of Aging and Disability Services)	401 Hungerford Drive, 3rd Floor Rockville Montgomery County 20850	240-777-3000	www.montgomerycountymd.gov/hhs-program/ads/adsadsresourceunit-p179.html

(*continued*)

Maryland (*continued*)

Prince George's County	Maryland Access Point of Prince George's County (Prince George's County Department of Family Services, Aging Services Division)	6420 Allentown Road Camp Springs Prince George's County 20748	301-265-8450	www.princegeorgescountymd.gov/1718/Information-Assistance
Queen Anne's County	Maryland Access Point of Queen Anne's County (Queen Anne's County Department of Community Services)	104 Powell Street Centreville Queen Anne's County 21617	410-758-1040, ext. 2715	www.qac.org/default.aspx?pageid=68&template=3&toplevel=34
St. Mary's County	Maryland Access Point of St. Mary's County (St. Mary' County Department of Aging)	41780 Baldridge Street P.O. Box 653 Leonardtown St. Mary's County 20650	301-475-4200, ext. 1050	www.co.saint-marys.md.us/aging/index.asp
Talbot County	Maryland Access Point of the Upper Shore (Upper Shore Aging, Inc.)	400 Brookletts Ave. Easton Talbot County 21601	410-822-2869, ext. 255	www.uppershoreaging.org
Washington County	Maryland Access Point of Washington County (Washington County Commission on Aging, Inc.)	140 W. Franklin Street 4th Floor Hagerstown Washington County 21740	301-790-0275	www.wccoaging.org/InformationAndAssistance.aspx?MAP

(*continued*)

Maryland (*continued*)

Worcester County	Worcester County	4767 Snow Hill Road Snow Hill Worcester County21863	410-632-9915 ext. 183 410-632-9915 ext. 170	www.worcesterhealth.org
	Maryland Access Point of Garrett County (Garrett County Community Action Committee)	104 East Center Street Oakland Garrett County 21550	301-533-9000 1-888-877-8403	www.garrettcac.org/aging-and-nutrition-services/maryland-access-point-map
	Maryland Access Point of Calvert County (Calvert County Office on Aging)	450 West Dares Beach Road Prince Frederick Calvert County 20678	410-535-4606	www.co.cal.md.us/residents/health/aging

Massachusetts

ADRC of Central Massachusetts	Montachusett Home Care Corporation	680 Mechanic Street - Suite 120 Leominster Worcester County 01453-4402	978-537-7411	www.montachusetthomecare.com
ADRC of Greater North Shore	ADRC of Greater North Shore	300 Rosewood Drive Suite 260 Danvers Essex County 01923	978-406-4614	www.adrcgns.org
ADRC of the Greater North Shore	Greater Lynn Senior Services	8 Silsbee St. Lynn Essex County 01901	781-599-0110	www.glss.nevvv
ADRC of the Greater North Shore	North Shore Elder Services	300 Rosewood Drive Suite 200 Danvers Essex County01923	978-750-4540	www.nselder.org

(*continued*)

Massachusetts (*continued*)

ADRC of the Greater North Shore	Senior Care, Inc.	49 Blackburn Center Gloucester Essex County 01930	978-281-1750 978-281-1750	www.seniorcareinc.org
ADRC OF Merrimack Valley	Elder Services of the Merrimack Valley	280 Merrimack Street Suite 400 Lawrence Essex County 01843	978-683-7747 800-892-0890	www.esmv.org
ADRC of Southeastern Massachusetts	Bristol Elder Services	1 Father DeValles Blvd., Unit 8 Fall River Bristol County 02723	508-675-2101	www.bristolelder.org
ADRC of Southeastern Massachusetts	Bristol Elder Services, Inc.	1 Father DeValles Blvd. Unit 8 Fall River Bristol County 02773	508-675-2101	www.bristolelder.org
Berkshire County	Berkshire County ADRC, Elder Services of Berkshire County	877 South Street Suite 4E Pittsfield Berkshire County 01201	413-499-0524	www.esbci.org
Boston ADRC	City of Boston Commission on the Affairs of the Elderly	1 City Hall Square, Room 271 Boston Suffolk County 02201-2010	617.635.4366	www.cityofboston.gov/elderly
Boston ADRC	Ethos, Inc.	555 Amory Street Jamaica Plain Suffolk County 02130-2672	617 522-6700	www.ethocare.org

(*continued*)

Massachusetts (*continued*)

Boston ADRC	City of Boston, Commission on the Affairs of the Elderly	Boston City Hall Room 271 Boston Suffolk County 02201	617-635-4375	www.cityofboston.gov/elderly
Central Massachusetts ADRC	Center for Living & Working, Inc. (CLW)	484 Main Street Suite S-345 Worcester Worcester County 01608	508-798-0350	www.centerlw.org
Central Massachusetts ADRC	Tri Valley Elder Services	10 Mill Street Dudley Worcester County 01570	508-949-6640	www.trivalleyinc.org
MetroWest ADRC	BayPath Elder Services, Inc.	33 Post Road West Marlborough Middlesex County 01752	508-573-7200	www.baypath.org
MetroWest ADRC	MetroWest Center for Independent Living	280 Irving Street Framingham Middlesex County 01702	508-875-7853	www.mwcil.org
MetroWest ADRC	HESSCO Elder Services-Health and Social Services Consortium	One Merchant Street Sharon Norfolk County 02067	781-784-4944	www.hessco.org
Merrimack Valley ADRC	NILP	20 Ballard Road Lawrence Essex County 01843	978-687-4288	www.nilp.org

(*continued*)

Massachusetts (*continued*)

Pioneer Valley ADRC	Stavros Center for Independent Living	210 Old Farm Road Amherst Hampshire County 01002	413-256-0473	www.stavros.org
Pioneer Valley ADRC	WestMass Elder Care, Inc.	4 Valley Mill Road Holyoke Hampden County 01040	413-538-9020	www.wmeldercare.org
Pioneer Valley ADRC	Franklin County Home Care Corporation	330 Montague City Rd., Suite 1 Turner Falls Franklin County 01376-2530	413-773-5555	https://resources.caregiver.com/listing/adrc-of-pioneer-valley-54c2c0d1da6bc.html
Pioneer Valley ADRC	Greater Springfield Senior Services	66 Industry Ave Suite 9 Springfield Barnstable County 01104	413-781-8800	www.gsssi.org
Southeastern Massachusetts ADRC	Coastline Elderly Services	1646 Purchase St. New Bedford Bristol County 02740	508-999-6400	http://coastlineelderly.org
Southeastern Massachusetts ADRC	Southeast Center for Independent Living	66 Troy St. Fall River Bristol County 02720	508-679-9210	www.secil.org
Southern Massachusetts ADRC	Old Colony Elderly Services	144 Main St Brockton Plymouth County 02301	508-584-1561	www.oldcolonyelderservices.org

(*continued*)

Massachusetts (*continued*)

Southern Massachusetts ADRC	Independence Associated	100 Laurel St. Suite 122 East Bridgewater Bristol County 02333	508-583-2166	www.iacil.org
Southern Massachusetts ADRC	South Shore Elder Services, Inc.	1515 Washington St. Braintree Norfolk County 02184	781-848-3910	www.sselder.org

ADRC, Aging and Disability Resource Center; NILP, Northeast Independent Living Program.

Michigan

ADRC of Barry and Calhoun Counties	Disability Network Southwest Michigan	517 W. Crosstown Parkway Kalamazoo Kalamazoo County 49001	269-345-1516	www.dnswm.org
ADRC of Barry and Calhoun Counties	Region 3B Area Agency on Aging	200 W. Michigan Suite 102 Battle Creek Calhoun County 49017	269-966-2450	www.region3b.org
ADRC of GLS	The Disability Network	3600 S. Dort Hwy. Suite 54 Flint Genesee County 48507	810-742-1800 810-742-2400	www.disnetwork.org
ADRC of GLS	Shiawassee Council on Aging	300 N. Washington Owosso Shiawassee County 48867	989-723-8875	www.shiawasseecoa.org

(*continued*)

Michigan (*continued*)

ADRC of GLS and ADRC of the Thumb	Blue Water Center for Independent Living	1042 Griswold Street Port Huron St. Clair County 48060	810-987-9337	www.bwcil.org
ADRC of Northeast Michigan	Northeast Michigan Community Services Agency, Region 9 Area Agency on Aging	2375 Gordon Road Alpena Alpena County 49707	989-356-3474	www.nemcsa.org
ADRC of Northeast Michigan	Disability Network of Northern Michigan	415 East Eighth Street Traverse City Grand Traverse County 48686	231-922-0903	http://disabilitynetwork.org
ADRC of Northeast Michigan	Disability Network of Mid-Michigan	1705 S. Saginaw Road Midland Midland County 48640	989-835-4041	www.dnmm.org
ADRC of Northwest Michigan	Disability Network/ Northern Michigan	333 E. State Street Traverse City Grand Traverse County 49684	231-922-0903	https://disabilitynetwork.org
ADRCSEMI	Ann Arbor Center for Independent Living	3941 Research Park Drive Ann Arbor Washtenaw County 48108	734-971-0277	www.annarborcil.org/about
ADRCSEMI	Area Agency on Aging 1-B	29100 Northwestern Hwy. Suite 400 Southfield Oakland County 48034	248-357-2255 800-852-7795	www.aaa1b.com

(*continued*)

Michigan (*continued*)

ADRC of SWWC	The Senior Alliance (AAA 1-C)	3850 Second Street Suite 100 Wayne Wayne County 48184	734-722-2830	www.aaa1c.org
ADRC of the Lakeshore	Disability Network Lakeshore	426 Century Lane Holland Ottawa County 49423	616-396-5326	http://dnlakeshore.org
ADRC of the Lakeshore	Disability Connection of West Michigan	27 E. Cay Avenue Muskegon Muskegon County 49442	231-722-0088 866-322-4501	http://www.dcilmi.org
ADRC of the Thumb	Region VII Area Agency on Aging	1615 S. Euclid Ave. Bay City Bay County 48706	989-893-4506	http://region7aaa.org
ADRC of Western Michigan	DAKC	3600 Camelot SE Grand Rapids Kent County 49546	616-949-1100	www.disabilityadvocates.us/index.php
ADRC-Capital Area	Tri-County Office on Aging	5303 S. Cedar Street Suite 1 Lansing Ingham County 48911-3800	517-887-1440 517-887-1488	www.tcoa.org
ADRC-Capital Area	Capital Area Center for Independent Living	2812 N. MLK Jr. Blvd. Lansing Ingham County 48906	517-999-2760	www.cacil.org/index.php

(*continued*)

Michigan (*continued*)

ADRC of Central Michigan	Disability Network of Mid-Michigan	1705 S. Saginaw Road Midland Bay County 48640	989-835-4041	http://dnmm.org
ADRC of Central Michigan	Region VII Area Agency on Aging	1615 S. Euclid Ave. Bay City Bay County 48706	989-893-4506	http://region7aaa.org
ADRC of GLS	Valley Area Agency on Aging	225 E. Fifth Street Suite 200 Flint Genesee County 48502	810-239-7671	www.michigan.gov/adrc
ADRC of Hillsdale, Jackson, and Lenawee Counties	Region 2 Area Agency on Aging	102 N. Main Street Brooklyn Jackson County 49230	517-592-1974	www.r2aaa.net
ADRC of Hillsdale, Jackson, and Lenawee Counties	DisAbility Connections, Inc.	409 Linden Jackson Jackson County 49201	517-782-6054	www.disabilityconnect.org
ADRC of Kalamazoo	Region 3-A Area Agency on Aging	3299 Gull Road Kalamazoo Kalamazoo County 49048	269-373-5147	www.kalcounty.com/aaa
ADRC of Northwest Michigan	Area Agency on Aging of Northwest Michigan	1609 Park Drive Traverse City Grand Traverse County 49686	231-947-8920	www.aaanm.org

(*continued*)

Michigan (*continued*)

ADRCSEMI	Disability Network Oakland and Macomb	16645 15 Mile Road Clinton Township Macomb County 48035	586-268-4160	www.omcil.org/index.htm
ADRCSEMI	Blue Water Center for Independent Living	1042 Griswold Street Suite 2 Port Huron St. Clair County 48060	810-987-9337	www.bwcil.org
ADRCSEMI	Lynn Kellogg, CEO	2900 Lakeview Ave. St. Joseph St. Joseph County 49085	269-983-0177 800-654-2810	www.areaagencyonaging.org
ADRCSEMI and ADRC of Kalamazoo	Disability Network Southwest Michigan	517 Crosstown Parkway Kalamazoo Kalamazoo County 49001	269-985-0111 for Berrien/Cass 269-345-1516 for Kalamazoo Office	www.dnswm.org
ADRC of the Lakeshore	Senior Resources of West Michigan	560 Seminole Road Muskegon Muskegon County 49444	231-739-5858	www.seniorresourceswmi.org
ADRC of the Upper Peninsula	U.P. Area Agency on Aging UPCAP Services, Inc.	501 14th Avenue South P.O. Box 606 Escanaba Delta County 49829	906-786-4701 800-338-7227 (U.P. I & R only)	www.upcap.org

(*continued*)

Michigan *(continued)*

ADRC of the Upper Peninsula	SAIL	1200 Wright Street Suite A Marquette Marquette County 49855	906-228-5744	/www.upsail.com/contact.php
ADRC of Western Michigan	AAAWM	3215 Eaglecrest Drive, N.E. Grand Rapids Kent County 49503	616-456-5664	www.aaawm.org
ADRC-Detroit and Eastern Wayne County	Detroit Area Agency on Aging	1333 Brewery Park Blvd. Suite 200 Detroit Wayne County 48207-4544	313-446-4444	www.daaa1a.org
ADRC-Detroit and Eastern Wayne County and ADRC of Southern and Western Wayne	Disability Network-Wayne County-Detroit	5555 Corner Street Suite 2224 Detroit Wayne County 48213	313-923-1655	www.dnwayne.org

AAA, Area Agency on Aging; AAAWM, Area Agency on Aging of Western Michigan; ADRC, Aging and Disability Resource Center; ADRCSEMI, ADRC of Southeast Michigan; DAKC, Disability Advocates of Kent County; GLS, Genesee, Lapeer and Shiawassee; SAIL, Superior Alliance for Independent Living.

Minnesota

Services available statewide through website and toll-free linkage lines. In-person services currently	Minnesota Help Network (Senior LinkAge Line)	540 Cedar Street PO Box 64976 St. Paul Ramsey County 55164-0976	651-431-2605 Department of Health & Human Services 612 348-4500 Hennepin County Aging and Disability Services	www.MinnesotaHelp.info

(continued)

Minnesota (*continued*)

expanding statewide to all 87 counties			800-333-2433 for Senior Linkage Line 866-333-2466 for Disability Linkage Line 888-546-5838 for Veterans Linkage Line	

Mississippi

Canton MAC Center	Canton MAC Center	152 Watford Parkway Canton Madison County 39046	769-777-7666	www.MississippiAccessToCare.org
Greenville MAC Center	Greenville MAC Center	124 South Broadway Greenville Washington County 38706	662-537-2105	www.MississippiAccessToCare.org
Gulfport MAC Center	Gulfport MAC Center	9229 Highway 49 Gulfport Harrison County 39503	228-868-2312 844-822-4622	www.MississippiAccesstoCare.org
Hattiesburg MAC Center	Hattiesburg MAC Center	700 Hardy Street Hattiesburg Forrest County 39401	844-822-4622	www.MississippiAccessToCare.org
Newton MAC Center	Newton MAC Center	280 Commercial Drive Newton Newton County 39345	601-683-1226 844-822-4622	www.MississippiAccessToCare.org

(*continued*)

Mississippi (*continued*)

Pontotoc MAC Center	Pontotoc MAC Center	75 South Main Street Pontotoc Pontotoc County 38863	662-488-6983 844-822-4622	www. MississippiAccess ToCare.org

MAC, Mississippi Access to Care.

Missouri

Atchison, Nodaway, Worth, Gentry, Holt, Andrew, DeKalb, Buchanan, Clinton	MERIL	4420 South 40th Street St. Joseph Buchanan County 64503	816-279-8558 ext.1021 800-MERI-L4U	
Buchanan County	North West Area Agency on Aging			An ADRC has been designated in this county but local contact information has not been added to this database. Please contact Vickie Keller at Vicki.Keller@health.mo.gov for more information about services in this area
Harrison, Mercer, Daviess, Grundy, Caldwell, Ray, Carroll, Livingston	Access II Independent Living Center, Inc.	101 Industrial Parkway Gallatin Daviess County 64640	660-663-2423	
Maries, Gasconade, Franklin	Heartland Independent Living Center	1010 Hwy 28 W Owensville Gasconade County 65066	573-437-5100 866-322-3224	
Putnam, Schuyler, Scotland, Sullivan, Adair, Knox, Linn, Macon, Shelby, Chariton	RAIL	1100 S Jamison St Kirksville Adair County 63501	660-627-7245 888-295-6461	

MERIL, Midland Empire Resources for Independent Living; RAIL, Rural Advocates for Independent Living.

Montana

Ten counties surrounding Yellowstone County, and Northern Cheyenne and Crow Indian Reservations	Area II Agency on Aging	P O Box 127 Roundup Musselshell County 59072	406-323-1320 800-551-3191	www.midrivers.com/areatwo
Area VI Agency on Aging: Lincoln, Sanders, Mineral, and Lake counties	Western Montana AAA	110 Main St Ste #5 Polson Lake County 59860-2316	406-883-7284	
Beaverhead, Deer Lodge, Granite, Madison, Powell, Silver Bow	Area V Agency On Aging	PO Box 459 1015 S Montana St Butte Silver Bow County 59703	406-782-5555	
Billings/ Yellowstone County	Yellowstone County Council on Aging Resource Center	1603 Grand Ave, Ste E17 PO Box 20895 Billings Yellowstone County 59104	406-259-5212 800-551-3191	https://dphhs.mt.gov/SLTC/aging/adrc
Cascade County	Area VIII Agency on Aging	1801 Benefits Ct Great Falls Cascade County 59405	406-454-6990	www.co.cascade.mt.us
Carter, Custer, Daniels, Dawson, Fallon, Garfield, McCone, Phillips, Powder River, Prairie, Richland, Roosevelt, Rosebud, Sheridan, Treasure, Valley, Wibaux	Area I Agency On Aging—Action For Eastern MT	Po Box 1309 Glendive Dawson County 59330	406-377-3564	https://dphhs.mt.gov/SLTC/aging/adrc

(*continued*)

Montana (*continued*)

Hill County	Area X Agency on Aging	2 W 2nd St Havre Hill County 59501-3434	406-265-5464 406-265-5464	https://dphhs.mt.gov/SLTC/aging/adrc
Lewis & Clark, Broadwater, Jefferson, Meagher, Gallatin, and Park counties	Area IV Agency on Aging	648 Jackson St PO Box 1717 Helena Lewis and Clark County 59624-1717	406-447-1680	www.rmdc.net
Missoula County	Missoula Aging Services	337 Stephens Ave Missoula Missoula County 59801	406-728-7682 800-551-3191	www.missoulaagingservices.org
Ravalli County	Ravalli County Council on Aging	310 Old Corvallis Road Hamilton Ravalli County 59840	406-363-5690	www.ravalliccoa.org/index.html

AAA, Area Agency on Aging.

Nevada

Churchill and Pershing counties	Churchill County Senior Center	310 Court Street Fallon Churchill County 89406	775-423-7096	
Southern Nevada	Nevada Senior Services	901 N. Jones Blvd Las Vegas Clark County 89108	702-364-2273	www.nevadaseniorservices.com

(*continued*)

Nevada (*continued*)

Lyon County; Silver Springs, Fernley, Dayton, Smith Valley, Wellington, and Yerington	Lyon County Human Services	1075 Pyramid Street P.O. Box 1141 Silver Springs Lyon County 89429	775-577-5009	www.nevadaadrc.com
Northeastern Nevada	Access to Healthcare Network	405 Idaho Street Suite 214 Elko Elko County 89801	877-385-2345	www.accesstohealthcare.org
Northwestern Nevada	Access to Healthcare Network	4001 S. Virginia Street Reno Washoe County 89502	877-385-2345	www.accesstohealthcare.org

New Hampshire

Belknap County (Laconia)	ServiceLink Resource Center of Belknap County	67 Water Street Suite 105 Laconia Belknap County 03246	603-528-6945 866-634-9412	http://www.nh.gov/servicelink
Carroll County (Chocorua)	ServiceLink Resource Center of Carroll County	448 White Mountain Hwy. PO Box 420 Chocorua Carroll County 03817	(603) 323-2043 866-634-9412	http://www.nh.gov/servicelink
Coos County (Berlin)	ServiceLink Resource Center of Coos County	610 Sullivan St. Suite 6 Berlin Coos County 03570	603-752-6407 866-634-9412	http://www.nh.gov/servicelink
Grafton County (Lebanon, Littleton)	ServiceLink Resource Center of Grafton County	10 Campbell St. PO Box 433 Lebanon Grafton County 03766	603-448-1558 for Lebanon 603-444-4498 for Littleton 603-448-1558 866-634-9412	http://www.nh.gov/servicelink or http://www.gcscc.org

(*continued*)

New Hampshire (*continued*)

Hillsborough County (Manchester, Nashua)	ServiceLink Resource Center of Hillsborough County	555 Auburn St. Manchester Hillsborough County 03103	603-644-2240 for Manchester Office 603-598-4709 for Nashua Office 866-634-9412	www.nh.gov/servicelink
Merrimack County (Concord)	ServiceLink Resource Center of Merrimack County	2 Industrial Park Drive PO Box 1016 Concord Merrimack County 03302-1016	601-228-6625 603-228-6625 866-634-9412	www.nh.gov/servicelink
Monadnock Region (Keene)	ServiceLink Resource Center of the Monadnock Region	105 Castle St. Keene Cheshire County 03431	603-357-1922 866-634-9412	www.nh.gov/servicelink
Strafford County	ServiceLink Resource Center of Strafford County	1 Old Dover Road, Suite 6 Merchant Rochester Strafford County 03867	603-332-7398 866-634-9412	www.nh.gov/servicelink
Sullivan County	ServiceLink Resource Center of Sullivan County	224 Elm Street Claremont Sullivan County 03743	603-542-5177 603-542-2640 866-634-9412	www.nh.gov/servicelink
Rockingham County	ServiceLink Resource Center of Rockingham County (Portsmouth, Salem)	Seacoast: 30 International Drive, Suite 202, Portsmouth, NH 03801 38Salem Area: 8 Commerce Drive Unit 802, Atkinson 03811 Rockingham County	Seacoast: (603) 334-6594 Salem Area: 866-634-9412	www.nh.gov/servicelink

(*continued*)

New Jersey

Atlantic County (Northfield)	Atlantic County Aging and Disability Resource Connection (County Division of Intergenerational Services)	101 S. Shore Road Northfield Atlantic County 08225	609-645-7700, ext. 4700 800-426-9243	www.adrcnj.gov
Bergen County (Hackensack)	ADRC (County Division of Senior Services)	One Bergen County Plaza, 2nd Floor, Hackensack, NJ Bergen County 07601-7000	201-336-7400	www.adrcnj.gov
Burlington County	Burlington County Office on Aging/ADRC	49 Rancocas Road, P. O. Box 6000 Mount Holly Burlington County 08060	609-265-5069	www.adrcnj.gov
Cape May County	Cape May County Department of Aging and Disability Services/ADRC	4005 Route 9 South Rio Grande, NJ Cape May County 08242	609-886-2784	www.adrcnj.gov
Camden County	ADRC (County Division of Senior & Disabled Services)	512 Lakeland Road, 4th Floor PO Box 406 Blackwood Camden County 08102	856-858-3220	www.adrcnj.gov
Cumberland County	Cumberland County Office on Aging & Disabled/ADRC	800 E. Commerce Street Bridgeton, NJ Atlantic County 08302	856-453-2220	www.adrcnj.gov

(*continued*)

New Jersey (*continued*)

Essex County	Essex County Division of Senior Services	900 Bloomfield Ave. Verona, NJ Essex County 07044	973-395-8375	www.adrcnj.gov
Gloucester County	Gloucester Division of Senior Services	115 Budd Blvd. West Deptford, NJ Gloucester County 08096	856-384-6900	www.adrcnj.gov
Hudson County	Hudson County Office on Aging/ADRC	595 County Ave., Bldg. 2 Secaucus, NJ Hudson County 07094	201-369-4313	www.adrcnj.gov
Hunterdon County (Flemington)	ADRC (County Division of Senior Services)	PO Box 2900 Flemington, NJ Hunterdon County 08822-2900	908-788-1361	www.adrcnj.gov
Mercer County (Trenton)	ADRC (County Office on Aging)	PO Box 8068, 640 South Broad Street Trenton, NJ Mercer County 08650	609-989-6661	www.adrcnj.gov
Middlesex County	Middlesex County Office on Aging and Disabled Services/ADRC	New Brunswick, NJ Middlesex County 08901	732-745-3295	www.adrcnj.gov
Monmouth County	Monmouth County Division on Aging, Disabilities & Veterans Services/ADRC	3000 Kozloski Road Freehold Monmouth County 07728	732-431-7450	www.adrcnj.gov

(*continued*)

New Jersey (*continued*)

Morris County (Morristown)	ADRC (County Division on Aging, Disabilities and Veterans	340 West Hanover Avenue, Ground Floor, PO Box 900 Morristown, NJ Morris County 07963-0900	973-285-6848	www.adrcnj.gov
Ocean County	Ocean County Offices of Senior Services/ADRC	P. O. Box 2191 Toms River, NJ Ocean County 08754	732-929-2091	www.adrcnj.gov
Passaic County	Passaic County Dept. of Senior Services, Disabilities and Veterans	930 Riverview Dr. Suite 200 Totowa, Passaic County 07512	973-569-4060	www.adrcnj.gov
Salem County	Salem County Office on Aging/ADRC	98 Market St. Salem, NJ Salem County 08079	856-339-8622	www.adrcnj.gov
Somerset County	Somerset County Aging and Disability Services/ADRC	27 Warren St. 1st Floor, P. O. Box 3000 Somerville, NJ Somerset County 08876	908-704-6346	www.adrcnj.gov
Sussex County	Sussex County Office on Aging/ADRC	1 Spring St., 2nd Floor Sussex County 07860	973-579-0555	www.adrcnj.gov
Union County	Union County Division on Aging/ADRC	Adm. Bldg. Elizabeth, NJ Union County 07207	908-527-4870	www.adrcnj.gov
Warren County (Belvidere)	ADRC (County Division of Aging & Disability Services)	165 County Road, 519 South Belvidere Warren County 07823-1949	908-475-6591 877-222-3737	www.adrcnj.gov

ADRC, Aging and Disability Resource Connection.

(*continued*)

New York

Albany County	New York Connects: Albany County			An ADRC has been designated in this county but local contact information has not been added to this database. Please contact NY Connects, http://www.nyconnects.ny.gov for more information about services in this area.
Allegany County	New York Connects: Allegany County	6085 State Route 19 North Belmont Allegany County 14813	1-866-268-9390	
Broome County	New York Connects: Broome County	60 Hawley Street Binghamton Broome County	607-778-2420	gobroomecounty.com/casa
Madison County	New York Connects Madison County	138 Dominic Bruno Blvd. Canastota 13032	315-697-5700	www.ofamadco.org
Oneida County	New York Connects: Oneida County	120 Airline St Oriskany Oneida County 13424	315-798-5456	http://www.ocgov.net/ofa
Schuyler County	Schuyler County Office for the Aging/ New York Connects	323 Owego Montour Falls Schuyler County 14865	607-535-7108	
St. Regis Mohawk		412 State Rt 37 Hogansburg 13655	518-358-2963	

(*continued*)

New York (*continued*)

Tompkins County	New York Connects: Tompkins County
Ulster County	New York Connects: Ulster County
Warren/ Hamilton	New York Connects: Warren/Hamilton
Washington County	New York Connects: Washington County
Wayne County	New York Connects: Wayne County
Westchester County	New York Connects: Westchester County
Wyoming County	New York Connects: Wyoming County
Yates County	New York Connects: Yates County

North Carolina

Cabarrus County—AAA Region F	Cabarrus Community Resource Connections	P.O. Box707 Concord, NC Cabarrus County 28026	704-920-3484	www.cabarruscounty.us/resources/community-resource-connections
Centralina: Gaston, Iredell, Lincoln, Rowan, Stanly, and Union Counties	Centralina CRC Connector			www.centralinacounty.us/resources/community-resource-connections
Cherokee, Clay, Graham, and Swain Counties	Western CRC	125 Bonnie Lane Sylva Jackson County 28779	828-586-1962	www.regiona.org

(*continued*)

North Carolina (*continued*)

Eastern Carolina	Eastern Carolina CRC Development Project			
Forsyth County—AAA Region G	Forsyth County CRC	2895 Shorefair Drive Winston-Salem Forsyth County 27105	336-725-0907 366-725-0907	www.seniorservicesinc.org
Guilford, Rockingham, Montgomery, Alamance, Caswell, Davidson, Randolph Counties—AAA Region G	Piedmont Triad CRC for Aging and Disabilities	P.O. Box 21993 Greensboro, NC Guilford County 27420	336-641-4680 336-373-4816	
Haywood, Jackson, and Macon Counties—AAA Region A	CRC of the Great Smokies	2251 Old Balsam Rd Waynesville, NC Haywood County 28786	828-712-4003	www.mountainprojects.org
High Country—AAA Region D	High Country CRC	180 Chattyrob Lane West Jefferson, NC Ashe County 28694	336-246-2461 ext. 225 336-246-4347	www.asheaging.org
Lumber River region	Lumber River CRC Development Project			www.nc211.org/aging-and-disability-resource-centers
Mecklenburg County	Aging and Disabilities Community Resource Connections—Mecklenburg	5801 Executive Center Drive, Suite 101 Charlotte, NC Mecklenburg County 28212	704-432-1111	
Northwest Piedmont CRC	Surry County			

(*continued*)

North Carolina (*continued*)

Pitt and Beaufort Counties—AAA Region Q	Mid East CRC	1011 Anderson Street Greenville, NC Pitt County 27858	252-412-4278 252-758-4357	www.realcrisis.org or www.pittresource.org
Transylvania County	Land of Sky CRC	106 E. Morgan Street Brevard, NC Transylvania County 28712	828-884-3174 Ext 278	www.landofsky.org
Wake County—AAA Region J	Wake County CRC	401 E Whitaker Mill Rd Raleigh, NC Wake County 27608	919-856-5980	

AAA, Area Agency on Aging.

North Mariana Islands

Territory wide	Central North Mariana Islands Aging and Disability Resource Center	P. O. Box 502178 China Town Saipan Northern Islands 96950	670-664-2598 670-664-2598

North Dakota

North Dakota Region II	North Dakota DHS—Aging Services Division	1237 West Divide Avenue Suite 6 Bismarck 58501	701-328-4601 1-855-462-5465	https://carechoice.nd.assistguide.net/site/371/find_organizations.aspx
North Dakota, Region VII	Burleigh County Senior Adults Program	315 North 20th St. Bismarck Adams County 58501	701-255-4648 1-855-462-5465	www.carechoice.nd.gov

Ohio

Central Ohio	Central Ohio Area Agency on Aging	174 E Long St Columbus Franklin County 43215-1809	614-645-7250 1-800-589-7277	www.coaaa.org

(*continued*)

Ohio *(continued)*

East Central Ohio	Area Agency on Aging Region 9	60788 Southgate Rd, SR 209S Byesville Guernsey County 43723-9533	740-439-4478 1-800-945-4250	www.aaa9.org
Greater Akron-Canton Area	Area Agency on Aging 10B	1550 Corporate Woods Pkwy Uniontown Summit County 44685-7856	330-896-9172	www.services4aging.org
Greater Cleveland Area	Western Reserve Aging and Disability Resource Network	925 Euclid Ave., STE 550 Cleveland Cuyahoga County 44115	216-621-0303 2-1-1 800-626-7277 216-621-0303 or 2-1-1 800-626-7277	www.ConnectMeOhio.org
Miami Valley (Greater Dayton)	Dayton/Miami Valley Area Agency on Aging, PSA 2	40 West Second St, Ste 400 Dayton Montgomery County 45402-1873	937-341-3000 937-341-3000	www.info4seniors.org
North Central Ohio	Ohio District 5 Area Agency on Aging, Inc.	780 Park Ave West Mansfield Richland County 44906-3009	419-524-4144 1-800-860-5799	www.agingnorthcentralohio.org
Northeast Ohio	Area Agency on Aging 11	5555 Youngstown-Warren Rd Niles Trumbull County 44446-4820	330-505-2300 1-800-686-7367	www.aaa11.org

(continued)

Ohio (*continued*)

Northwestern Ohio	Area Office on Aging of Northwestern Ohio	2155 Arlington Ave Toledo Lucas County 43609-0624	419-382-0624	www.areaofficeonaging.com
Southeastern Ohio	Buckeye Hills Area Agency on Aging PSA8	1400 Pike St Marietta Washington County 45750-5196	740-373-6400 1-800-331-2644	www.help4seniors.org/Programs-Services/Aging-Disability-Resource-Center.aspx
Southern Ohio	Area Agency on Aging, District 7	160 Dorsey Dr Rio Grande Gallia County 45674-0500	740-245-5306 1-800-582-7277	www.aaa7.org
Southwestern Ohio	Council on Aging of Southwestern Ohio	175 Tri-County Parkway Cincinnati Hamilton County 45246	513-721-1025 1-800-252-0155	www.help4seniors.org
West Central Ohio/Lima	PSA3 Agency on Aging	200 E High St, Ste. 2A Lima Allen County 45801-4465	419-222-7723	www.psa3.org

Oklahoma

Central Oklahoma	Areawide Aging Agency, Inc.	4104 Perimeter Center Drive, Suite 310 Oklahoma City Oklahoma County 73112	405-942-8500	
Central Oklahoma	Central Oklahoma Economic Development District	400 N. Bell P.O. Box 3398 Shawnee, OK Pottawatomie County 74802-3398	405-273-6401	www.coedd.net

(*continued*)

Oklahoma *(continued)*

Central Oklahoma	Progressive Independence, Inc.	121 North Porter Road Norman Cleveland County 73071	405-321-3203	www.progind.org
Central Oklahoma	Sandra Beasley Independent Living Center	705 S. Oakwood, Suite B1 Enid Garfield County 73703	580-237-8508	www.sbilc.com
Creek, Osage, Rogers, Tulsa, and Wagoner Counties	Ability Resources			An ADRC has been designated in this county but local contact information has not been added to this database. Please contact Sherry Crosthwait at Sherry.Crosthwait@okdhs.org for more information about services in this area
Eastern Oklahoma	Eastern Oklahoma Development District	1012 N. 38th St. P.O. Box 1367 Muskogee Muskogee County	918-682-7891 1-800-211-2116	www.eoddok.org
North East Oklahoma	Dynamic Independence	4100 SE Adams Rd Bartlesville 74006	918- 335-1314	www.dynind.org
North Eastern Oklahoma	Grand Gateway Economic Development Association	333 S. Oak St. P.O. Box Drawer B Big Cabin, OK Craig County 74332-0502	918-783-5793 1-800-482-4594	www.grandgateway.org

(continued)

Oklahoma *(continued)*

North West Oklahoma	Kiamichi Economic Development District of Oklahoma	002 Hwy. 2 North Vo-Tech Administration Addition Wilburton Latimer County 74578	918-465-2367 1-800-211-2116	www.keddo.org
Northern Oklahoma	Long-Term Care Authority of Enid	202 West Broadway Enid Garfield County 73701	580-237-2236	
Panhandle of Oklahoma	Oklahoma Economic Development Authority	330 Douglas Ave. P.O. Box 668 Beaver Beaver County 73932-0668	580-625-4531	www.oeda.org
South Central Oklahoma	Association of South Central Oklahoma Governments	802 Main St. P.O. Box 1647 Duncan Stephens County 73534-1647	580-252-0595 ext. 39	www.ascog.org
South East Oklahoma	Oklahomas for Independent Living	601 East Carl Albert Parkway McAlester Pittsburg County 74501	918 426-6220 ext. 112	www.oilok.org
Southern Oklahoma	South Oklahoma Development Association	2704 N. 1st Street Durant Bryan County 74701-4759	580-920-1388 580-920-1388	www.soda-ok.org

(continued)

Oklahoma *(continued)*

Southwestern Oklahoma	Southwestern Oklahoma Development Authority	Building 420, Sooner Dr. P.O. Box 569 Burns Flat Washita County 73624-0569	580-562-4882	www.swoda.org
Tulsa and surrounding counties	INCOG AAA	2 West Second Street, Suite 800 Tulsa Tulsa County 74103	918-584-7526 918-584-7526	www.incog.org

AAA, Area Agency on Aging; INCOG, Indian Nations Council of Governments.

Oregon

Lane County	Lane County Seniors and Disabled Services	1015 Willamette, Suite 200 PO Box 11336 Eugene Lane County 97440	800-441-4038	www.lcog.org/332/Aging-Disability-Resource-Connection-ADR
Linn, Benton, Lincoln	Oregon Cascades West Senior and Disability Services	1400 Queen Ave SE Suite 206 Albany Linn County 97322	1-800-638-0510	www.ADRCofOregon.org
Marion, Polk, Yamhill, Clatsop, and Tillamook	North West Senior and People with Disabilities	3410 Cherry Ave NE Salem Marion County 97309	1-866-206-4799	www.ADRCofOregon.org
Rogue Valley	Rogue Valley Council of Governments	155 N. First St Central Point Jackson County 97502-2209	541-664-6674	https://rvcog.org/empowerment/adrc/

Pennsylvania

All Counties	Pennsylvania Link to Aging and Disability Resources		1-800-753-8827	www.dhs.pa.gov/cs/groups/webcontent/documents/document/c_084067.pdf
Allegheny County	Allegheny Link	1 Smithfield Street, 2nd Floor Pittsburgh Allegheny County 15222	866-730-2368	http://www.alleghenylink.org
Cumberland County	Cumberland Link to Aging and Disability Resources (Cumberland County Office of Aging and Community Services)	1100 Claremont Road Carlisle Cumberland County 17015	717-240-7887	www.ccpa.net/CumberlandLink

Rhode Island

Statewide (Providence)	THE POINT, Rhode Island Resource Place for Seniors and Adults with Disabilities	50 Valley Street Providence Providence County 02909	401-462-4444 2-1-1	www.ThePointRI.org or www.dhs.ri.gov/askrhody/ or www.211ri.org

South Carolina

Appalachia Region	Appalachia ADRC	30 Century Circle Post Office Drawer 6668 Greenville Greenville County 29606	864-242-9733 800-434-4036	www.scaccesshelp.org

(continued)

South Carolina (*continued*)

Catawba Region	Catawba ADRC	2051 Ebenezer Road, Suite B PO Box 4618 Rock Hill York County 29732	803-329-9670 800-662-8330	www. scaccesshelp. org
Central Midlands	Central Midlands ADRC	236 Stoneridge Drive Columbia Richland County 29210	803-376-5390 866-394-4166	www. scaccesshelp. org
Lowcountry Region	Lowcountry ADRC	634 Campground Road Yemassee Beaufort County 29945	843-726-536 877-846-8148	www. scaccesshelp. org
Lower Savannah Region	Lower Savannah ADRC	2748 Wagener Road PO Box 850 Aiken Aiken County 29802	803-649-7981 866-845-1550	www. scaccesshelp. org
Pee Dee Region	Pee Dee ADRC	147 West Carolina Ave. Post Office Box 999 Hartsville Darlington County 29551	843-383-8632 866-505-3331	www. scaccesshelp. org
Santee Lynches Region	Santee Lynches ADRC	36 W. Liberty Street P. O. Box 1837 Sumter Sumter County 29151	803-775-7381 800-948-1042	www. santeelynchescog. org
Trident Region	Trident ADRC	4450 Leeds Place West Suite B Charleston County 29405	843-554-2275 800-894-0415	www. scaccesshelp. org

(*continued*)

South Carolina *(continued)*

Upper Savannah Region	Upper Savannah ADRC	222 Phoenix Avenue PO Box 1366 Greenwood Greenwood County 29648	864-941-8053 800-922-7729	www.scaccesshelp.org
Waccamaw Region	Waccamaw ADRC	1230 Highmarket Street Georgetown Georgetown County 29440	843-546-8502 800-302-7550	www.scaccesshelp.org

South Dakota

Aberdeen	Adult Services and Aging Aberdeen Office	3401 10th Avenue SE Aberdeen Brown County 57401	855-315-1987	https://dss.sd.gov/formsandpubs/docs/ELDERLY/ADRC.pdf
Belle Fourche	Adult Services and Aging Belle Fourche Office	609 5th Avenue Belle Fourche Butte County 57717	605-892-2731	https://dss.sd.gov/formsandpubs/docs/ELDERLY/ADRC.pdf
Brookings	Adult and Aging Services Brookings Office	1310 S. Maine, Suite 101 Brookings Brookings County	855-315-1987	https://dss.sd.gov/formsandpubs/docs/ELDERLY/ADRC.pdf
Chamberlain	Aging and Adult Services Chamberlain Office	320 Sorenson Drive Chamberlain Brule County 57325	888-749-0007	https://dss.sd.gov/formsandpubs/docs/ELDERLY/ADRC.pdf
Custer	Aging and Adult Services Custer Office	1164 Mt. Rushmore Rd., #3 Custer Custer County 57730	877-463-0006	https://dss.sd.gov/formsandpubs/docs/ELDERLY/ADRC.pdf

(continued)

South Dakota *(continued)*

Hot Springs	Adult Services and Aging Hot Springs Office	2500 Minnekahta Avenue Hot Springs Fall River County 57747	855-315-1986	https://dss.sd.gov/formsandpubs/docs/ELDERLY/ADRC.pdf
Huron	Adult Services and Aging Huron Office	110 3rd Street, Suite 200 Huron Beadle County 57350	855-315-1987	https://dss.sd.gov/formsandpubs/docs/ELDERLY/ADRC.pdf
Lake Andes	Aging and Adult Services Lake Andes Office	3rd and Lake PO Box 190 Lake Andes Charles Mix County 57356	877-656-0023	https://dss.sd.gov/formsandpubs/docs/ELDERLY/ADRC.pdf
Madison	Aging and Adult Services Madison Office	223 S. Van Eps. STE 201 Madison Lake County 57042	877-412-0022	https://dss.sd.gov/formsandpubs/docs/ELDERLY/ADRC.pdf
Mission	Adult Services and Aging Mission Office	671 N. Marge Street PO Box 279 Mission Todd County 57580	888-280-0021	https://dss.sd.gov/formsandpubs/docs/ELDERLY/ADRC.pdf
Mitchell	Adult Services and Aging Mitchell Office	116 E. 11th Street Mitchell Davison County 57301	855-315-1988	https://dss.sd.gov/formsandpubs/docs/ELDERLY/ADRC.pdf
Mobridge	Aging and Adult Services Mobridge Office	920 W. 6th Mobridge Walworth County 57601	877-431-3978	https://dss.sd.gov/formsandpubs/docs/ELDERLY/ADRC.pdf

(continued)

South Dakota (*continued*)

Olivet	Aging and Adult Services Olivet Office	Hutchinson Co. Courthouse 140 E. Euclid, RM 127 Olivet Hutchinson County 57052		https://dss.sd.gov/formsandpubs/docs/ELDERLY/ADRC.pdf
Pierre	Adult Services and Aging Pierre Office	912 E. Sioux Pierre Hughes County 57501	605-773-3612	https://dss.sd.gov/formsandpubs/docs/ELDERLY/ADRC.pdf
Rapid City	Adult Services and Aging Rapid City Office	510 N. Cambell Rapid City Pennington County 57701	855-315-1986	https://dss.sd.gov/formsandpubs/docs/ELDERLY/ADRC.pdf
Redfield	Aging and Adult Services Redfield Office	210 E. 7th Avenue Redfield Walworth County 57469	877-372-0010	https://dss.sd.gov/formsandpubs/docs/ELDERLY/ADRC.pdf
Sioux Falls	Aging and Adult Services Sioux Falls Office	811 E. 10th Street, Dept. 4 Sioux Falls Minnehaha County 57103		https://dss.sd.gov/formsandpubs/docs/ELDERLY/ADRC.pdf
Sisseton	Aging and Adult Services Sisseton Office	119 Cherry Street East Sisseton Roberts County 57262	888-747-0017	https://dss.sd.gov/formsandpubs/docs/ELDERLY/ADRC.pdf
Sturgis	Adult Services and Aging Sturgis Office	2200 W. Main Sturgis Meade County 57785	1-888-476-0036	https://dss.sd.gov/formsandpubs/docs/ELDERLY/ADRC.pdf

(*continued*)

South Dakota (*continued*)

Vermillion	Aging and Adult Services Vermillion Office	114 Market Street, Suite 102 Vermillion Clay County 57069	800-730-0153	https://dss.sd.gov/formsandpubs/docs/ELDERLY/ADRC.pdf
Watertown	Aging and Adult Services Watertown Office	2001 9th Avenue SW, Suite 300 Watertown Codington County 57201	855-315-1987	https://dss.sd.gov/formsandpubs/docs/ELDERLY/ADRC.pdf
Winner	Aging and Adult Services Winner Office	649 W. 2nd Street PO Box 31 Winner Tripp County 57580	866-913-0031	https://dss.sd.gov/formsandpubs/docs/ELDERLY/ADRC.pdf
Yankton	Aging and Adult Services Yankton Office	3113 N. Spruce, Suite 200 Yankton Yankton County 57078	855-315-1988	https://dss.sd.gov/formsandpubs/docs/ELDERLY/ADRC.pdf

Tennessee

1	First Tennessee Area Agency on Aging & Disability	First Tennessee Development District 3211 North Roan Street Johnson City Washington County 37601-1213	423-928-0224 423-928-3258 866-836-6678	www.ftaaad.org
2	East Tennessee Area Agency on Aging & Disability	East Tennessee Human Resource Agency 9111 Cross Park Drive, Suite 100 Knoxville Knox County 37923-4517	865-691-2551 ext. 4216 866-836-6678	www.ethra.org
3	Southeast Tennessee Area Agency on Aging & Disability	Southeast Tennessee Developmental District 1000 Riverfront Pkwy. Chattanooga Hamilton County 37402-2103	423-266-5781 866-836-6678	www.sedev.org

(*continued*)

Tennessee (*continued*)

4	Upper Cumberland Area Agency on Aging & Disability	Upper Cumberland Developmental District 1225 South Willow Avenue Cookeville Putnam County 38506-4194	931-432-4111 866-836-6678	www.ucdd.org
5	Greater Nashville Area Agency on Aging & Disability	Greater Nashville Regional Council 501 Union Street, 6th Floor Nashville Davidson County 37219-1705	615-862-8828 615-255-1010 866-836-6678	www.gnrc.org
6	South Central Area Agency on Aging & Disability	South Central Tennessee Development District 815 South Main Street Mt. Pleasant Maury County 38474	931-379-2940 866-836-6678	www.sctdd.org
7	Northwest Area Agency on Aging & Disability	Northwest Tennessee Developmental District 124 Weldon Drive Martin Weakley County 38237-1308	731-587-4213 866-836-6678	www.nwtdd.org
8	Southwest Tennessee Area Agency on Aging & Disability	Southwest Tennessee Developmental District 27 Conrad Drive, Suite 150 Jackson Madison County 38305-2850	731-668-6403 866-836-6678	www.swtdd.org
9	Aging Commission of the Mid-South	Aging Commission of the Mid-South 2670 Union Avenue Extended, Suite 1000 Memphis Shelby County 38112-4416	901-222-4100 866-836-6678	www.agingcommission.org

Texas

Atascosa, Bandera, Bexar, Comal, Frio, Gillespie, Guadalupe, Karnes, Kerr, Kendall, McMullen, Medina, and Wilson Counties	Alamo Service Connection	8700 Tesoro Drive Suite 700 San Antonio Bexar County 78217-6228	210-477-3275 1-866-231-4922	www.askasc.org
Austin, Brazoria, Chambers, Colorado, Fort Bend, Galveston, Harris, Liberty, Matagorda, Montgomery, Walker, Waller, and Wharton Counties	Care Connection ADRC—Gulf Coast	4802 Lockwood Drive Houston Harris County 77026	832-393-4415 1-877-393-1090	www.careconnection.org
Bell, Coryell, Hamilton, Lampasas, Milam, Mills, and San Saba Counties	Central Texas ADRC	2180 North Main Street Belton Bell County 76513	254-770-2342 1-800-447-7169	http://www.centraltexasadrc.org
Brazos, Burleson, Grimes, Leon, Madison, Robertson, and Washington Counties	Brazos Valley ADRC	3991 E. 29th Bryan Brazos County 77802	979-595-2801 ext. 2013 979-595-2800	www.bvcog.org/programs/aging-and-disability-resource-center
Tarrant County	ADRC of Tarrant County	1300 Circle Drive Fort Worth Tarrant County 76119	888-730-ADRC (2372) 888-730-ADRC (2372)	www.tarrantcountyadrc.org

(*continued*)

Texas (*continued*)

This ADRC serves Coke, Concho, Crockett, Irion, Kimble, Mason, McCulloch, Menard, Reagan, Schleicher, Sterling, Sutton, and Tom Green Counties	Concho Valley ADRC	2809 Southwest Blvd San Angelo Anderson County 76904	325-227-6624	www.dcciltx.org
This project serves Aransas, Bee, Brooks, Duval, Jim Wells, Kenedy, Kleberg, Live Oak, McMullen, Nueces, Refugio, and San Patricio Counties	Coastal Bend ADRC	2910 Leopard Street Corpus Christi Nueces County 78408-3614	361-883-3935 1-800-817-5743	
This project serves Brown, Callahan, Coleman, Comanche, Eastland, Fisher, Haskell, Jones, Kent, Knox, Mitchell, Nolan, Runnels, Scurry, Shackelford, Stephen, Stonewall, Taylor, and Throckmorton Counties	West Central Texas ADRC	3702 Loop 322 Abilene Taylor County 79602	325-793-8440	www.wctadrc.org
This project serves Cameron, Hidalgo, and Willacy Counties	RIO-Net ADRC	255 S. Kansas Weslaco Hidalgo County 78596	956-682-3481 ext. 408 800-365-6131	www.lrgv.tx.networkofcare.org

(*continued*)

Texas (*continued*)

The project serves Anderson, Camp, Cherokee, Gregg, Harrison, Henderson, Marion, Panola, Rains, Rusk, Smith, Upshur, Van Zandt, and Wood Counties	East Texas ADRC	Community Healthcore P. O. Box 6800 Longview Gregg County 75608	903-237-2341 877-237-2268	http://www.etxadrc.org
The project serves Lubbock County	Lubbock County ADRC	P. O. Box 2828 Lubbock Lubbock County 79408	806-767-1740 800-687-7581	http://www.lubbockadrc.org
This project serves Collin, Denton, Hood, and Somervell Counties	North Central Texas ADRC	616 Six Flags Drive Arlington Tarrant County 76011	877-229-9084 877-229-9084	www.nctadrc.org
This project serves Dallas County (Dallas Metropolitan Area)	Connect to Care ADRC	1380 River Bend Drive Dallas Dallas County 75247	214-743-1258	https://www.connecttocaredallas.org
This project serves El Paso, Culberson, Hudspeth, Brewster, Jeff Davis, and Presidio Counties	El Paso and Far West Texas ADRC	1359 Lomaland Suite 400 El Paso El Paso County 79935	915-298-7307 877-413-ADRC (2372)	http://www.projectamistad.org/adrc.php

Utah

Central Utah	Mountainland Area on Aging	586 E 800 N Orem Utah County 84097	801-229-3804	www.mountainland.org/aging

(*continued*)

Utah (*continued*)

Central Utah	Ability First (formerly CUCIL)	491 North Freedom Blvd. Provo Utah County 84601	801-373-5044	http://abilityfirstutah.org
North Central	Roads to Independence (formerly known as Tri-County Independent Living Center)	3355 Washington Blvd. Ogden Weber County 84401	801-612-3215	www.RoadsToIndependence.org
Northern Utah	Bear River AAA	170 N Main Logan Cache County 84321	435-752-7242	http://www.brag.utah.gov/aging.html
Salt Lake City and surrounding	Salt Lake County Aging Services	2001 South State Street S1500 Salt Lake City Salt Lake County 84114-4575	385-468-3210 (3200)	http://aging.slco.org
Southeastern Utah	Active Re-Entry Moab	182 N 500 W Moab Grand County 84532	435-259-0245	http://www.arecil.org
Southern Utah	Five County AAA	1070 West 1600 South Bldg B St. George Washington County 84770	435-673-3548	http://www.fivecounty.utah.gov/programs/aging/Website.htm

AAA, Area Agency on Aging; ADRC, Aging and Disability Resource Center; CUCIL, Central Utah Center for Independent Living.

Vermont

Addison, Chittenden, Franklin, and Grand Isle Counties	Champlain Valley Agency on Aging—ADRC	76 Pearl Street, Suite 201 Essex Junction Chittenden County 05452	802-865-0360 800-642-5119	http://www.cvaa.org

(*continued*)

Vermont (*continued*)

Bennington and Rutland	Southwestern Vermont Council on Aging	East Ridge Professional Building 1085 U.S. Route 4 East, Unit 2B Rutland Rutland County 05701-9039	802-786.5990 1-800-642-5119	http://www.svcoa.org
Caledonia, Essex, Orleans Counties	Northeastern Vermont Area Agency on Aging—ADRC	481 Summer Street, Suite 101 St. Johnsbury Caledonia County 05819	802-748-5182 800-642-5119	http://www.nevaaa.org
Lamoille, Orange (except town of Thetford), Washington Counties, including towns of Bethel, Granville, Hancock, Pittsfield, Rochester, Royalton, Sharon, and Stockbridge	Central Vermont Council on Aging	30 Washington Street, Suite 1 Barre Washington County 05641	1-802-479-0531 1-800-642-5119	http://www.cvcoa.org
Statewide	Brain Injury Association of Vermont—ADRC	P.O. Box 482 92 S. Main Street Waterbury Washington County 05676	802-324-2601 877-856-1772	www.biavt.org
Statewide	Vermont 2-1-1-ADRC	United Ways of Vermont 412 Farrell Street, Suite 200 South Burlington Chittenden County 05492	1-866-652-4636 1-802-652-4636 2-1-1	http://www.vermont211.org/index.php

(*continued*)

Vermont (*continued*)

Statewide	VCIL—ADRC	11 East State Street Montpelier Washington County 05602	802-229-0501 800-639-1522	http://www.vcil.org
Statewide	Green Mountain Self-Advocates	2 Prospect Street Suite 6 Montpelier Washington County 05602	802-229-2600	http://www.gmsavt.org
Statewide	Vermont Family Network—ADRC	600 Blair Park Road Suite 240 Williston Chittenden County 05495	802-876-5315	http://www.vtfn.org
Windham and Windsor Counties	Council on Aging for Southeastern Vermont	56 Main St. Suite 202 Springfield Windsor County 05156	802-885-2655 1-800-642-5119	http://www.coasevt.org

ADRC, Aging and Disability Resource Center; VCIL, Vermont Center for Independent Living.

Virginia

Alexandria	Alexandria Office of Aging and Adult Services	4480 King Street Alexandria Alexandria city 22302	703-746-5999	http://www.easyaccess.virginia.gov
Appalachian Region	Appalachian Agency for Senior Citizens	216 College Ridge Road, Wardell Industrial Park P.O. Box 765 Cedar Bluff 24609-0765	276-964-4915	http://www.aasc.org
Arlington	Arlington Agency on Aging	c/o Department of Human Services 2100 Washington Boulevard, 4th Floor Arlington Arlington County 22204	703-228-1709 703-228-1709	http://www.arlingtonva.us/aging

(*continued*)

Virginia (*continued*)

Bay Aging	Bay Aging	5306 Old Virginia Street PO Box 610 Urbanna 23175-0610	804-758-2386 804-758-2386	http://www.bayaging.org
Central Shenandoah Valley Region	Valley Program for Aging Services, Inc.	325 Pine Avenue PO Box 817 Waynesboro Accomack County 22980-0603	540-949-7141 800-868-8727	https://www.vadars.org
Central Virginia	Central Virginia Area Agency on Aging, Inc.	PO Box 1390 Lynchburg 24505	434-385-9070	http://www.cvaaa.com
Charlottesville Area	Jefferson Area Board For Aging	674 Hillsdale Drive Suite 9 Charlottesville Accomack County 22901-1799	434-817-5222	http://www.jabacares.org
Crater District	Crater District Area Agency on Aging	23 Seyler Drive Petersburg Accomack County 23805-9243	804-732-7020	http://www.cdaaa.org
District Three	District Three Senior Services	4453 Lee Highway Marion 24354-4269	276-783-8157 276-783-8158 1-800-541-0933	http://www.district-three.org
Eastern Shore	Eastern Shore Agency on Aging	Community Action Agency, Inc. PO Box 415 Belle Haven 23306-0415	757-442-9652 800-452-5977	
Greater/ Central Richmond	Senior Connections—The Capital Area Agency on Aging, Inc.	24 East Cary Street Richmond Accomack County 23219-3796	804-343-3000 800-989-2286	http://www.seniorconnections-va.org

(*continued*)

Virginia (*continued*)

Loudoun County	Loudoun County Area Agency on Aging	20145 Ashbrook Place, Suite 170 Ashburn Loudoun County 20147	703-777-0257	www.loudoun.gov/index.aspx?NID=1123
MEOC	MEOC	1501 Third Avenue E. PO Box 888 Big Stone Gap Wise County 24219-0888	276-523-4202 800-252-6362	http://www.meoc.org
New River Valley	New River Valley Agency on Aging	141 East Main Street Suite 500 Pulaski Pulaski County 24301-5029	540-980-7720 1-866-260-4417	http://www.nrvaoa.org
Peninsula—Williamsburg Region	Peninsula Agency on Aging	739 Thimble Shoals Blvd, Executive Center Building 1000, Suite 1006 Newport News Newport News city 23606-3562	757-873-0541 (Toll-free for Peninsula Area Residents)	http://www.paainc.org
Piedmont	Piedmont Senior Resources Area Agency on Aging	5539 Colonial Trail Highway PO Box 398 Burkeville Nottoway County 23922	434-767-5588 800-995-6918	
Prince William Area	Prince William Area Agency on Aging	5 County Complex Court, Suite 240 Woodbridge Prince William County 22192	703-792-6400 703-792-6374	www.pwcgov.org/aoa

(*continued*)

Virginia *(continued)*

Rappahannock	Rappahannock Area Agency on Aging	171 Warrenton Road Fredericksburg Spotsylvania County 22405-1343	540-371-3375 800-262-4012	http://www.raaa16.org
Rappahannock/ Rapidan	Rappahannock Rapidan Community Services	15361 Bradford Road PO Box 1568 Culpeper Accomack County 22701-1568	540-825-3100	http://www.rrcsb.org
Roanoke Area	Local Office on Aging	PO Box 14205 706 Campbell Avenue, SW Roanoke Roanoke city 24038	540-345-0451	http://www.loaa.org
Shenandoah Region	Shenandoah Area Agency on Aging	207 Mosby Lane Front Royal Warren County 22630	540-635-7141	www.shenandoahaaa.com
South Central Virginia	Lake Country Area Agency on Agency	1105 West Danville Street South Hill Accomack County 23970-3501	434-447-7661 800-252-4464	http://www.lcaaa.org
Southeastern Virginia/ Hampton Roads	Senior Services of Southeastern Virginia	5 Interstate Corporate Center 6350 Center Drive, Suite 101 Norfolk Accomack County 23502	757-461-9481	http://www.ssseva.org
Southern Henry County	Southern Area Agency on Aging, Inc.	204 Cleveland Avenue Martinsville Henry County 24112-2020	276-632-6442 800-468-4571	http://www.southernaaa.org

Washington

PSA 9 Asotin County	Aging and Disability Resource Center	744 5th St #C Clarkston, WA Asotin County 99403	509-758-2355 1-877-961-2582	www. altcwashington. com
PSA 9 Columbia County	Aging and Disability Resource Center	410 E. Main St. PO Box 44 Dayton, WA Columbia County 99328	509-382-4787	www. altcwashington. com
PSA 11—Eastern Washington	Aging and Long Term Care of Eastern Washington	1222 N. Post Spokane Spokane County 99201-2518	509-458-2509	http://www. altcew.org
PSA 9 Garfield County	Garfield County Aging and Disability Resource Center	695 Main St PO Box 23 Pomeroy WA Garfield County 99347	509-843-3563	www. altcwashington. com
PSA 2—Northwest Washington	Northwest Regional Council	600 Lakeway Drive Suite 100 Bellingham Whatcom County 98225	360-676-6749 360-738-2500	www.nwrcwa. org
PSA 5—Pierce County	Pierce County Aging & Disability Resources	1305 Tacoma Avenue Suite 104 Tacoma Pierce County 98402	253-798-4500 (4600)	www. PierceADRC.org
PSA 9—Southeast Washington	SE ALTC Aging and Disability Resource Center	1710 S. 24th Ave Ste 100 Yakima Yakima County 98902	509-469-0500 1-866-891-2582	www. altcwashington. com
PSA 9 Walla Walla County	Aging and Disability Resource Center	125 E. Cherry St. Ste A Walla Walla, WA Walla Walla County 99362	509-529-6470 1-888-769-2582	www. altcwashington. com

West Virginia

Region I	West Virginia Aging and Disability Resource Center	PO Box 2086 105 Bridge Street Wheeling Ohio County 26003	304-830-2779	http://www.wvnavigate.org
Region I	West Virginia Aging and Disability Resource Center	521 Market Street, #18 Parkersburg Wood County 26101	304-865-1172	http://www.wvnavigate.org
Region I	West Virginia Aging and Disability Resource Center	9541 Middletown Mall Fairmont Marion County 26554	304-363-1595	http://www.wvnavigate.org
Region II	West Virginia Aging and Disability Resource Center	1 Dunbar Plaza Suite 102 Dunbar Kanawha County 25064	304-720-6861 866-981-2372	http://www.wvnavigate.org
Region II	West Virginia Aging and Disability Resource Center	1 Perry Morris Square Milton Cabell County 25541	304-390-0075 866-981-2372	http://www.wvnavigate.org
Region III	West Virginia Aging and Disability Resource Center	PO Box 869 8 Airport Road Petersburg Grant County 26847	304-257-2847	http://www.wvnavigate.org
Region III	West Virginia Aging and Disability Resource Center	1200 Harrison Avenue, Suite 113 Elkins Randolph County 26241	304-630-2207	http://www.wvnavigate.org
Region III	West Virginia Aging and Disability Resource Center	115 Aikens Center, Suite 18 Martinsburg Berkeley County 25404	304-263-3943 800-296-5341	http://www.wvnavigate.org

(*continued*)

West Virginia (*continued*)

Region IV	West Virginia Aging and Disability Resource Center	1460 Main Street, Box 8 Princeton Mercer County 24740	304-425-2040	http://www.wvnavigate.org
Region IV	West Virginia Aging and Disability Resource Center	75 Seneca Trail Greenbrier Valley Mall, Suite 15 Lewisburg Greenbrier County 24901	304-645-4770	http://www.wvnavigate.org

Wisconsin

Adams County	ADRC of Adams, Green Lake, Marquette, and Waushara Counties	108 East North Street PO Box 619 Friendship Adams County 53934-0619	877-883-5378	www.adrcinformation.org
Ashland County	ADRC of the North (serving Iron, Ashland, Bayfield, Price, and Sawyer Counties)	630 Sanborn Ave Ashland Ashland County 54891	715-682-7004 866-663-3607	
Barron County, Wisconsin	ADRC of Barron, Rusk & Washburn Counties	335 Monroe Avenue Barron Barron County 54812	715-537-6225 888-538-3031	www.adrcconnections.org
Bayfield County	ADRC of the North (serving Iron, Ashland, Bayfield, Price, and Sawyer Counties)	117 E 5th Street Washburn Bayfield County 54891	715-373-6144 866-663-3607	www.adrc-n-wi.org

(*continued*)

Wisconsin *(continued)*

Brown County	ADRC of Brown County	300 South Adams Street Green Bay Brown County 54301	920-448-4300 866-473-2372	www.adrcofbrowncounty.org
Buffalo County	ADRC of Buffalo, Clark, and Pepin Counties	407 South Second Street PO Box 517 Alma Buffalo County 54610	608-685-6307	www.adrc-bcp.com
Burnett County	ADRC of Northwest Wisconsin (serving Burnett, Polk, and St. Croix Chippewa Indians of Wisconsin)	7410 County Road K #180 Siren Burnett County 54872	866-485-2372	www.adrcnwwi.org
Calumet County	ADRC of Calumet, Outagamie, and Waupaca Counties	206 Court Street Chilton Calumet County 53014	920-849-1400	www.youradrcresource.org
Clark County	ADRC of Buffalo, Clark, and Pepin Counties	517 Court Street Room 202 Neillsville Clark County 54456	715-743-5166	http://adrc-bcp.com
Columbia County	ADRC of Columbia County	2652 Murphy Road PO Box 136 Portage Columbia County 53901	608-742-9233	www.co.columbia.wi.us/columbiacounty/adrc/ADRCHomePage/tabid/1497/Default.aspx
Chippewa County	ADRC of Chippewa County	711 N. Bridge Street, Room 118 Chippewa Falls Chippewa County 54729	715-726-7777	www.co.chippewa.wi.us/adrc

(*continued*)

Wisconsin (*continued*)

Crawford, Juneau, Richland, Sauk Counties	ADRC of Eagle Country	225 N Beaumont Rd Suite 118 Prairie du Chien Crawford County 53821	608-326-0235	http://www.adrceagle.org
Dane County	ADRC of Dane County	2865 N. Sherman Avenue Madison Dane County 53704	608-240-7400	www.daneadrc.org
Dodge County	ADRC of Dodge County	199 County Road DF, 3rd Floor Juneau Dodge County 53039	920-386-3580	www.dhs.wisconsin.gov/adrc/consumer/dodge.htm
Door County	ADRC of Door County	The Senior & Community Center 421 Nebraska Street Sturgeon Bay Door County 54235	920-746-2372	http://adrcdoorcounty.org
Douglas County	ADRC of Douglas County	1316 North 14th Street Suite 337 Superior Douglas County 54880	715-395-1234	www.douglascountywi.org/adrc
Douglas County	ADRC of Douglas County	1316 North 14th Street Superior Douglas County 54880	715-395-1234	www.douglascountywi.org/adrc
Dunn County	ADRC of Dunn County	808 Main Street PO Box 470 Menomonie Dunn County 54751	715-232-4006	http://duncountywi.govoffice2.com
Eau Claire County	ADRC of Eau Claire County	721 Oxford Avenue Room 1550 Eau Claire Eau Claire County 54703	715-839-4735	www.co.eau-claire.wi.us/adrc

(*continued*)

Wisconsin (*continued*)

Florence County	ADRC of Florence County	501 Lake Avenue, Lower Level Florence Florence County 54121	715-528-4890	www.florencecountywi.com
Fond du Lac County	ADRC of Fond du Lac County	50 N. Portland Street Fond du Lac Fond du Lac County 54936-1196	920-929-3466 888-435-7335	http://www.fdlco.wi.gov/Index.aspx?page=318
Forest County	ADRC of the Northwoods (Serving Forest, Oneida, Taylor, and Vilas Counties and Forest County Potawatomi, Lac du Flambeau, and Sokaogon Chippewa Tribes)	300 South Lake Street Crandon Forest County 54520	715-478-2162 800-699-6704	http://adrcofthenorthwoods.org
Grant County	ADRC of Southwest Wisconsin (serving Grant, Green, Iowa, and Lafayette Counties)	8820 Hwy 35/61 South Lancaster Grant County 53813	608-328-9499	http://adrcswwi.org
Green County	ADRC of Southwest Wisconsin (serving Grant, Green, Iowa, and Lafayette Counties)	N3152 State Road 81 Monroe Green County 53566	608-328-9499	http://adrcswwi.org

(*continued*)

Wisconsin (*continued*)

Green Lake	ADRC of Adams, Green Lake, Marquette, and Waushara Counties	571 County Road A PO Box 588 Green Lake Green Lake County 54941-0588	877-883-5378 920-294-4122	www.adrcinformation.org
Iowa County	ADRC of Southwest Wisconsin (serving Grant, Green, Iowa, and Lafayette Counties)	303 W. Chapel Street, Suite 1300 Dodgeville Iowa County 53533	608-328-9499	http://adrcswwi.org
Iron County	ADRC of the North (serving Iron, Ashland, Bayfield, Price, and Sawyer Counties)	300 Taconite St Suite 201 Hurley Iron County 54534	866-663-3607	http://www.adrc-n-wi.org
Jackson County	ADRC of Western Wisconsin (serving La Crosse, Jackson, Monroe, and Vernon Counties)	420 Highway 54 West P. O. Box 457 Black River Falls Jackson County 54615	715-284-4301 800-500-3910	www.adrcww.org
Jefferson County	ADRC of Jefferson County	1541 Annex Road Jefferson Jefferson County 53549	920-674-8734	www.jeffersoncountywi.gov
Juneau County	ADRC of Eagle Country (serving Crawford, Juneau, Richland, and Sauk Counties)	220 E. LaCrosse Street Mauston Juneau County 53948	608-847-9371	http://www.adrceagle.org

(*continued*)

Wisconsin (*continued*)

Kenosha County	ADRC of Kenosha County	8600 Sheridan Road Suite 500 Kenosha Kenosha County 53143-6514	262-605-6646 800-472-8008	http://adrc.kenoshacounty.org
Kewaunee County	ADRC of the Lakeshore	810 Lincoln Street Kewaunee Kewaunee County 54216	877-416-7083 877-416-7083	http://www.manitowocadrc.org
La Crosse County	ADRC of Western Wisconsin (serving La Crosse, Jackson, Monroe, and Vernon Counties)	300 4th Street North La Crosse La Crosse County 54601	608-785-5700 800-500-3910	www.adrcww.org
Lafayette County	ADRC of Southwest Wisconsin (serving Grant, Green, Iowa, and Lafayette Counties)	627 Main Street Darlington Lafayette County 53530	608-328-9499	http://adrcswwi.org
Langlade County	ADRC of Central Wisconsin	1225 Langlade Road Antigo Langlade County 54409	715-627-6232	http://www.adrc-cw.com
Lincoln County	ADRC of Central Wisconsin (Serving Langlade, Lincoln, Marathon and Wood Counties)	607 N Sales Street Suite 206 Merrill Lincoln County 54452	715-536-0311	http://www.adrc-cw.com
Manitowoc County	ADRC of the Lakeshore	4319 Expo Drive PO Box 935 Manitowoc Manitowoc County 54221	877-416-7083 877-416-7083	www.manitowocadrc.org

(*continued*)

Wisconsin (*continued*)

Marathon County	ADRC of Central Wisconsin (Serving Langlade, Lincoln, Marathon, and Wood Counties)	1000 Lakeview Drive Wausau Marathon County 54401	715-261-6070 in Wausau, 715-384-8479 in Marshfield, 715-421-0014 in Wisconsin Rapids 888-486-9545	
Marinette County	ADRC of Marinette County	2500 Hall Avenue Marinette Marinette County 54143	715-732-3850	http://www.marinettecounty.com
Menominee, Oconto and Shawano Counties and Stockbridge Munsee Tribe	ADRC of the Wolf River Region	7436 Rea Rd Oconto Falls Oconto County 54153	855-492-2372	www.adrcwrr.org
Milwaukee County	Disability Resource Center of Milwaukee County	1220 W. Vliet Street Suite 300 Milwaukee Milwaukee County 53205	414-289-6660	http://county.milwaukee.gov/dsd.htm
Milwaukee County	Aging Resource Center of Milwaukee County	1220 West Vliet Street Suite 300 Milwaukee Milwaukee County 53205	414-289-6874	http://county.milwaukee.gov/ResourceCenter12673.htm
Monroe County	ADRC of Western Wisconsin (serving La Crosse, Jackson, Monroe and Vernon Counties)	14305 County Hwy B Building B Sparta Monroe County 54656	608-269-8900	https://adrcgreencounty.org

(*continued*)

Wisconsin (*continued*)

Oneida County	ADRC of the Northwoods (Serving Forest, Oneida, Taylor and Vilas Counties and Forest County Potawatomi, Lac du Flambeau, and Sokaogon Chippewa Tribes)	100 W Keenan Street Rhinelander Oneida County 54501	800-699-6704	http://adrcofthenorthwoods.org
Outagamie County	ADRC Calumet, Outagamie, and Waupaca Counties	401 S. Elm St. Appleton Outagamie County 54911	920-832-5178 866-739-2372	www.yourADRCresource.org
Ozaukee County	ADRC of Ozaukee County	121 W. Main Street Port Washington Ozaukee County 53074	262-284-8120 866-537-4261	http://www.co.ozaukee.wi.us/ADRC
Pepin County	ADRC of Buffalo, Clark and Pepin Counties	740 7th Avenue West Durand Pepin County 54736	715-672-8945	https://adrcgreencounty.org
Pierce County	ADRC of Pierce County	412 W Kinne Street Ellsworth Pierce County 54011	715-273-6780	www.co.pierce.wi.us
Polk County	ADRC of Northwest Wisconsin (serving Burnett, Polk, and St. Croix Chippewa Indians of Wisconsin)	100 Polk County Plaza #60 Balsam Lake Polk County 54810	715-485-8449	www.adrcnwwi.org

(*continued*)

Wisconsin (*continued*)

Portage County	ADRC of Portage County	1519 Water Street Stevens Point Portage County 54481	715-346-1401 866-920-2525	http://www.co.portage.wi.us/adrc
Price County	ADRC of the North (serving Iron, Ashland, Bayfield, Price, and Sawyer Counties)	104 S. Eyder Ave Phillips Price County 54555	866-663-3607	http://www.adrc-n-wi.org
Racine County	ADRC of Racine County	14200 Washington Ave Sturtevant Racine County 53177	262-833-8777	www.adrc.racinecounty.com
Richland County	ADRC of Eagle Country (serving Crawford, Juneau, Richland, and Sauk Counties)	221 West Seminary Street Richland Center Richland County 53581	608-647-4616	http://adrcswwi.org
Rock County	ADRC of Rock County	1900 Center Avenue Janesville Rock County 53546	608-741-3600 855-741-3600	www.co.rock.wi.use/adrc
Rusk County	ADRC of Barron, Rusk, and Washburn Counties	311 Miner Avenue East Suite C260 Courthouse Bldg Ladysmith Rusk County 54848	715-532-2176	www.adrcconnections.org
Sauk County	ADRC of Eagle Country (serving Crawford, Juneau, Richland, and Sauk Counties)	505 Broadway, Room 102 Baraboo Sauk County 53913	608-355-3289	http://adrcswwi.org

(*continued*)

Wisconsin *(continued)*

Sawyer County	ADRC of the North (serving Iron, Ashland, Bayfield, Price, and Sawyer Counties)	10610 Main Street Hayward Sawyer County 54843	866-663-3607	http://www.adrc-n-wi.org
Serving Menominee, Oconto, and Shawano Counties and Stockbridge Munsee Tribe	ADRC of the Wolf River Region	W3272 Wolf River Road Keshena Menominee County 54135	855-492-2372	www.adrcwrr.org
Sheboygan County	ADRC of Sheboygan County	650 Forest Ave Sheboygan Falls Sheboygan County 53085	920-467-4100 800-596-1919	www.co.sheboygan.wi.us
St. Croix County	ADRC of St. Croix County	1101 Carmichael Road Hudson St. Croix County 54017	715-381-4360	
Taylor County	ADRC of the Northwoods (Serving Forest, Oneida, Taylor, and Vilas Counties and Forest County Potawatomi, Lac du Flambeau, and Sokaogon Chippewa Tribes)	845 B East Broadway Medford Taylor County 54451	800-699-6704	http://adrcofthenorthwoods.org

(continued)

Wisconsin (*continued*)

Trempealeau County	ADRC of Trempealeau County	Government Center, 36245 Main Street P. O. Box 67 Whitehall Trempealeau County 54773-0067	715-538-2001 800-273-2001	http://www.tremplocounty.com/adrc
Vernon County	ADRC of Western Wisconsin (serving La Crosse, Jackson, Monroe, and Vernon Counties)	402 Courthouse Square Viroqua WI Vernon County 54665	800-500-3910	www.adrcww.org
Vilas County	ADRC of the Northwoods (Serving Forest, Oneida, Taylor, and Vilas Counties and Forest County Potawatomi, Lac du Flambeau, and Sokaogon Chippewa Tribes)	521 Wall Street Eagle River Vilas County 54521	800-699-6704	http://adrcofthenorthwoods.org
Walworth County	ADRC of Walworth County	W4051 County Road NN PO Box 1005 Elkhorn Walworth County 53121	262-741-3400	www.co.walworth.wi.us
Washburn County	ADRC of Barron, Rusk & Washburn Counties	850 W Beaverbrook Avenue Spooner Washburn County 54801	715-635-4460	www.adrcconnections.org

(*continued*)

Wisconsin (*continued*)

Washington County	ADRC of Washington County	333 E. Washington St., Suite 1000 West Bend Washington County 53095	262-335-4497 877-306-3030	www.co.washington.wi.us
Waukesha County	ADRC of Waukesha County	500 Riverview Ave Waukesha Waukesha County 53188	262-548-7848	www.waukeshacounty.gov/adrc
Waupaca County	ADRC of Calumet, Outagamie, and Waupaca Counties	811 Harding Street Waupaca Waupaca County 54981	715-258-6400	www.yourADRCresource.org
Waushara County	ADRC of Adams, Green Lake, Marquette, and Waushara Counties	209 South Saint Marie Street PO Box 621 Wautoma Waushara County 54982	877-883-5378	http://www.adrcinformation.org
Winnebago County	ADRC of Winnebago County	220 Washington Ave Oshkosh Winnebago County 54903	877-886-2372	www.co.winnebago.wi.us/adrc
Wolf River Region (Shawano, Menominee, and Oconto Counties as well as the Stockbridge-Munsee Community)	ADRC of the Wolf River Region	607 E. Elizabeth St Shawano Shawano County 54166	855-492-2372	www.adrcwrr.org

(*continued*)

Wisconsin (*continued*)

Wood County	ADRC of Central Wisconsin (Serving Langlade, Lincoln, Marathon, and Wood Counties)	220 3rd Avenue South, Suite 1 Wisconsin Rapids Wood County 54495	715-421-0014	http://www.adrc-cw.com

ADRC, Aging and Disability Resource Center.

Wyoming

Statewide	WyADRC—SW-WRAP	PO Box 189 280 Monroe Ave Green River Sweetwater County 82935	307-875-2196 877-435-7851

Appendix F: Overview of *ICD-10* and *ICF*: Application to People with Disabilities and Older Adults

Patricia Welch Saleeby, PhD, MSSA
Southern Illinois University, Carbondale School of Social Work

GENERAL INTRODUCTION TO *ICD* AND *ICF*

Trends such as global aging along with increased prevalence of chronic conditions and disability continues worldwide. Consequently, a greater number of social workers are faced with addressing aging and/or disability issues in their diverse practice settings including schools, hospitals, health clinics, mental health agencies, and community organizations. Additionally, social workers are impacted through disability and aging-related policy initiatives. This situation heightens the need for increased training of social workers to address both aging and disability-related issues inside and outside schools of social work.

Knowledge of two important international classifications are essential for social workers and other professionals working in gerontology and disability fields—(a) the *International Classification of Diseases* (*ICD*) and (b) the *International Classification of Functioning, Disability, and Health* (*ICF*). Governed by the World Health Organization (WHO), these complementary classifications provide an effective system to facilitate the understanding of diseases, disability, health, and functioning across the individual life span. Clinical social workers are required health professionals to use the *ICD-10* when identifying mental health disorders. The *ICF* is increasingly being considered the standard diagnostic tool for health management, epidemiology, and clinical purposes.

INTERNATIONAL CLASSIFICATION OF DISEASES

The *International Classification of Diseases* (*ICD*) was developed by the WHO and endorsed by its World Health Assembly in 1990. The *ICD* is widely used in countries to classify and report mortality data, a primary indicator of health status, by doctors, insurers, and other providers. It is used to classify diseases and health problems recorded on health and vital records such as death certificates. This information is used for clinical, epidemiological, and quality purposes. The *ICD* is available in six official languages endorsed by the WHO including Arabic, Chinese, English, French, Russian, and Spanish as well as over 30 other languages.

The *ICD-10* (the tenth Edition of the *ICD*) was mandated for use in the United States beginning on October 1, 2015.

An upcoming version, *ICD*-11, will be presented in May 2019 and will be used for reporting health data in 2022. Essentially there is an increased need to integrate the ICD into an electronic system., The ICD-11 version will be a digitally-enabled version that will be linked to other terminologies. The newest version will support electronic health records.

Table A.F1 Comparison of *ICD-10* and *ICD-9* Classifications

ICD-10	*ICD-9*
21 Chapters	19 Chapters
Approximately 68,000 codes	Approximately 14,000 codes
Three to seven digits	Three to five digits
First digit is alpha only and second digit is numeric	First digit is alpha or numeric
Digits three to seven are alpha or numeric	Digits two to five are numeric

Although the *ICD* has been used since the 1970s, the previous version, *ICD-9*, contained outdated terms and it was inconsistent with current health practices. Additionally, it did not allow for updates in the modern healthcare industry. Therefore, the updated *ICD*-10 has several advantages over its predecessor including increased specificity, updated medical terminology, enhanced accuracy in processing claims, and overall improved capability to measure healthcare services. It is important to note that the *ICD-10* affects diagnosis and inpatient procedure coding for everyone covered by the Health Insurance Portability and Accountability Act (HIPAA), not just those who submit Medicare or Medicaid claims.

Several countries have developed additional systems based on the ICD for use outside coding and classifying mortality data, which is the primary purpose of ICD. For instance, the United States version developed two modifications: the *ICD-10-CM* or Clinical Modification; and the *ICD-10-PCS* or Procedure Coding System. The *ICD-10-CM* is used in all healthcare settings for medical diagnoses made by healthcare personnel. Diagnosis coding under *ICD-10-CM* uses three to seven digits instead of the three to five digits used with *ICD-9-CM*, but the format of the code sets is similar. The *ICD-10-PCS* is used in inpatient hospital settings only. *ICD-10-PCS* uses seven alphanumeric digits instead of the three or four numeric digits used under *ICD-9-CM* procedure coding. Coding under *ICD-10-PCS* is much more specific and substantially different from *ICD-9-CM* procedure coding (Table A.F1).

INTERNATIONAL CLASSIFICATION OF FUNCTIONING, DISABILITY, AND HEALTH

Released in 2001 by the WHO, the *ICF* is considered a health-related classification and standardized framework for describing health. The *ICF* represents a revision of an earlier version known as the *International Classification of Impairments, Disabilities, and Handicaps* (*ICIDH*; WHO, 1980). The *ICIDH* revision process that led to the *ICF* embraced various timely changes occurring in the disability community. For example, a significant change was the removal of the obsolete "handicap" term and the inclusion of more neutral terminology throughout the classification. Moreover, the *ICF* framework became more dynamic and interactive in nature than the linear model of the *ICIDH*. In fact, the *ICF* biopsychosocial approach depicts a much more realistic view of disability and functioning.

Figure A.F1 depicts the *ICF* conceptual framework and the underlying foundation of its classification system (WHO, 2008). The *ICF* system is presented along a continuum of functioning to disability. Functioning is considered the umbrella term for all body functions and structures, activities, and participation while disability is considered the umbrella term for impairments, activity limitations, and participation restrictions. Contextual factors including both personal factors and environmental factors play an important role in the *ICF* framework. Although there is an environment section in the classification, personal factors were purposefully not included due to wide variability globally.

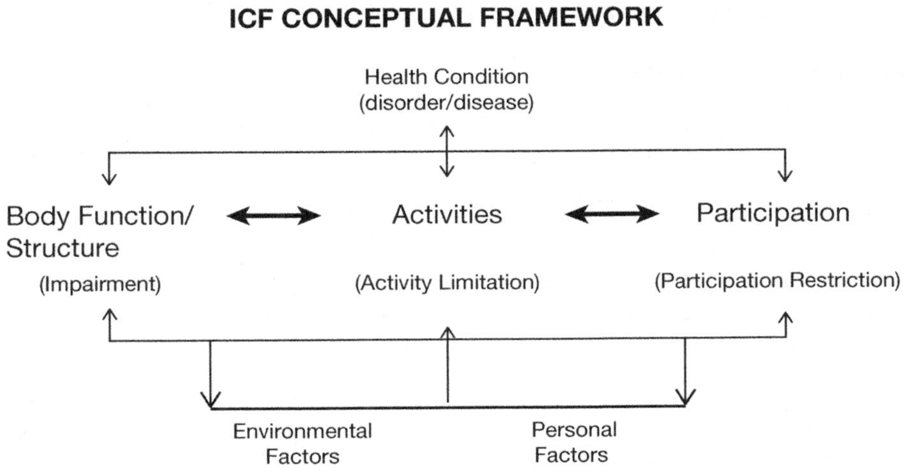

Figure A.F1 *ICF* conceptual framework.

ICF, International classification of functioning, disability, and health.

Source: World Health Organization. (2001). *International classification of functioning, disability and health.* Geneva, Switzerland: Author.

Impairments are defined as the loss or abnormality of body function or structure. Activities are defined as the execution of tasks or activities by an individual while activity limitations are difficulties individuals may have in executing activities. Participation is defined as the involvement in a life situation while participation restrictions are problems individuals may experience in involvement in life situations. The domains for body functions and structures, activities and participation, and the environment are outlined in Table A.F2.

APPLICATIONS OF THE *ICD-10* AND *ICF* IN SOCIAL WORK

There is a great need for valid, reliable statistics on disability as well as functioning among older adults and persons with disabilities. Together, the *ICD* and *ICF* enable the collection of such disability and health data at national and international levels. Improved comparable statistics at a national and international level will lead to the development or better programs and policies (Welch Saleeby, 2011). In fact, the National Committee on Vital and Health Statistics has recognized the need for functional status information and the lack of action on it in the health information policy area (National Committee on Vital and Health Statistics [NCVHS], 2001). In its report, it recommends the *ICF* for consideration as a standardized format for coding functional status data. And the United Nations Statistics Division has recommended the *ICF* conceptual framework as the basis for measuring disability (United Nations, 2002).

ICD-10 AND *ICF* RESOURCES

Centers for Medicare and Medicaid Services (CMS) website for *ICD*: www.cms.gov/Medicare/Coding/ICD10/index.html

Centers for Disease Control and Prevention (CDC) website for *ICD* and *ICF*: www.cdc.gov/nchs/icd/index.htm

WHO website for *ICD*: www.who.int/classifications/icd/en

WHO website for *ICF*: www.who.int/entity/classifications/icf/en

Table A.F2 *ICF* Body Functions and Structures, Activities and Participation, and Environment

Body Functions	***Body Structures***	***Activities and Participation***	***Environmental Factors***
Mental Functions	Structures of the Nervous System	Learning and Applying Knowledge	Products and Technology
Sensory Functions and Pain	The Eye, Ear and Related Structures	General Tasks and Demands	Natural Environment and Human-made Changes to Environment
Voice and Speech Functions	Structures involved in Voice and Speech	Communication	Support and Relationships
Functions of the Cardiovascular, Haematological, Immunological and Respiratory Systems	Structure of the Cardiovascular, Immunological and Respiratory Systems	Mobility	Attitudes
Functions of the Digestive, Metabolic, Endocrine Systems	Structures Related to the Digestive, Metabolic and Endocrine Systems	Self-Care	Services, Systems, and Policies
Genitourinary and Reproductive Functions	Structure Related to Genitourinary and Reproductive Systems	Domestic Life	
Neuromusculoskeletal and Movement-Related Functions	Structures Related to Movement	Interpersonal Interactions and Relationships	
Functions of the Skin and Related Structures	Skin and Related Structures	Major Life Areas	
		Community, Social and Civic Life	

REFERENCES

National Committee on Vital and Health Statistics. (2001). *Classifying and reporting functional health status.* Washington, DC: Department of Health and Human Services.

United Nations (2002). Guidelines and principles for the development of disability statistics. New York: United Nations.

Welch Saleeby P. (2011). Using the International Classification of Functioning, Disability and Health in Social Work Settings. Health and Social Work, 36(4). 303–305. doi:10.1093/hsw/36.4.303

World Health Organization. (1980). *International classification of impairments, disabilities and handicaps (ICIDH).* Geneva, Switzerland: Author.

World Health Organization. (2001). *International classification of functioning, disability and health.* Geneva, Switzerland: Author.

Index

Made in the USA
Coppell, TX
30 December 2021

70485299R00306